Drug Metabolism and Pharmacokinetics

Drug Metabolism and Pharmacokinetics

Editor: Erica Helmer

AMERICAN
MEDICAL PUBLISHERS
www.americanmedicalpublishers.com

AMERICAN
MEDICAL PUBLISHERS
www.americanmedicalpublishers.com

Cataloging-in-Publication Data

Drug metabolism and pharmacokinetics / edited by Erica Helmer.
p. cm.
Includes bibliographical references and index.
ISBN 979-8-88740-078-5
1. Drugs--Metabolism. 2. Pharmacokinetics. 3. Pharmacology. 4. Chemical kinetics. I. Helmer, Erica.
RM301.55 .D78 2023
615.7--dc23

American Medical Publishers,
41 Flatbush Avenue,
1st Floor, New York,
NY 11217, USA

ISBN 979-8-88740-078-5 (Hardback)

Contents

Preface

Over the recent decade, advancements and applications have progressed exponentially. This has led to the increased interest in this field and projects are being conducted to enhance knowledge. The main objective of this book is to present some of the critical challenges and provide insights into possible solutions. This book will answer the varied questions that arise in the field and also provide an increased scope for furthering studies.

Drug metabolism refers to the conversion of a drug molecule into other related compounds throughout the body. There are drug modifying enzymes (DME) such as cytochrome P450 which are involved in the modification of an administered drug during the process of drug metabolism. The liver is the primary organ involved in the modification and removal of drug compounds, along with numerous other locations within the body. The therapeutic efficacy of a drug is influenced by many factors, including pharmacokinetics. It refers to the passage of a drug through the body's biological system. There are four different phases in the passage of a drug in the human body, which includes absorption, distribution, metabolism, and excretion (ADME). These pharmacokinetic qualities collectively provide deeper insights into the performance of a drug and help to establish the optimal dosage. This book provides significant information to help develop a good understanding of drug metabolism and pharmacokinetics. It presents researches and studies performed by experts across the globe. This book aims to equip students and experts with the advanced topics and upcoming concepts in this area of study.

I hope that this book, with its visionary approach, will be a valuable addition and will promote interest among readers. Each of the authors has provided their extraordinary competence in their specific fields by providing different perspectives as they come from diverse nations and regions. I thank them for their contributions.

Editor

1

Pharmacokinetics and Brain Distribution of the Active Components of DA-9805, Saikosaponin A, Paeonol and Imperatorin in Rats

Mi Hye Kwon [1], Jin Seok Jeong [2], Jayoung Ryu [2], Young Woong Cho [2] and Hee Eun Kang [1,*]

1 College of Pharmacy and Integrated Research Institute of Pharmaceutical Sciences, The Catholic University of Korea, 43 Jibong-ro, Wonmi-gu, Bucheon 14662, Korea; mihye8699@hanmail.net

2 Research Center, Dong-A ST Co., Ltd., 21 Geumhwa-ro, 105beon-gil, Giheung-gu, Yongin 17073, Korea; treadwheel@donga.co.kr (J.S.J.); jyryu@donga.co.kr (J.R.); herojoe@donga.co.kr (Y.W.C.)

* Correspondence: kanghe@catholic.ac.kr

Abstract: DA-9805 is a botanical anti-Parkinson's drug candidate formulated from ethanol extracts of the root of *Bupleurum falcatum*, the root cortex of *Paeonia suffruticosa*, and the root of *Angelica dahurica*. The pharmacokinetics (PKs) and brain distribution of active/representative ingredients of DA-9805, Saikosaponin a (SSa; 1.1–4.6 mg/kg), Paeonol (PA; 14.8–59.2 mg/kg), and Imperatorin (IMP; 1.4–11.5 mg/kg) were evaluated following the intravenous or oral administration of each pure component and the equivalent dose of DA-9805 in rats. All three components had greater dose-normalized areas under the plasma concentration-time curve (AUC) and slower clearance with higher doses, following intravenous administration. By contrast, dose-proportional AUC values of SSa, PA, and IMP were observed following the oral administration of each pure component (with the exception of IMP at the highest dose) or DA-9805. Compared to oral administration of each pure compound, DA-9805 administration showed an increase in the AUC of SSa (by 96.1–163%) and PA (by 155–164%), possibly due to inhibition of their metabolism by IMP or other component(s) in DA-9805. A delay in the absorption of PA and IMP was observed when they were administered as DA-9805. All three components of DA-9805 showed greater binding values in brain homogenates than in plasma, possibly explaining why the brain-to-plasma ratios were greater than unity following multiple oral administrations of DA-9805. By contrast, their levels in cerebrospinal fluid were negligible. Our results further our understanding of the comprehensive PK characteristics of SSa, PA, and IMP in rats and the comparative PKs between each pure component and DA-9805.

Keywords: DA-9805; saikosaponin a; paeonol; imperatorin; pharmacokinetics; brain distribution

1. Introduction

Recently, the potential role of herbal products in the treatment of Parkinson's disease has emerged [1]. Neuroprotective or neurorestorative agents for the treatment of this disease by either inhibiting primary neurodegenerative events or boosting compensatory and regenerative mechanisms in the brain remain an unmet medical need [2]. DA-9805, a novel botanical neuroprotective anti-Parkinson's drug candidate, was formulated from ethanol extracts of the mixture (1:1:1, *w/w/w*) of three herbal drugs, the root of *Bupleurum falcatum* L. (Apiaceae), the root cortex of *Paeonia suffruticosa* Andrews (Paeoniaceae), and the root of *Angelica dahurica* Benth et Hook (Umbelliferae). An investigational new drug application for DA-9805 for a phase II clinical study was recently submitted to the U.S. Food and Drug Administration. The neuroprotective effects of each of the three herbal constituents in DA-9805 have been reported in various in vitro and animal models. Ethanol extracts of the root of *B. falcatum* have been shown to inhibit neuroinflammation in murine microglial cells [3], improve behavioral defects after spinal-cord injury [4], and alleviate stress-induced memory impairment [5]. Extracts from the root cortex of *P. suffruticosa* have been found to have neuroprotective effects in an 1-methyl-4-phenyl-1,2,3,6-tetrahydropyridine (MPTP)-induced Parkinson's disease model [6]. Extracts from *A. dahurica* reduce apoptotic cell death and improve functional recovery after spinal cord injury [7].

Saikosaponin a (SSa, [3β,4α,16β]-13,28-epoxy-16,23-dihydroxyolean-11-en-3-yl-6-deoxy-3-*O*-β-D -glucopyranosyl-β-D-galactopyranoside; Figure 1A), originated from the root of *B. falcatum*, is a representative component of DA-9805, for which it is used as a quality control (QC) ingredient (at >0.297%). The quantity of SSa is listed in the Chinese Pharmacopeia for QC of a traditional Chinese medicine (TCM) prescribed with Radix Bupleuri [8]. Its pharmacological activity and structure are similar to those of steroids [9], and its antiepileptic [10] and neuroprotective effects [11] have recently been reported. However, its toxicity, including an ability to cause hemolysis and liver damage, has also been reported [12]. The pharmacokinetics (PKs) of SSa following intravenous administration of 15 mg/kg [8] and oral administration of the extract of the dried roots of *B. chinense* DC (equivalent to ~40 mg/kg SSa) [13] have been reported.

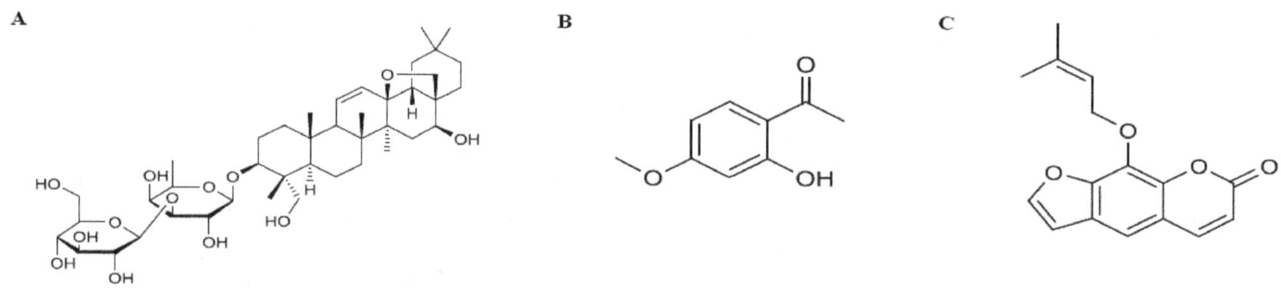

Figure 1. Chemical structures of three active/representative components in DA-9805: (**A**) saikosaponin a (SSa); (**B**) paeonol (PA); (**C**) imperatorin (IMP).

Paeonol (PA; 1-[2-hydroxy-4-methoxyphenyl]ethanone; Figure 1B), a marker component of the root cortex of *P. suffruticosa* [14], is the most abundant active compound in DA-9805 (at >2.802%). It has various pharmacological activities [15–17] and neuroprotective effects in various murine models [18–20]. Its PKs and/or tissue distribution have been reported after intravenous (2.5–10 mg/kg) [21] and oral administration (35–140 mg/kg) [14,22], as well as after oral administration of herbal products containing PA or TCM prescriptions (equivalent to 17.5–100 mg/kg PA) [23,24].

Imperatorin (IMP, 9-[3-methylbut-2-enoxy]-7-furo[3,2-g]chromenone; Figure 1C), an active ingredient in the root of *A. dahurica*, is another representative component of DA-9805 (at >0.512%). It has anti-inflammatory effects [25,26] and other favorable effects in the central nervous system (CNS) including neuroprotective, anticonvulsant, anxiolytic, and procognitive activities [27–29]. Its PKs following intravenous and oral administration (6.25–25 mg/kg or 80 mg/kg) in rats have been reported [30,31], as has its brain distribution after oral administration of 20 mg/kg of IMP [32] or ~26 mg/kg in an extract [33].

The efficacy and safety of herbal medicines remain major issues of concern. Up to now, a widely accepted approach for evaluating in vivo efficacy of an herbal medicine is that the efficacy of mixed herbal preparation can be correlated with pharmacokinetic behavior of one or several known active ingredients [34]. PKs studies of these three active/representative ingredients of DA-9805 are essential for botanical drug development to evaluate not only the efficacy of the drug but also its potential drug interactions and toxicity. Despite the promising neuroprotective activities of DA-9805 as an anti-Parkinson's agent, the PKs of its active/representative ingredients at relatively low doses have not been characterized comprehensively. Moreover, PKs of each active ingredient following DA-9805 administration may be altered by the multiple components in DA-9805.

In this study, the PKs of pure SSa, PA, and IMP and their dose dependency were evaluated following the intravenous and oral administration of each pure component. The PKs of each marker compound following the oral administration of DA-9805 were also compared to those following the respective equivalent dose of the pure marker components. Moreover, the distribution of the three active components in the brain, which is the site of action, was evaluated following multiple oral administrations of DA-9805.

2. Materials and Methods

2.1. Materials and Reagents

DA-9805 (Lot No. PD15702; containing 0.456% SSa, 5.919% PA, and 0.576% IMP, as determined by HPLC-UV) was obtained from Dong-A ST (Yongin, Korea). SSa (98.32% purity) and IMP (99.17% purity) were products from Letopharm, Ltd. (Shanghai, China), and PA (99.8% purity) was obtained from Sigma-Aldrich (St. Louis, MO, USA). Internal standard (IS) for SSa, PA, and IMP (dexamethasone, bumetanide, indomethacin, respectively), hydroxypropyl-methylcellulose (HPMC), dimethylsulfoxide (DMSO), Tween® 80, and Solutol® HS 15 were purchased from Sigma-Aldrich (St. Louis, MO, USA). Other chemicals were of reagent or HPLC grade.

2.2. Animals

Animal-study protocols were approved by the Department of Laboratory Animals, Institutional Animal Care and Use Committee on the Sungsim Campus of the Catholic University of Korea (Approval No. 2015-011; Bucheon, Korea). Male Sprague-Dawley rats, 7–8 weeks old and weighing 195–300 g, were purchased from Young Bio (Sungnam, Korea). The procedures used for the housing and handling of rats were similar to those previously described [35].

2.3. Intravenous Drug Administration

For intravenous administration, the carotid artery and jugular vein were cannulated using previously reported procedures [35]. Thereafter, each pure active component of DA-9805 was infused for 1 min via the jugular vein: SSa (dissolved in 2:1:7 [*v*/*v*/*v*] DMSO:Tween 80:distilled water (DW)) at doses of 2.3 and 4.6 mg (2 mL)/kg (n = 5 and 4, respectively); PA (dissolved in 2:2:6 [*v*/*v*/*v*] DMSO:Tween 80:20% Solutol in DW) at doses of 14.8, 29.6, and 59.2 mg (2 mL)/kg (n = 5, 5, and 6, respectively); and IMP (dissolved in 2:2:6 [*v*/*v*/*v*] DMSO:Tween 80: DW) at doses of 2.9, 5.8, and 11.5 mg (2 mL)/kg (n = 5, 6 and 5, respectively). A blood sample of ~200 µL was collected via the carotid artery at time 0 (prior to dosing), 1 (at the end of the infusion), and 5, 15, 30, 60, 90, 120, 180, 240, 360, and 480 min after the start of infusion. After centrifugation (13,000× g for 2 min), 100 µL aliquots of plasma were collected and stored at −20 °C until liquid chromatography-tandem mass spectrometry (LC-MS/MS) analyses. The preparation and handling of 24 h urine samples (Ae_{0-24h}) and gastrointestinal tract (GI) samples (including their contents at 24 h and feces during 0–24 h) at 24 h (GI_{24h}) were similar to a previously reported method [35].

2.4. Oral Drug Administration

DA-9805 (dissolved in 2:7.75, 2:7.5, and 2:7 [*v*/*v*] DMSO:DW with 2% HPMC, respectively) at doses of 250, 500, and 1000 mg (10 mL)/kg was administered orally using a gastric gavage tube (n = 5 each). Equivalent doses of each pure SSa, PA, and IMP (dissolved in 2:7.75:0.25, 2:7.5:0.5, and 2:7:1 [*v*/*v*/*v*] DMSO:DW with 2% HPMC:ethanol with dose elevation) were also administered orally (n = 4 or 5 each). Doses of 1.1, 2.3, and 4.6 mg (10 mL)/kg pure SSa; 14.8, 29.6, and 59.2 mg (10 mL)/kg pure PA; and 1.4, 2.9, and 5.8 mg (10 mL)/kg pure IMP were orally administered. A blood sample of ~200 µL was collected via the carotid artery at 0, 5, 15, 30, 45, 60, 90, 120, 180, 240, 360, 480, and 600 min after oral administration. Other procedures for the oral study were similar to those used for the intravenous study.

2.5. *Brain Distribution of Saikosaponin A(SSa), Paeonol (PA), and Imperatorin (IMP) Following Multiple Oral Doses of DA-9805*

DA-9805 (dissolved in 2:7 [*v*/*v*] DMSO:DW with 2% HPMC and diluted 2-fold with DW to a final concentration of 250 mg/5 mL) at a dose of 250 mg (5 mL)/kg/day was orally administered for 8 days. At 2 and 6 h after the final oral dose, the rats were euthanized ($n = 3$ at each time point) by carbon-dioxide asphyxiation, and cerebrospinal fluid (CSF) was collected from each rat. Blood samples were collected via cardiac puncture. Next, the mixed brain (whole of left hemisphere), frontal cortex, striatum, hippocampus, and cerebellum (from the right hemisphere) were excised and blotted on tissue paper. Each tissue sample was homogenized (Minilys®; Bertin Technologies, Montigny le Bretonneux, France) with 3 volumes (3 mL/g tissue) of methanol and centrifuged at 9000 g for 10 min. Two 100 μL aliquots of the supernatant and plasma samples were collected and stored at −70 °C until subsequent LC-MS/MS analyses.

2.6. *Measurement of the Protein Binding of SSa, PA, and IMP in Rat Plasma and Brain Homogenates*

The protein-binding abilities of SSa, PA, and IMP in fresh rat plasma and brain homogenates were measured using a single-use rapid equilibrium dialysis device (molecular weight cutoff of 8 kDa; Thermo Scientific, Rockford, IL, USA) in accordance with the manufacturer's instructions. For binding studies with rat plasma, SSa, PA, and IMP were spiked into each 1200 μL blank plasma sample ($n = 6$) to produce a final concentration of 0.5, 2, and 0.5 μg/mL, respectively. A triplicate of the above samples (each containing 300 μL) was placed into each sample chamber to minimize potential errors during sample processing, and was dialyzed against 500 μL isotonic phosphate buffer (pH 7.4) in each buffer chamber. After 4 h incubation in a water bath shaker (37 °C, 50 oscillations/min), the plasma and buffer samples were collected, and each 100 μL sample was used for LC-MS/MS analyses of SSa, PA, and IMP. For the binding study with rat brain (hippocampus, striatum, mixed brain) homogenates, each brain tissue sample was homogenized (Minilys®; Bertin Technologies, Montigny le Bretonneux, France) with 3 volumes (3 mL/g tissue) of isotonic phosphate buffer (pH 7.4). SSa, PA, and IMP were spiked into each blank brain homogenate to produce a final concentration of 0.2, 1, and 0.2 μg/mL, respectively. One (for the hippocampus and striatum) and a duplicate (for the mixed brain) of the above homogenate samples (each 200 μL) were transferred into each sample chamber and dialyzed against 350 μL isotonic phosphate buffer (pH 7.4) in each buffer chamber. Other procedures were the same as those used in the plasma protein-binding study. The unbound fraction (f_u) in plasma was calculated as follows:

$$f_u = 1 - (C_p - C_b)/C_p, \tag{1}$$

where C_p is the drug concentration in the protein-containing compartment and C_b is the drug concentration in the buffer compartment. Because the brain homogenates were diluted during the homogenization process, it was necessary to correct the f_u value measured in a diluted sample ($f_{u\,measured}$) to generate the undiluted f_u value ($f_{u\,brain}$) using the following equation (Kalvass and Maurer, 2002):

$$f_{u\ brain} = \frac{1/D}{\{(1/f_{u\ measured}) - 1\} + 1/D} \tag{2}$$

where D is the dilution factor (=4) of the brain homogenates.

2.7. *LC-MS/MS Analyses of SSa, PA, and IMP*

The LC-MS/MS system comprised the Agilent 1260 LC System and the Agilent 6460 Triple Quadrupole Tandem Mass Spectrometer (Agilent, Waldbronn, Germany). Instrument control and data acquisition were performed using the Agilent MassHunter Workstation software (Version B.

04. 01). The concentrations of SSa, PA, and IMP in the samples were determined according to the LC-MS/MS method recently published from our laboratory [36]. The calibration curves were linear in a concentration range of 0.5–1000 ng/mL for SSa, 20–10,000 ng/mL for PA, and 0.2–1000 ng/mL for IMP. The mean intra- and interday coefficients of variation of the analyses on 5 consecutive days were below 15.0%, and the assay accuracies ranged from 95.8 to 113%.

2.8. Pharmacokinetic Analyses

The total area under the plasma concentration–time curve from time zero to infinity (AUC_{0-inf}) or up to the last measured time (t) in plasma (AUC_{0-t}) was calculated using the trapezoidal rule-extrapolation method [37]. Calculation of the following PK parameters was performed using non-compartmental analyses (WinNonlin®; Pharsight Corporation, Mountain View, CA, USA): the time-averaged total body, renal, and nonrenal clearances (CL, CL_R, and CL_{NR}, respectively), terminal half-life, mean residence time (MRT), and apparent volume of distribution at steady state (V_{ss}) [38]. The maximum plasma concentration (C_{max}) and time to reach C_{max} (T_{max}) were directly read from the experimental data. For comparison, the extent of absolute oral bioavailability (F) was calculated by dividing the AUC value after oral administration by the AUC value after intravenous administration of equivalent doses of the pure component.

2.9. Statistical Analyses

The Statistical Package for Social Sciences program (SPSS Inc., Chicago, IL, USA) was used for statistical analyses. To compare two means of unpaired data, the t-test was used. To compare 3 means of unpaired data, the data were compared using one-way analysis of variance (ANOVA) and the post hoc Tukey test (for a homogenous subset), or Dunnett's T3 multiple-comparison test (for a non-homogenous subset). For data that were not normally distributed, nonparametric analyses (Kruskal-Wallis test) were used. A p value < 0.05 was considered statistically significant. All of the data are expressed as the means $\pm$ standard deviations (SD), except the median (range) for T_{max}.

3. Results

3.1. PKs of SSa, PA, and IMP after Intravenous Administration of Each Pure Compound

The mean arterial plasma concentration-time profiles and relevant PK parameters of SSa, PA, and IMP following intravenous administration of each pure compound are shown in Figure 2 and Table 1, respectively. The dose-normalized AUC values of SSa, PA, and IMP following intravenous administration tended to increase with dose elevation because of slower CL (particularly CL_{NR}) of the drugs in the higher dose group(s). A significantly greater (by 77.9%) dose-normalized AUC value of SSa following intravenous administration of 4.6 mg/kg SSa was observed with significantly slower CL (by 43.2%), CL_R (by 81.2%), and CL_{NR} (by 40.3%) than those of the 2.3 mg/kg dose group. A significantly smaller V_{ss} (by 19.0%), longer MRT (by 42.9%), and smaller Ae_{0-24h} (by 68.0%) of SSa were observed in the higher dose group. PA showed significantly greater (by 38.0%) dose-normalized AUC with slower CL (by 27.0%) and CL_{NR} (by 27.5%) in the highest intravenous dose (59.2 mg/kg) group than in the lowest dose (14.8 mg/kg) group. IMP also showed significantly greater (by 124% and 98.5%) dose-normalized AUC following the highest intravenous dose (11.5 mg/kg) with slower CL (by 56.4% and 50.5%) and CL_{NR} (by 56.4% and 50.5%) than the lower dose (2.9 and 5.8 mg/kg) groups. A significantly longer MRT (by 96.6% and 60.2%) was observed in the highest dose (11.5 mg/kg) IMP group than in the lower dose (2.9 and 5.8 mg/kg) groups. The 24 h urinary excretion of IMP was almost negligible (<0.1% of the intravenous dose).

Table 1. Pharmacokinetic parameters of Saikosaponin a (SSa), paeonol (PA), and imperatorin (IMP) after intravenous administration of each drug to rats (mean ± standard deviations (SD)).

Parameters	SSa			PA		IMP		
	2.3 mg/kg (n = 5)	4.6 mg/kg (n = 4)	14.8 mg/kg (n = 5)	29.6 mg/kg (n = 5)	59.2 mg/kg (n = 6)	2.9 mg/kg (n = 5)	5.8 mg/kg (n = 6)	11.5 mg/kg (n = 5)
Body weight (g)	290 ± 7.91	288 ± 8.66	262 ± 7.58	263 ± 12.5	258 ± 7.58	274 ± 10.7	280 ± 10.5	289 ± 11.9
AUC_{0-inf} (μg·min/mL) [a]	517 ± 64.3	1840 ± 349 [b]	511 ± 65.3	1250 ± 250	2820 ± 400 [f]	55.9 ± 12.4	126 ± 23.9	496 ± 66.5 [h]
CL (mL/min/kg)	4.51 ± 0.583	2.56 ± 0.418 [c]	29.3 ± 3.60	24.4 ± 4.03	21.4 ± 3.29 [g]	53.9 ± 11.9	47.5 ± 9.85	23.5 ± 3.07 [i]
CL_R (μL/min/kg)	321 ± 177	60.2 ± 34.2 [d]	587 ± 535	232 ± 110	556 ± 382	39.4 ± 9.33	42.5 ± 27.7	13.8 ± 4.35
CL_{NR} (mL/min/kg)	4.19 ± 0.492	2.50 ± 0.387 [c]	28.7 ± 3.75	24.2 ± 3.98	20.8 ± 3.16 [g]	53.9 ± 11.9	47.5 ± 9.87	23.5 ± 3.07 [i]
V_{ss} (mL/kg)	126 ± 11.1	102 ± 8.16 [e]	1130 ± 290	1290 ± 327	1100 ± 429	1760 ± 595	1600 ± 333	1470 ± 254
MRT (min)	28.2 ± 4.33	40.3 ± 4.73 [e]	38.5 ± 8.43	53.5 ± 14.0	51.4 ± 18.9	32.1 ± 5.46	39.4 ± 15.2	63.1 ± 12.1 [i]
Terminal half-life (min)	93.9 ± 18.7	91.5 ± 16.0	81.5 ± 17.4	157 ± 53.7	214 ± 111	77.8 ± 5.58	75.1 ± 18.2	77.7 ± 36.0
Ae_{0-24h} (% of dose)	6.94 ± 3.67	2.22 ± 1.16 [d]	2.06 ± 1.87	0.941 ± 0.362	2.55 ± 1.78	0.0750 ± 0.0191	0.0986 ± 0.0785	0.0605 ± 0.0223
GI_{24h} (% of dose)	0.701 ± 1.17	0.481 ± 0.219	0.182 ± 0.124	0.186 ± 0.223	0.153 ± 0.165	0.0105 ± 0.00709	0.0103 ±0.00265	0.0153 ± 0.0106

[a] Dose-normalized values were compared when statistical analysis was performed. [b] Dose-normalized value was significantly different from 2.3 mg/kg group ($p < 0.01$, t-test). [c] The value was significantly different from 2.3 mg/kg group ($p < 0.001$, t-test). [d] The value was significantly different from 2.3 mg/kg group ($p < 0.05$, t-test). [e] The value was significantly different from 2.3 mg/kg group ($p < 0.01$, t-test). [f] Dose-normalized value was significantly different from 14.8 mg/kg group ($p < 0.05$, one-way analysis of variance (ANOVA) with post hoc Tukey test). [g] The value was significantly different from 14.8 mg/kg group ($p < 0.05$, one-way ANOVA with post hoc Tukey test). [h] Dose-normalized value was significantly different from 2.9 and 5.8 mg/kg groups ($p < 0.05$, one-way ANOVA with post hoc Tukey test). [i] The value was significantly different from 2.9 and 5.8 mg/kg groups ($p < 0.05$, one-way ANOVA with post hoc Tukey test).

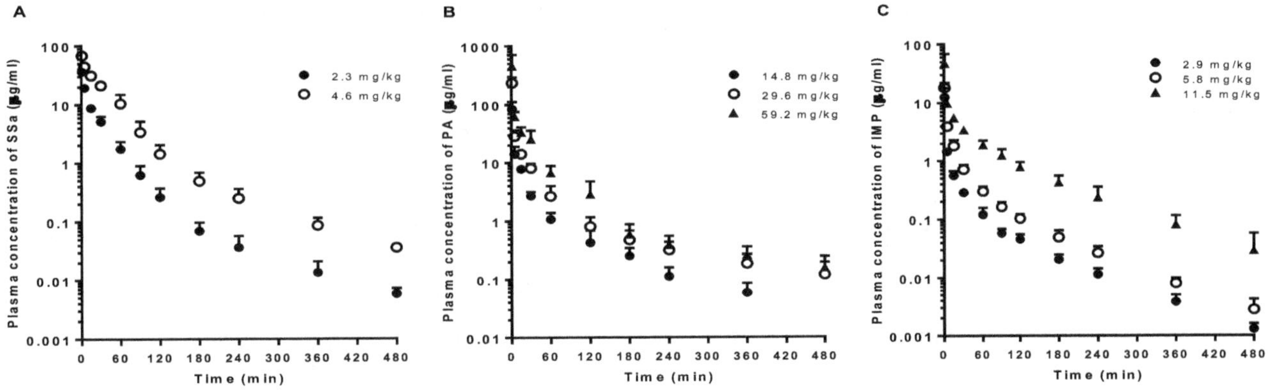

Figure 2. Mean arterial plasma concentration-time profiles of (**A**) SSa, (**B**) PA, and (**C**) IMP following 1-min intravenous administration of each pure compound at various doses (2.3 ($n = 5$) and 4.6 ($n = 4$) mg/kg of SSa; 14.8 ($n = 5$), 29.6 ($n = 5$), and 59.2 ($n = 6$) mg/kg of PA; and 2.9 ($n = 5$), 5.8 ($n = 6$), and 11.5 ($n = 5$) mg/kg of IMP) to rats. Vertical bars represent SD.

3.2. PKs of SSa after the Oral Administration of Pure SSa and DA-9805

The mean arterial plasma concentration-time profiles of SSa after oral administration in rats of pure SSa at doses of 2.3 and 4.6 mg/kg and DA-9805 at doses of 0.25, 0.5, and 1 g/kg (equivalent to 1.1, 2.3, and 4.6 mg/kg, respectively, as SSa) are shown in Figure 3. The relevant PK parameters are also listed in Table 2. Most of the plasma concentrations of SSa following oral administration of pure SSa at the lowest dose (1.1 mg/kg) were less than the lower limit of quantification (LLOQ; 0.5 ng/mL); thus, the data were excluded for PK analyses. The AUC and C_{max} values of SSa were dose-proportional following oral administration of pure SSa and DA-9805. Interestingly, the $AUC_{0–8h}$ values of SSa following oral administration of DA-9805 were significantly greater (by 96.1% and 163%) than those following oral administration of each equivalent dose of pure SSa, whereas the C_{max} values were comparable between pure SSa and DA-9805. Therefore, the F values were greater (by 96.2% and 163%) following DA-9805 administration than after pure SSa administration. The F values of SSa following oral administration were extremely low (<0.1% of oral dose). Interestingly, the recovery from the GI tract ($GI_{24\,h}$ values) was significantly higher (24.5- and 3.1-fold) in rats with DA-9805 administration than in rats with pure SSa administration.

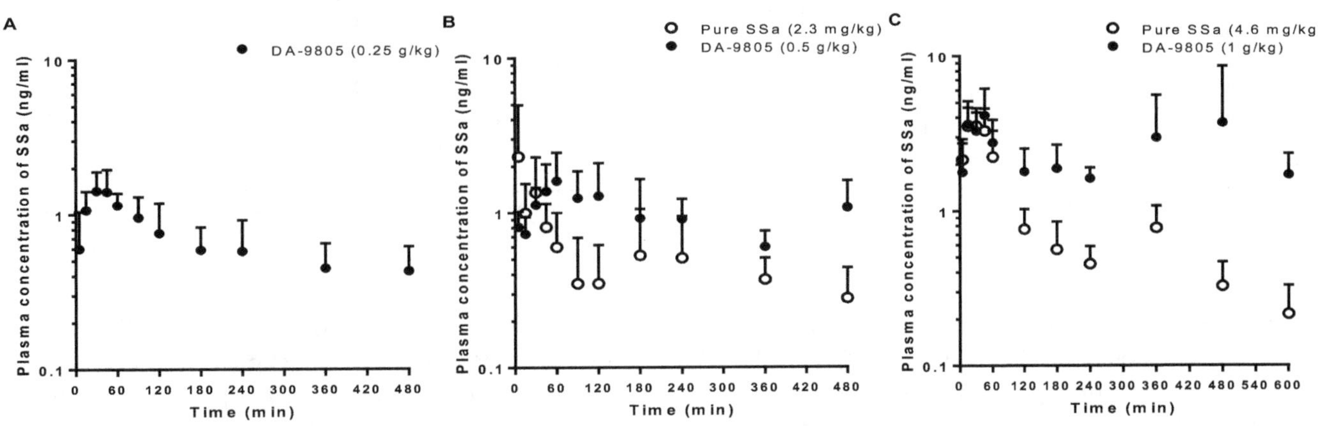

Figure 3. Mean arterial plasma concentration–time profiles of SSa following oral administration of DA-9805 (closed circle) at doses of 0.25 g/kg ((**A**); 1.1 mg/kg as SSa, $n = 5$), 0.5 g/kg ((**B**); 2.3 mg/kg as SSa, $n = 5$), and 1 g/kg ((**C**); 4.6 mg/kg as SSa, $n = 5$) and pure SSa (open circle) at doses of 2.3 mg/kg ((**B**); $n = 4$) and 4.6 mg/kg ((**C**); $n = 5$) to rats. Vertical bars represent SD.

Table 2. Pharmacokinetic parameters of SSa after oral administration of pure SSa or DA-9805 at doses equivalent to 1.1, 2.3, and 4.6 mg/kg of SSa to rats (mean ± SD).

Parameters	Oral Doses				
	1.1 mg/kg as SSa	2.3 mg/kg as SSa		4.6 mg/kg as SSa	
	DA-9805 0.25 g/kg (n = 5)	Pure SSa 2.3 mg/kg (n = 4)	DA-9805 0.5 g/kg (n = 5)	Pure SSa 4.6 mg/kg (n = 5)	DA-9805 1 g/kg (n = 5)
Body weight (g)	257 ± 5.70	249 ± 6.29	252 ± 6.71	204 ± 9.62	212 ± 5.70
AUC_{0-8h} (μg·min/mL) [a]	0.285 ± 0.0948	0.206 ± 0.129	0.404 ± 0.0839 *	0.460 ± 0.0451	1.21 ± 0.586 *
AUC_{0-10h} (μg·min/mL) [a]				0.490 ± 0.0521	1.49 ± 0.769 *
C_{max} (μg/mL) [a]	1.61 ± 0.248	3.00 ± 2.22	1.91 ± 0.808	4.67 ± 0.883	6.70 ± 3.46
T_{max} (min) [b]	45 (15–60)	17.5 (5–30)	60 (60–120)	30 (15–45)	45 (15–480)
GI_{24h} (% of dose)	2.19 ± 5.47	1.99 ± 1.49	26.5 ± 6.99 ***	14.2 ± 12.4	44.4 ± 7.17 ***
F (%)		0.0399	0.0783	0.0251	0.0659

[a] Dose-normalized values were compared when statistical analysis was performed. [b] T_{max} is expressed as median (range). * The value was significantly different from each same equivalent dose of pure SSa groups (* $p < 0.05$, *** $p < 0.001$; t-test).

3.3. PKs of PA after the Oral Administration of Pure PA and DA-9805

The mean arterial plasma concentration-time profiles of PA in rats after oral administration of pure PA at doses of 14.8, 29.6, and 59.2 mg/kg and equivalent doses of DA-9805 are shown in Figure 4. The relevant PK parameters are listed in Table 3. The AUC and C_{max} values of PA were proportional to PA doses following oral administration of pure PA and DA-9805. The AUC values of PA following oral administration of 0.5 and 1 g/kg of DA-9805 were significantly greater (by 164% and 155%) than those following the oral administration of each equivalent dose of pure PA, whereas the C_{max} values were comparable between pure PA and DA-9805 or even less than those in the pure PA group. Again, greater F values of PA were observed following DA-9805 administration than after pure PA administration (28.7–41.7% vs. 12.2–16.4%). Following the administration of DA-9805, slow absorption of PA supported by delayed T_{max} was observed compared to pure PA administration.

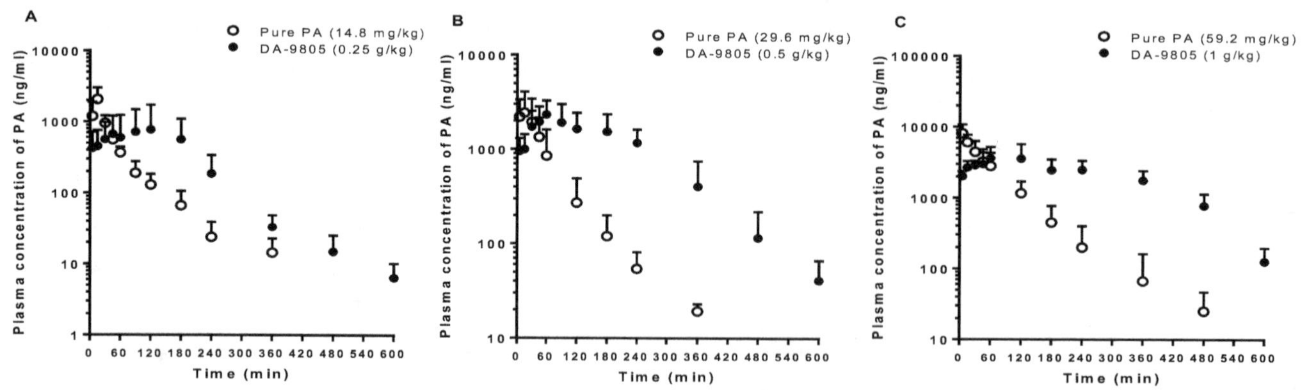

Figure 4. Mean arterial plasma concentration–time profiles of PA following oral administration of DA-9805 (closed circle) at doses of 0.25 g/kg (**A**; 14.8 mg/kg as PA, n = 5), 0.5 g/kg (**B**; 29.6 mg/kg as PA, n = 5), and 1 g/kg (**C**; 59.2 mg/kg as PA, n = 5) mg/kg and equivalent doses of pure PA (open circle; 14.8 mg/kg (**A**; n = 4), 29.6 mg/kg (**B**; n = 5), and 59.2 mg/kg (**C**; n = 4)) to rats. Vertical bars represent SD.

Table 3. Pharmacokinetic parameters of PA after oral administration of pure PA or DA-9805 at doses equivalent to 14.8, 29.6, and 59.2 mg/kg of PA to rats (mean ± SD).

Parameters	Oral Doses					
	14.8 mg/kg as PA		**29.6 mg/kg as PA**		**59.2 mg/kg as PA**	
	Pure PA 14.8 mg/kg (n = 4)	**DA-9805 0.25 g/kg** (n = 5)	**Pure PA 29.6 mg/kg** (n = 5)	**DA-9805 0.5 g/kg** (n = 5)	**Pure PA 59.2 mg/kg** (n = 4)	**DA-9805 1 g/kg** (n = 5)
Body weight (g)	251 ± 12.5	257 ± 5.70	247 ± 6.71	252 ± 6.71	204 ± 7.50	212 ± 5.70
$AUC_{0\text{-}inf}$ (μg·min/mL) [a]	82.4 ± 11.5	147 ± 129	153 ± 101	404 ± 83.9 *	462 ± 142	1180 ± 341 **
Terminal half-life (min)	79.1 ± 51.7	98.8 ± 56.1	70.5 ± 29.7	66.8 ± 15.6	50.5 ± 13.4	84.2 ± 55.4
C_{max} (μg/mL) [a]	2.05 ± 0.956	1.05 ± 0.855	2.78 ± 1.46	2.48 ± 0.853	8.20 ± 2.63	4.17 ± 1.53 *
T_{max} (min) [b]	15 (15)	30 (15–120)	15 (5–30)	60 (60–180)	5 (5–15)	120 (30–120)
GI_{24h} (% of dose)	0.406 ± 0.212	0.511 ± 1.01	0.0572 ± 0.0426	1.24 ± 1.39	0.119 ± 0.143	0.167 ± 0.128
F (%)	16.1	28.7	12.2	40.5	16.4	41.7

[a] Dose-normalized values were compared when statistical analysis was performed. [b] T_{max} is expressed as median (range). * The value was significantly different from each same equivalent dose of pure PA groups (* $p < 0.05$, ** $p < 0.01$; t-test).

3.4. PKs of IMP after the Oral Administration of Pure IMP and DA-9805

The mean arterial plasma concentration-time profiles of IMP after oral administration in rats of pure IMP at doses of 1.4, 2.9, and 5.8 mg/kg and equivalent doses of DA-9805 are shown in Figure 5. The relevant PK parameters are listed in Table 4. Following the oral administration of pure IMP, the dose-normalized AUC and C_{max} values of IMP at the highest level (5.8 mg/kg) were significantly greater (by 471% and 513%) than those in the lower dose groups (1.4 and 2.9 mg/kg). By contrast, DA-9805 showed dose-proportional AUC and C_{max} values of IMP in the equivalent oral dose range (0.25–1 g/kg; 1.4–5.8 mg/kg as IMP). Comparable AUC values of IMP were observed between the DA-9805 and pure IMP administration groups. Significantly delayed T_{max} values and/or lowered C_{max} values were observed following DA-9805 administration compared to those after each equivalent dose of pure IMP administration.

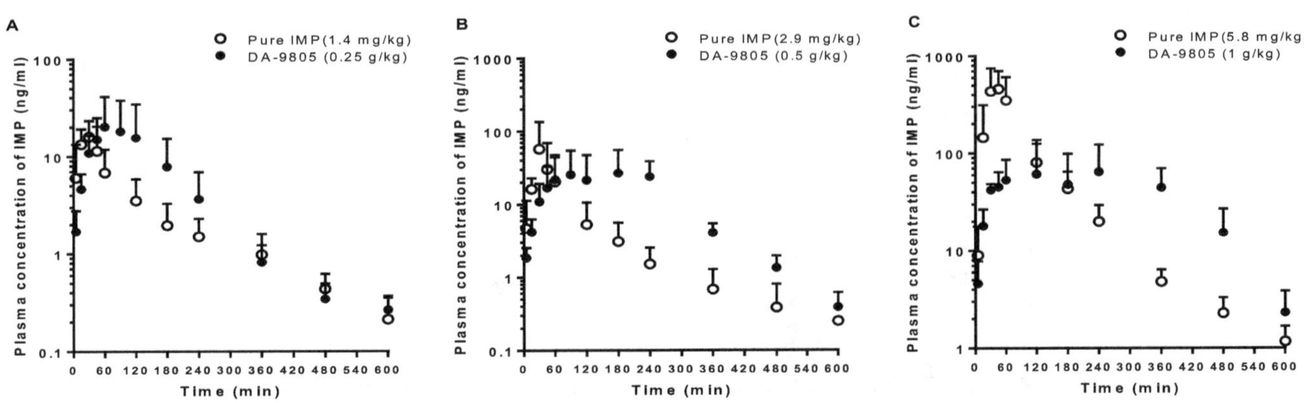

Figure 5. Mean arterial plasma concentration–time profiles of IMP following oral administration of DA-9805 (closed circle) at doses of 0.25 g/kg (**A**; 1.4 mg/kg as IMP, n = 5), 0.5 g/kg (**B**; 2.9 mg/kg as IMP, n = 5), and 1 g/kg (**C**; 5.8 mg/kg as IMP, n = 5) mg/kg and equivalent doses of pure IMP (open circle; 1.4 mg/kg (**A**; n = 6), 2.9 (**B**; n = 6), and 5.8 mg/kg (**C**; n = 5)) to rats. Vertical bars represent SD.

Table 4. Pharmacokinetic parameters of IMP after oral administration of pure IMP or DA-9805 at doses equivalent to 1.4, 2.9, and 5.8 mg/kg of DA-9805 to rats (mean ± SD).

Parameters	Oral Doses					
	1.4 mg/kg as IMP		2.9 mg/kg as IMP		5.8 mg/kg as IMP	
	Pure IMP 1.4 mg/kg (n = 6)	DA-9805 0.25 g/kg (n = 5)	Pure IMP 2.9 mg/kg (n = 6)	DA-9805 0.5 g/kg (n = 5)	Pure IMP 5.8 mg/kg (n = 5)	DA-9805 1 g/kg (n = 5)
Body weight (g)	258 ± 10.8	257 ± 5.70	253 ± 6.12	252 ± 6.71	204 ± 11.9	212 ± 5.70
$AUC_{0\text{-}inf}$ (μg·min/mL) [a]	1.53 ± 0.851	3.02 ± 2.38	2.95 ± 3.13	6.74 ± 5.29	36.2 ± 18.1 #	22.5 ± 12.6
Terminal half-life (min)	121 ± 38.3	120 ± 51.1	99.9 ± 31.5	73.8 ± 24.7	101 ± 29.2	56.5 ± 7.26 *
C_{max} (μg/mL) [a]	17.7 ± 6.79	28.4 ± 20.8	58.6 ± 76.4	33.5 ± 25.7	568 ± 312 #	88.2 ± 46.2 **
T_{max} (min) [b]	22.5 (5–45)	60 (30–120)	30 (15–30)	240 (90–240)	30 (15–60)	240 (30–360)
GI_{24h} (% of dose)	0.0285 ± 0.0152	2.19 ± 5.47	0.153 ± 0.228	0.846 ± 0.854	1.37 ± 1.09	6.30 ± 2.89
F (%)			5.27	12.1	28.7	17.8

[a] Dose-normalized values were compared when statistical analysis was performed. [b] T_{max} is expressed as median (range). # The dose-normalized value was significantly different from lower dose groups (# $p < 0.05$; Kruskal-Wallis test). * The value was significantly different from each same equivalent dose of pure IMP group (* $p < 0.05$, ** $p < 0.01$; *t*-test).

3.5. Protein Binding of SSa, PA, and IMP in Rat Plasma and Brain-Tissue Homogenates

The unbound fraction of SSa, PA, and IMP in rat plasma and brain-tissue homogenates are shown in Figure 6. The plasma protein-binding values of SSa, PA, and IMP were 97.3 ± 0.516% (free fraction of 2.7%), 28.5 ± 15.4% (free fraction of 71.5%), and 96.5 ± 0.744% (free fraction of 3.5%), respectively. Nonspecific binding of SSa, PA, and IMP to the equilibrium dialysis devices was negligible because their recovery after incubation was almost complete (>94.7%). The binding values of all three compounds were higher in brain homogenates than in plasma. The binding values of SSa in each brain tissue (striatum, hippocampus, and mixed brain) homogenate were 99.4 ± 0.138%, 99.4 ± 0.099%, and 99.3 ± 0.124% (free fraction of 0.618, 0.582, and 0.719%), respectively. The binding values of PA in the striatum, hippocampus, and mixed brain homogenates were 96.3 ± 0.957%, 91.9 ± 2.49%, and 90.5 ± 0.996% (free fraction of 3.75%, 8.10%, and 9.53%), respectively; and the corresponding IMP values were 99.0 ± 0.10%, 98.9 ± 0.037%, and 98.8 ± 0.068% (free fraction of 1.04%, 1.12%, and 1.22%), respectively.

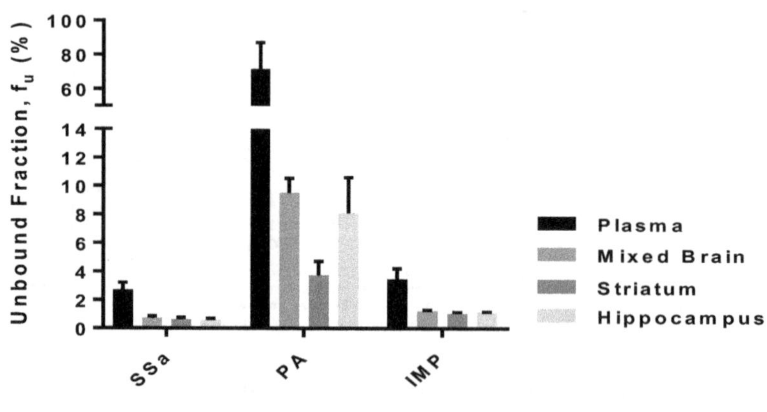

Figure 6. Mean unbound fraction (f_u, %) of SSa, PA, and IMP in rat plasma and brain (mixed brain, striatum, hippocampus) homogenates (n = 6 each). Vertical bars represent SD.

3.6. Brain and CSF Distribution of SSa, PA, and IMP after the Oral Administration of DA-9805

The mean plasma, brain regional (frontal cortex, striatum, hippocampus, and cerebellum), and CSF concentration–time profiles and tissue-to-plasma (T/P) ratios of SSa, PA, and IMP after multiple oral administration of DA-9805 (250 mg/kg/day for 8 days) are shown in Figure 7. The T/P ratios of SSa in each brain region were greater than unity (1.26–6.73) at 2 and 6 h, whereas the concentrations of

SSa in CSF were less than the LLOQ. For PA, the T/P ratios in each brain region were slightly greater than unity (1.13–1.98) at 2 h after the final DA-9805 oral dose, whereas the values, with the exception of those for the cerebellum, became smaller than unity at 6 h. The PA levels in the CSF were notably lower than those in the brain tissues and plasma. The T/P ratios of IMP in each brain region were greater than unity (1.24–3.04) at 2 h after the final dose, whereas the values became smaller than unity at 6 h. The concentrations of IMP in CSF were below the LLOQ.

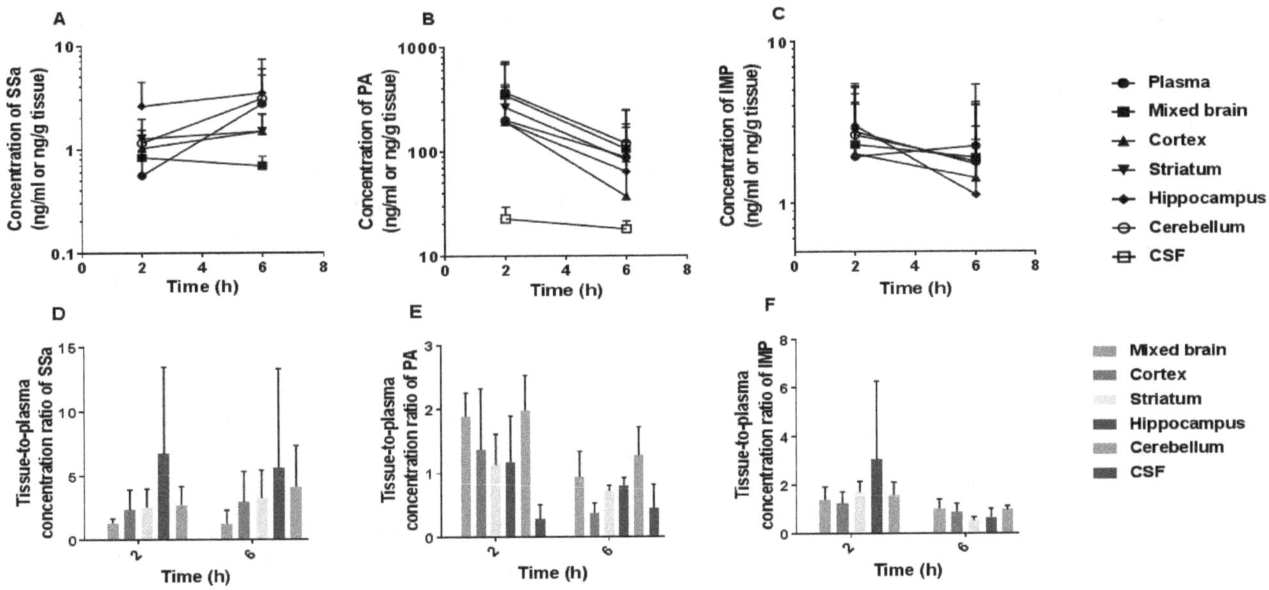

Figure 7. Mean plasma and brain regional concentration–time profiles of (**A**) SSa, (**B**) PA, and (**C**) IMP and their tissue-to-plasma (T/P) concentration ratios (**D**, **E**, and **F** for SSa, PA, and IMP, respectively) following multiple oral administration of DA-9805 (250 mg/kg/day for 8 days) at 2 h (n = 5) and 6 h (n = 4) after the final dose. Vertical bars represent SD.

4. Discussion

The effective oral dose of DA-9805 is 10–30 mg/kg/day in mice, and the planned dose regimen in the clinical study would be 30 mg or 60 mg three times a day (internal reports). However, the PKs of DA-9805 at this effective dose range could not be investigated due to the extremely low concentrations (<1%) of the two representative ingredients, SSa and IMP, in DA-9805. The doses of SSa (1.1–4.6 mg/kg), PA (14.8–59.2 mg/kg), and IMP (1.4–11.5 mg/kg) used in this study were determined based on the maximal tolerated dose of DA-9805, their concentrations in DA-9805, and assay sensitivity of each substance. Based on the relationship between the dose and PK parameters, the PKs of each component of DA-9805 in the effective dose range could be estimated.

The plasma concentrations of SSa after its intravenous administration at doses of 2.3 and 4.6 mg/kg decreased in a polyexponential fashion (Figure 2A). Based on the slower CL (primarily CL_{NR}) of SSa and greater dose-normalized AUC in the higher dose group, SSa was eliminated via a saturable process. The CL values of SSa were relatively slow compared to those of PA and IMP. Although the contribution of CL_R to CL was small (2.22–6.94%), renal excretion of SSa seemed to also be saturated in the higher dose group based on the slowed CL_R. The CL_R of SSa as the free (unbound to plasma proteins) fraction ($CL_{R,fu}$) was estimated based on the CL_R (Table 1) and free fraction of SSa in plasma. The estimated value was 2.23–11.9 mL/min/kg, similar to the reported glomerular filtration rate in rats at 5.24 mL/min/kg [39]. The V_{ss} values of SSa (102–126 mL/kg) were relatively small considering that the total body water in rats is 668 mL/kg [39]; hence, the distribution of SSa in tissues might be restricted due to its hydrophilicity, large molecular weight, and high binding affinity to plasma protein.

Interestingly, SSa showed linear PKs following the oral administration of pure SSa and DA-9805 based on the dose-proportional AUC and C_{max} values. This is because of the linear elimination of SSa at much lower plasma concentrations of SSa following oral administration in contrast to the saturation of SSa elimination following intravenous administration. The dose-normalized AUC of SSa following oral administration of 4.6 mg/kg of pure SSa is also similar to the dose-normalized value in previous reports with a much higher dose in TCM (~42 mg/kg as SSa) [13]. Note that the F values of SSa following oral administration were extremely low (<0.1%). Slow SSa CL (Table 1) suggested that its first-pass metabolism is not considerable. Therefore, the extremely low F value of SSa was most likely due to incomplete absorption. The low permeability of SSa because of its large molecular weight (>700 Da) and hydrophilicity may contribute to incomplete absorption. Considering the extremely low F values of SSa, its recovery from the GI tract ($GI_{24\,h}$ values, Table 2) seems incomplete due to possible decomposition in the GI tract. SSa, which includes an unstable allyl oxide linkage, could be converted into diene saponin by gastric juice [40]. In addition, both the SSa and diene-transformed saikosaponins could be stripped of their sugar moieties by intestinal flora [40,41]. Therefore, the decomposition of SSa in the GI tract could also be one of the possible reasons for the incomplete absorption.

The plasma concentrations of PA after its intravenous administration at dose ranges of 14.8–59.2 mg/kg also decreased in a polyexponential fashion (Figure 2B). PA showed slower CL (primarily CL_{NR}) and greater dose-normalized AUC values at the highest dose than at the lowest dose. This indicates that the elimination of PA is saturated at the highest dose. Intravenous PA over the lower dose range of 2.5–10 mg/kg showed linear PKs supported by constant CL (49.3–53.2 mL/min/kg) and dose-proportional AUC values [21]. The CL values of PA (21.4–29.3 mL/min/kg) obtained in this study (dose range of 14.8–59.2 mg/kg), which are slower than those from a previous report, again suggest the saturation of elimination at a higher dose range in this study. The CL_R of PA as a free (unbound to plasma proteins) fraction ($CL_{R,fu}$) was estimated based on the CL_R (Table 1) and free fraction of PA in plasma. Thus, the $CL_{R,fu}$ values estimated were 0.324–0.821 mL/min/kg, slower than the reported glomerular filtration rate in rats (5.24 mL/min/kg) [39]. The above data indicate that PA was primarily reabsorbed from the renal tubules in rats. Because the contribution of CL_R of PA to CL was negligible (0.941–2.55%), nonrenal elimination was concluded to be the major elimination route of PA. The V_{ss} values of PA (1100–1290 mL/kg) are greater than the reported total body water in rats (668 mL/kg) [39]. Unlike following intravenous administration, PA showed linear PKs following the oral administration of pure PA and DA-9805 at a dose range of 14.8–59.2 mg/kg as PA. The linear oral PKs of PA have been reported with a pure PA dose range of 35 to 140 mg/kg in rats [22].

The plasma concentrations of IMP after its intravenous administration at a dose range of 2.9–11.5 mg/kg also decreased in a polyexponential fashion (Figure 2C). Slowed CL (primarily CL_{NR}) and increased dose-normalized AUC values of IMP in the highest dose group suggested the saturation of its elimination at the highest dose. The almost negligible recovery from urine (Ae_{0-24h}) and CL_R of IMP (Table 1) indicates that the major elimination route of IMP is a nonrenal process. IMP showed the greatest V_{ss} values among the three components of DA-9805, which suggests that it has the highest affinity to tissue(s). Following oral administration of pure IMP, the significantly greater dose-normalized AUC and C_{max} values of IMP at the highest level (5.8 mg/kg) than those in the lower-dose groups (1.4 and 2.9 mg/kg) could be a result of the saturation of first-pass metabolism of IMP at the highest dose.

When the PKs of each component following oral administration of DA-9805 were compared to the administration of each equivalent dose of pure component, several significant and interesting differences were found. First, following the oral administration of DA-9805, significantly higher plasma concentrations, and hence, greater AUC and F values of SSa and PA, were observed than those following oral administration of each equivalent dose of pure SSa and PA. This suggests the significant influence of DA-9805 component(s) on the PKs of SSa and PA. Among the components of DA-9805, IMP shows inhibitory effects on CYP1A2 and 2B6 in both human and rat liver microsomes [42]. It also has weaker inhibitory effects on other major human (2C19, 2C9, 2D6, and 3A4) and rat (2D2 and 3A1/2)

CYP isozymes. O-demethylation of PA is the major in vivo metabolic pathway in rats [22], and the major isoform responsible for O-demethylation of PA in human liver microsomes is CYP1A2 [43]. Therefore, it is likely that IMP in DA-9805 inhibits the hepatic metabolism of PA via CYP1A2 and results in greater AUC values of PA following DA-9805 administration than after pure PA administration. SSa is also mainly metabolized in a Phase I manner [44]. Although the enzymes responsible for this Phase I metabolism of SSa have not been reported, the inhibition of SSa metabolism by IMP or other component(s) in DA-9805 could result in increased AUCs following DA-9805 administration.

Second, significantly more SSa was recovered from the GI tract at 24 h (including feces collected for 24 h) after the oral dose ($GI_{24\,h}$ values in Table 2) when DA-9805 was administered compared to pure SSa administration. This may not be due to decreased absorption of SSa when DA-9805 was administered compared to when pure SSa was administered because even greater AUC and F values of SSa were observed in rats with DA-9805 administration. Possibly, other saikosaponins and sugar-containing glycosides in DA-9805 could competitively prevent the decomposition of SSa in the GI lumen such as the hydrolysis of sugar moieties by intestinal flora.

Finally, the absorption of PA and IMP seemed to be delayed following oral administration of DA-9805 supported by their delayed T_{max} values compared to the administration of each pure component. Multiple components in DA-9805 might influence the absorption rate of each component. One of the possible reasons for the slowed absorption of PA and IMP could be slowed GI motility following DA-9805 administration because both Radix Paeoniae [45,46] and Radix Bupleuri [47] have antispasmodic effects on the GI tract. Because of the delayed absorption of IMP following DA-9805 administration, the C_{max} value of IMP is lowered and might not reach the level to cause saturation of its first-pass metabolism. This explains linear PKs of IMP up to the highest oral dose, when DA-9805 was administered. By contrast, following the highest oral dose (5.8 mg/kg) of pure IMP, possible saturation of its first-pass metabolism may result in greater dose-normalized AUCs than the lower dose groups.

Enhanced exposure of SSa and PA and delayed absorption of PA and IMP when administered as DA-9805 resulted in favorable PK profiles (i.e., elevated and sustained plasma concentrations of the three active components). The different PKs of the active components when administered as DA-9805 suggest possibly superior efficacy of DA-9805 over each pure component or their simple mixture.

The binding values of SSa and IMP to plasma protein were considerable (97.3% and 96.5%, respectively), whereas PA has relatively low binding values. However, the binding values of SSa, PA, and IMP were all considerable (>90.5%) in mixed brain, striatum, and hippocampus homogenates. Note that all three components of DA-9805 showed greater binding values (smaller free fraction) in brain homogenates than in plasma, possibly enabling their higher concentrations in the brain than in plasma. This result is consistent with the tissue-to-plasma ratios of the three components being greater than unity in most brain tissues at 2 h following multiple oral administrations of DA-9805. PA and IMP pass through the blood–brain barrier [14,32]. The concentrations of IMP in the striatum and hippocampus are higher than those in other regions [32]; our results are consistent with those findings. Notably, a brain-to-plasma ratio greater than unity of SSa suggests the possibility that SSa passes through the blood–brain barrier, despite its high polarity and large molecular weight, in line with previous studies reporting pharmacological activities of SSa in CNS [10,11]. By contrast, extremely low concentrations of the three components in the CSF suggest that the distribution of the three components in the CSF is negligible.

5. Conclusions

Following the intravenous administration of each pure component of DA-9805 (SSa, PA, and IMP), all three components showed dose-dependent PKs because of the saturation of elimination at a higher dose. By contrast, the dose-proportional AUC values of SSa, PA, and IMP were observed following oral administration of each pure component (except IMP at the highest dose) or DA-9805. Compared to the oral administration of each pure compound, oral administration as DA-9805 showed an increase in the AUC of SSa and PA, possibly due to inhibition of their metabolism by IMP or other component(s) in DA-9805. A delay in the absorption of PA and IMP was also observed when they were administered as DA-9805. The binding values of SSa and IMP to plasma protein or brain homogenates were considerable, whereas PA had relatively low binding values in plasma. All three components showed greater binding values in brain homogenates than in plasma, possibly explaining the observed brain-to-plasma ratios being greater than unity following multiple oral administrations of DA-9805 in contrast to their negligible levels in the CSF. This study furthers our understanding of the comprehensive PKs of SSa, PA, and IMP in rats and comparative oral PKs between each pure component and DA-9805.

Author Contributions: Conceptualization, J.S.J., J.R., Y.W.C. and H.E.K.; funding acquisition, H.E.K.; methodology, H.E.K.; formal analysis, M.H.K. and H.E.K.; investigation, M.H.K. and H.E.K.; resources, J.S.J., J.R. and Y.W.C.; Writing-Original draft preparation, M.H.K.; Writing-Review and editing, H.E.K.

Abbreviations

Ae_{0-24h}	the percentage of the dose excreted in the urine during 24 h
AUC	area under the plasma concentration–time curve
CL	time-averaged total body clearance
CL_{NR}	time-averaged nonrenal clearance
CL_R	time-averaged renal clearance
C_{max}	maximum plasma concentration
F	the extent of absolute oral bioavailability
f_u	unbound fraction
$GI_{24\ h}$	the percentage of the dose recovered from the gastrointestinal tract at 24 h (including their contents and feces during 24 h)
IMP	imperatorin
IS	internal standard
LC-MS/MS	liquid chromatographic–tandem mass spectrometry
LLOQ	lower limit of quantification
MRT	mean residence time
PA	paeonol
PKs	pharmacokinetics
SD	standard deviation
SSa	saikosaponin a
T_{max}	time to reach C_{max}
V_{ss}	apparent volume of distribution at steady state

References

1. Amro, M.S.; Teoh, S.L.; Norzana, A.G.; Srijit, D. The potential role of herbal products in the treatment of Parkinson's disease. *Clin. Ter.* **2018**, *169*, e23–e33. [PubMed]
2. Francardo, V.; Schmitz, Y.; Sulzer, D.; Cenci, M.A. Neuroprotection and neurorestoration as experimental therapeutics for Parkinson's disease. *Exp. Neurol.* **2017**, *298*, 137–147. [CrossRef] [PubMed]
3. Park, W.H.; Kang, S.; Piao, Y.; Pak, C.J.; Oh, M.S.; Kim, J.; Kang, M.S.; Pak, Y.K. Ethanol extract of *Bupleurum falcatum* and saikosaponins inhibit neuroinflammation via inhibition of NF-κB. *J. Ethnopharmacol.* **2015**, *174*, 37–44. [CrossRef] [PubMed]
4. Lee, J.Y.; Kim, H.S.; Oh, T.H.; Yune, T.Y. Ethanol extract of *Bupleurum falcatum* improves functional recovery by inhibiting matrix metalloproteinases-2 and -9 activation and inflammation after spinal cord injury. *Exp. Neurobiol.* **2010**, *19*, 146–154. [CrossRef] [PubMed]
5. Lee, B.; Shim, I.; Lee, H.; Hahm, D.H. Effect of *Bupleurum falcatum* on the stress-induced impairment of spatial working memory in rats. *Biol. Pharm. Bull.* **2009**, *32*, 1392–1398. [CrossRef] [PubMed]

6. Kim, H.G.; Park, G.; Piao, Y.; Kang, M.S.; Pak, Y.K.; Hong, S.P.; Oh, M.S. Effects of the root bark of *Paeonia suffruticosa* on mitochondria-mediated neuroprotection in an MPTP-induced model of Parkinson's disease. *Food Chem. Toxicol.* **2014**, *65*, 293–300. [CrossRef] [PubMed]
7. Moon, Y.J.; Lee, J.Y.; Oh, M.S.; Pak, Y.K.; Park, K.S.; Oh, T.H.; Yune, T.Y. Inhibition of inflammation and oxidative stress by *Angelica dahuricae* radix extract decreases apoptotic cell death and improves functional recovery after spinal cord injury. *J. Neurosci. Res.* **2012**, *90*, 243–256. [CrossRef] [PubMed]
8. Tang, Y.H.; Zhang, Y.Y.; Zhu, H.Y.; Huang, C.G. A high-performance liquid chromatographic method for saikosaponin a quantification in rat plasma. *Biomed. Chromatogr.* **2007**, *21*, 458–462. [CrossRef] [PubMed]
9. Chen, M.F.; Huang, C.C.; Liu, P.S.; Chen, C.H.; Shiu, L.Y. Saikosaponin a and saikosaponin d inhibit proliferation and migratory activity of rat HSC-T6 cells. *J. Med. Food* **2013**, *16*, 793–800. [CrossRef] [PubMed]
10. Ye, M.; Bi, Y.F.; Ding, L.; Zhu, W.W.; Gao, W. Saikosaponin a functions as anti-epileptic effect in pentylenetetrazol induced rats through inhibiting mTOR signaling pathway. *Biomed. Pharmacother.* **2016**, *81*, 281–287. [CrossRef] [PubMed]
11. Mao, X.; Miao, G.; Tao, X.; Hao, S.; Zhang, H.; Li, H.; Hou, Z.; Tian, R.; Lu, T.; Ma, J.; et al. Saikosaponin a protects TBI rats after controlled cortical impact and the underlying mechanism. *Am. J. Transl. Res.* **2016**, *8*, 133–141. [PubMed]
12. Liu, Y.; Li, Z.; Liu, X.; Pan, R. Review on the toxic effects of Radix Bupleuri. *Curr. Opin. Complement. Alternat. Med.* **2014**, *1*, 3–7.
13. Xu, L.; Song, R.; Tian, J.X.; Tian, Y.; Liu, G.Q.; Zhang, Z.J. Analysis of saikosaponins in rat plasma by anionic adducts-based liquid chromatography tandem mass spectrometry method. *Biomed. Chromatogr.* **2012**, *26*, 808–815. [CrossRef] [PubMed]
14. Li, H.; Wang, S.; Yang, Q.; Xie, Y.; Cao, W.; Zhang, B.; Wang, J.; Wang, J.; Wang, M. LC tissue distribution study of paeonol in rats after oral administration. *Chromatographia* **2011**, *73*, 495–500. [CrossRef]
15. Li, Y.J.; Bao, J.X.; Xu, J.W.; Murad, F.; Bian, K. Vascular dilation by paeonol—A mechanism study. *Vasc. Pharmacol.* **2010**, *53*, 169–176. [CrossRef] [PubMed]
16. Lee, B.; Shin, Y.W.; Bae, E.A.; Han, S.J.; Kim, J.S.; Kang, S.S.; Kim, D.H. Antiallergic effect of the root of *Paeonia lactiflora* and its constituents paeoniflorin and paeonol. *Arch. Pharm. Res.* **2008**, *31*, 445–450. [CrossRef] [PubMed]
17. Tsai, H.Y.; Lin, H.Y.; Fong, Y.C.; Wu, J.B.; Chen, Y.F.; Tsuzuki, M.; Tang, C.H. Paeonol inhibits RANKL-induced osteoclastogenesis by inhibiting ERK, p38 and NF-kappaB pathway. *Eur. J. Pharmacol.* **2008**, *588*, 124–133. [CrossRef] [PubMed]
18. Hsieh, C.L.; Cheng, C.Y.; Tsai, T.H.; Lin, I.H.; Liu, C.H.; Chiang, S.Y.; Lin, J.G.; Lao, C.J.; Tang, N.Y. Paeonol reduced cerebral infarction involving the superoxide anion and microglia activation in ischemia-reperfusion injured rats. *J. Ethnopharmacol.* **2006**, *106*, 208–215. [CrossRef] [PubMed]
19. Wu, J.B.; Song, N.N.; Wei, X.B.; Guan, H.S.; Zhang, X.M. Protective effects of paeonol on cultured rat hippocampal neurons against oxygen-glucose deprivation-induced injury. *J. Neurol. Sci.* **2008**, *264*, 50–55. [CrossRef] [PubMed]
20. Zhong, S.Z.; Ge, Q.H.; Qu, R.; Li, Q.; Ma, S.P. Paeonol attenuates neurotoxicity and ameliorates cognitive impairment induced by D-galactose in ICR mice. *J. Neurol. Sci.* **2009**, *277*, 58–64. [CrossRef] [PubMed]
21. Tsai, T.H.; Chou, C.J.; Chen, C.F. Pharmacokinetics of paeonol after intravenous administration in rats. *J. Pharm. Sci.* **1994**, *83*, 1307–1309. [CrossRef] [PubMed]
22. Xie, Y.; Zhou, H.; Wong, Y.F.; Xu, H.X.; Jiang, Z.H.; Liu, L. Study on the pharmacokinetics and metabolism of paeonol in rats treated with pure paeonol and an herbal preparation containing paeonol by using HPLC-DAD-MS method. *J. Pharm. Biomed. Anal.* **2008**, *46*, 748–756. [CrossRef] [PubMed]
23. Xie, Y.; Jiang, Z.H.; Zhou, H.; Ma, W.Z.; Wong, Y.F.; Liu, Z.Q.; Liu, L. The pharmacokinetic study of sinomenine, paeoniflorin and paeonol in rats after oral administration of a herbal product Qingfu Guanjiesu capsule by HPLC. *Biomed. Chromatogr.* **2014**, *28*, 1294–1302. [CrossRef] [PubMed]
24. Xiao, Y.; Zhang, Y.H.; Sheng, Y.X.; Zhang, J.L. LC-MS determination and pharmacokinetic studies of paeonol in rat plasma after administration of different compatibility of Su-Xiao-Xin-Tong prescriptions. *Biomed. Chromatogr.* **2008**, *22*, 527–534. [CrossRef] [PubMed]

25. Abad, M.J.; de las Heras, B.; Silvan, A.M.; Pascual, R.; Bermejo, P.; Rodriquez, B.; Villar, A.M. Effects of furocoumarins from *Cachrys trifida* on some macrophage functions. *J. Pharm. Pharmacol.* **2001**, *53*, 1163–1168. [CrossRef] [PubMed]
26. Ban, H.S.; Lim, S.S.; Suzuki, K.; Jung, S.H.; Lee, S.; Lee, Y.S.; Shin, K.H.; Ohuchi, K. Inhibitory effects of furanocoumarins isolated from the roots of *Angelica dahurica* on prostaglandin E2 production. *Planta Med.* **2003**, *69*, 408–412. [PubMed]
27. Wang, N.; Wu, L.; Cao, Y.; Wang, Y.; Zhang, Y. The protective activity of imperatorin in cultured neural cells exposed to hypoxia re-oxygenation injury via anti-apoptosis. *Fitoterapia* **2013**, *90*, 38–43. [CrossRef] [PubMed]
28. Budzynska, B.; Boguszewska-Czubara, A.; Kruk-Slomka, M.; Skalicka-Wozniak, K.; Michalak, A.; Musik, I.; Biala, G.; Glowniak, K. Effects of imperatorin on nicotine-induced anxiety- and memory-related responses and oxidative stress in mice. *Physiol. Behav.* **2013**, *122*, 46–55. [CrossRef] [PubMed]
29. Luszczki, J.J.; Glowniak, K.; Czuczwar, S.J. Time-course and dose-response relationships of imperatorin in the mouse maximal electroshock seizure threshold model. *Neurosci. Res.* **2007**, *59*, 18–22. [CrossRef] [PubMed]
30. Zhao, G.; Peng, C.; Du, W.; Wang, S. Simultaneous determination of imperatorin and its metabolites in vitro and in vivo by a GC-MS method: Application to a bioavailability and protein binding ability study in rat plasma. *Biomed. Chromatogr.* **2014**, *28*, 947–956. [CrossRef] [PubMed]
31. Zhang, J.; Zhang, M.; Fu, S.; Li, T.; Wang, S.; Zhao, M.; Ding, W.; Wang, C.; Wang, Q. Simultaneous determination of imperatorin and its metabolite xanthotoxol in rat plasma by using HPLC-ESI-MS coupled with hollow fiber liquid phase microextraction. *J. Chromatogr. B Anal. Technol. Biomed. Life Sci.* **2014**, *945–946*, 185–192. [CrossRef] [PubMed]
32. Zhang, X.; Xie, Y.; Cao, W.; Yang, Q.; Miao, S.; Wang, S. Brain distribution study of imperatorin in rats after oral administration assessed by HPLC. *Chromatographia* **2011**, *74*, 259–265. [CrossRef]
33. Lili, W.; Yehong, S.; Qi, Y.; Yan, H.; Jinhui, Z.; Yan, L.; Cheng, G. In vitro permeability analysis, pharmacokinetic and brain distribution study in mice of imperatorin, isoimperatorin and cnidilin in Radix *Angelicae dahuricae*. *Fitoterapia* **2013**, *85*, 144–153. [CrossRef] [PubMed]
34. Li, Y.; Wang, Y.; Tai, W.; Yang, L.; Chen, Y.; Chen, C.; Liu, C. Challenges and solutions of pharmacokinetics for efficacy and safety of traditional Chinese medicine. *Curr. Drug Metab.* **2015**, *16*, 765–776. [CrossRef] [PubMed]
35. Kim, J.M.; Yoon, J.N.; Jung, J.W.; Choi, H.D.; Shin, Y.J.; Han, C.K.; Lee, H.S.; Kang, H.E. Pharmacokinetics of hederacoside C, an active ingredient in AG NPP709, in rats. *Xenobiotica* **2013**, *43*, 985–992. [CrossRef] [PubMed]
36. Kwon, M.H.; Jeong, J.S.; Ryu, J.; Cho, Y.W.; Kang, H.E. Simultaneous determination of saikosaponin a, paeonol, and imperatorin, components of DA-9805, in rat plasma by LC-MS/MS and application to a pharmacokinetic study. *J. Chromatogr. B Anal. Technol. Biomed. Life Sci.* **2017**, *1068–1069*, 289–296. [CrossRef] [PubMed]
37. Chiou, W.L. Critical Evaluation of the potential error in pharmacokinetic studies of using the linear trapezoidal rule method for the calculation of the area under the plasma level–time curve. *J. Pharmacokinet. Biopharm.* **1978**, *6*, 539–546. [CrossRef] [PubMed]
38. Gibaldi, M.; Perrier, D. *Pharmacokinetics*, 2nd ed.; Marcel-Dekker: New York, NY, USA, 1982; ISBN 9780824710422.
39. Davies, B.; Morris, T. Physiological parameters in laboratory animals and humans. *Pharm. Res.* **1993**, *10*, 1093–1095. [CrossRef] [PubMed]
40. Shimizu, K.; Amagaya, S.; Ogihara, Y. Structural transformation of saikosaponins by gastric juice and intestinal flora. *J. Pharmacobiodyn.* **1985**, *8*, 718–725. [CrossRef] [PubMed]
41. Kida, H.; Akao, T.; Meselhy, M.R.; Hattori, M. Metabolism and pharmacokinetics of orally administered saikosaponin b1 in conventional, germ-free and *Eubacterium* Sp. A-44-infected gnotobiote rats. *Biol. Pharm. Bull.* **1998**, *21*, 588–593. [CrossRef] [PubMed]

42. Cao, Y.; Zhong, Y.H.; Yuan, M.; Li, H.; Zhao, C.J. Inhibitory Effect of imperatorin and isoimperatorin on activity of cytochrome p450 enzyme in human and rat liver microsomes. *Zhongguo Zhong Yao Za Zhi* **2013**, *38*, 1237–1241. [PubMed]
43. Liu, H.X.; Hu, Y.; Liu, Y.; He, Y.Q.; Li, W.; Yang, L. CYP1A2 is the major isoform responsible for paeonol *O*-demethylation in human liver microsomes. *Xenobiotica* **2009**, *39*, 672–679. [CrossRef] [PubMed]
44. Liu, G.; Tian, Y.; Li, G.; Xu, L.; Song, R.; Zhang, Z. Metabolism of saikosaponin a in rats: Diverse oxidations on the aglycone moiety in liver and intestine in addition to hydrolysis of glycosidic bonds. *Drug Metab. Dispos.* **2013**, *41*, 622–633. [CrossRef] [PubMed]
45. Chen, L.C.; Chou, M.H.; Lin, M.F.; Yang, L.L. Effects of Paeoniae Radix, a traditional Chinese medicine, on the pharmacokinetics of phenytoin. *J. Clin. Pharm. Ther.* **2001**, *26*, 271–278. [CrossRef] [PubMed]
46. Kobayashi, M.; Ueda, C.; Aoki, S.; Tajima, K.; Tanaka, N.; Yamahara, J. Anticholinergic action of paeony root and its active constituents. *Yakugaku Zasshi* **1990**, *110*, 964–968. [CrossRef] [PubMed]
47. Jung, B.S.; Shin, M.K. *Korean Domestic Pharmaceutical Pharmacopoeia (Herbal Medicine)*; Yeongnimsa: Seoul, Korea, 2003; pp. 412–414. ISBN 9788985897044.

2

Automated Real-Time Tumor Pharmacokinetic Profiling in 3D Models: A Novel Approach for Personalized Medicine

Jan F. Joseph [1,†], Leonie Gronbach [2,†], Jill García-Miller [2], Leticia M. Cruz [2], Bernhard Wuest [3], Ulrich Keilholz [4], Christian Zoschke [2] and Maria K. Parr [5,*]

1 Core Facility BioSupraMol, Freie Universität Berlin, 14195 Berlin, Germany; jan.joseph@fu-berlin.de
2 Institute of Pharmacy (Pharmacology & Toxicology), Freie Universität Berlin, 14195 Berlin, Germany; leonie.gronbach@fu-berlin.de (L.G.); jillg94@zedat.fu-berlin.de (J.G.-M.); leticia.cruz@fu-berlin.de (L.M.C.); christian.zoschke@fu-berlin.de (C.Z.)
3 Agilent Technologies GmbH, 76337 Waldbronn, Germany; bernhard_wuest@agilent.com
4 Charité–Universitätsmedizin Berlin, corporate member of Freie Universität Berlin, Humboldt-Universität zu Berlin and Berlin Institute of Health, Comprehensive Cancer Center, 10117 Berlin, Germany; Ulrich.Keilholz@charite.de
5 Institute of Pharmacy (Pharmaceutical and Medicinal Chemistry), Freie Universität Berlin, 14195 Berlin, Germany
* Correspondence: maria.parr@fu-berlin.de
† These authors contributed equally to this work.

Abstract: Cancer treatment often lacks individual dose adaptation, contributing to insufficient efficacy and severe side effects. Thus, personalized approaches are highly desired. Although various analytical techniques are established to determine drug levels in preclinical models, they are limited in the automated real-time acquisition of pharmacokinetic profiles. Therefore, an online UHPLC-MS/MS system for quantitation of drug concentrations within 3D tumor oral mucosa models was generated. The integration of sampling ports into the 3D tumor models and their culture inside the autosampler allowed for real-time pharmacokinetic profiling without additional sample preparation. Docetaxel quantitation was validated according to EMA guidelines. The tumor models recapitulated the morphology of head-and-neck cancer and the dose-dependent tumor reduction following docetaxel treatment. The administration of four different docetaxel concentrations resulted in comparable courses of concentration versus time curves for 96 h. In conclusion, this proof-of-concept study demonstrated the feasibility of real-time monitoring of drug levels in 3D tumor models without any sample preparation. The inclusion of patient-derived tumor cells into our models may further optimize the pharmacotherapy of cancer patients by efficiently delivering personalized data of the target tissue.

Keywords: automatization; drug absorption; drug dosing; head-and-neck cancer; pharmacokinetics; real-time measurements; taxanes; tissue engineering; UHPLC-MS/MS

---

1. Introduction

Selecting clinically relevant doses for the evaluation of anticancer drugs remains challenging in preclinical drug development and contributes to the low translatability of effects in vitro to efficacy in patients. While the understanding of cancer biology advances as the complexity of tumor models and analytical techniques increases, the success rate of drug development in oncology remains the lowest among all therapeutic areas.

Historically, anticancer drug doses for clinical trials have been determined by extrapolating the maximum tolerated dose (MTD) in animals to the human patient. Taking the MTD as the starting point, the effective and safe dose for humans was anticipated in the range of −3 to +3, with three concentrations below and three concentrations above. The revision of this concept is urgently needed, since many nonoptimal doses were taken into late stages of drug development. Especially the testing of high-risk drugs requires a more conservative approach, using the minimum anticipated biological effect level (MABEL) in first-in-human trials [1,2].

Up to now, new concepts focused on the improved extrapolation from animal studies to clinical trials, e.g., by introducing drug metabolism and pharmacokinetic studies in early drug development [3]. In particular, model-based, adaptive/Bayesian approaches already helped to better find effective and safe dosage [4]. Nevertheless, animal models are affected by differences in the human pathophysiology and even xenograft models do not fully recapitulate the barriers of drug uptake into human solid tumors [5].

In fact, drug exposure of tumor cells depends on the architecture of solid tumors with cell density, the spatial arrangement of cells and extracellular matrix proteins, interstitial fluid pressure, and vascular supply [6–8]. While 2D monolayer cell culture cannot provide meaningful insights into the pharmacokinetic profiles of solid tumors, sophisticated 3D tumor models such as spheroids or multilayered tumor models could do this, eventually even in a patient-specific manner [9,10].

The introduction of in vitro tumor models into the dose selection for a particular patient requires adapting the protocols to high-content, high-throughput approaches to handle high numbers of tests, e.g., with different drugs and several combinations. However, analytical approaches to quantify drug amounts in tissues comprise imaging- and microdialysis-based methods. While imaging techniques and microdialysis closely map the drug distribution within (tumor) tissues, all methods share the high effort needed in sample preparation [11,12], restricting their use for personalized medicine.

Herein, the development of an in vitro approach for real-time pharmacokinetic investigations in human cell-based models of head-and-neck squamous cell carcinoma is reported. It aims for an automated measurement of docetaxel concentrations within the tumor tissue to quantify the drug absorption. Therefore, an UHPLC-MS/MS method was adapted from clinical practice and optimized for a maximum number of online measurements per time.

2. Materials and Methods

2.1. Materials

Oral fibroblasts and oral fibroblast medium were purchased from ScienCell (Carlsbad, CA, USA). Tongue cancer cells from the SCC-25 cell line (RRID:CVCL_1682) were a generous gift from Howard Green (Dana-Farber Cancer Institute; Boston, MA, USA) [13]. Collagen G was purchased from Biochrom (Berlin, Germany) and consumables for tumor oral mucosa model culture from Greiner bio-one (Leipzig, Germany). Docetaxel was purchased from Selleckchem (Houston, TX, USA). Acetonitrile, formic acid, methanol, and isopropanol, all LC-MS grade, were purchased from Sigma-Aldrich (München, Germany).

2.2. Cell Culture

Oral fibroblasts were precultured in oral fibroblast medium and SCC-25 cells in DMEM/F-12 Ham medium, supplemented with 9% fetal calf serum, 0.9% L-glutamine and 0.9% penicillin/streptomycin at 37 °C and 5% CO_2. The cancer cells were regularly checked by single nucleotide polymorphism authentication (Multiplexion; Heidelberg, Germany). The medium was changed three times a week and the cells were subcultivated after reaching a confluence of 80%. Cell culture was performed according to standard operating procedures and referred to good cell culture practice.

2.3. *Sample Port Integration into Tumor Oral Mucosa (TOM) Models*

Tumor oral mucosa (TOM) models were prepared as described elsewhere [14] but adopted to a 6-well-plate design to handle the integration of the sample port (Figure 1a). In brief, 0.3×10^6 oral fibroblasts were embedded in collagen G and 1×10^6 SCC-25 cells were seeded on top of these lamina propria equivalents one week after. The model growth medium was changed three times a week and replaced by model differentiation medium one week after seeding the tumor cells [14]. The sampling port was created by placing a 24-well insert (400 nm pore size) into the TOM model before the collagen started to solidify. The tumor cells proliferated and migrated into the collagen matrix around the sampling port for seven days, before docetaxel was applied. The 24-well insert was fixed by a custom-made metal support and filled with 600 µL serum-free growth medium. The top of the 6-well plate was sealed with aluminum foil (VWR, Darmstadt, Germany) instead of using the standard plastic lid. TOM models were incubated at 37 °C inside the autosampler of the UHPLC-MS/MS device (Agilent Technologies GmbH, Waldbronn, Germany) for the 96 h observation period in the final week of TOM model culture.

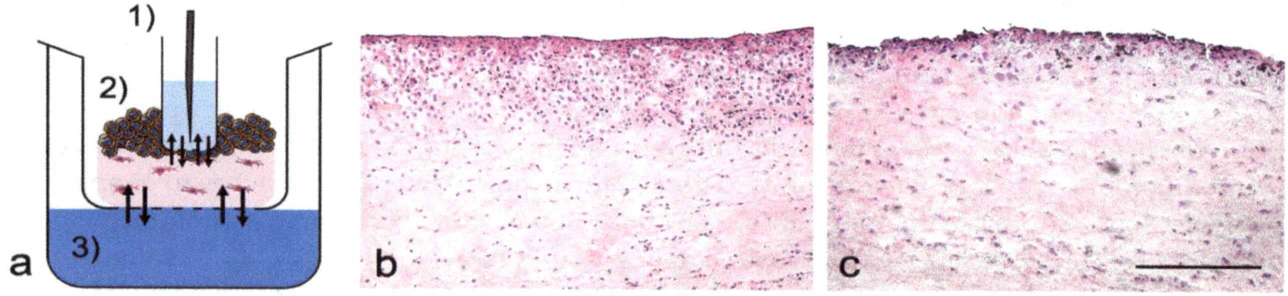

Figure 1. Experimental design and morphology of tumor oral mucosa (TOM) models. (**a**) Schematic cross-section of (1) sampling port with the needle of the autosampler, (2) TOM model with tumor cells (brown) and fibroblasts (magenta) within lamina propria, (3) Reservoir with differentiation medium, supplemented with docetaxel. The arrows indicate drug diffusion equilibria. Hematoxylin and eosin (H&E) staining of TOM models following two applications of (**b**) the vehicle control and (**c**) 7000 ng/mL docetaxel. Images were representative of four batches; scale bar = 250 µm.

2.4. *Docetaxel Treatment of TOM Models*

Docetaxel was dissolved in DMSO to a 70 mg/mL stock solution and diluted with construct differentiation medium to 7; 70; 700; 7000 ng/mL. DMSO, 0.01% in model differentiation medium, served as vehicle control since this was the maximum DMSO concentration among all samples (0.00001%; 0.0001%; 0.001%; and 0.01% DMSO for 7; 70; 700; 7000 ng/mL docetaxel). Docetaxel solutions were applied two times per construct with an application interval of 48 h.

2.5. *Morphological Analysis*

TOM models were snap frozen at the end of the 96 h observation period and cut into 7 µm thick slices using a cryotome (Leica CM 1510 S; Leica, Wetzlar, Germany). Cryosections were analyzed by hematoxylin and eosin (H&E) staining and pictures were taken with a microscope (BZ-8000; Keyence, Neu-Isenburg, Germany).

2.6. *UHPLC-MS/MS Analyses*

Method A: For automated real-time quantitation of docetaxel, an Agilent 1290 UHPLC coupled to an Agilent 6495 triple quadrupole tandem mass spectrometer equipped with a Jet Stream electrospray ionization (ESI) source was used (Agilent Technologies GmbH, Waldbronn, Germany). Separation of docetaxel was achieved on an Agilent Poroshell Phenyl Hexyl column (50 mm × 2.1 mm, 1.9 µm particle size) equipped with a corresponding guard column (5 mm × 2.1 mm, 1.9 µm particle size) using water (solvent A) and acetonitrile (solvent B) each containing 0.1% formic acid (*v/v*) as mobile phase. At a flow rate of 0.350 mL/min, the following gradient was applied: 5% B for 0.5 min, to 100% B at 4 min, 1 min hold, 5% B at 5.1 min, stop time 6.50 min. The column compartment was kept at 40 °C. The injection volume was 5 μL and the autosampler temperature was set to 37 °C. A needle wash (acetonitrile/methanol/isopropanol/water, 25% each, *v/v/v/v*) was applied for 20 s while an additional needle seat backflush using an Agilent Flex Cube was used to minimize carry over (15 s at 2 mL/min with needle wash solvent, pure isopropanol, and a mixture of water/acetonitrile (95/5, *v/v*) containing 0.1% formic acid). The total run time was 9.75 min.

The mass spectrometer was operated in multiple reaction monitoring (MRM) acquisition mode. Positive electrospray ionization mode (ESI+) yielded the sodium adduct of docetaxel $[M + Na]^+$ and was detected at *m/z* 830.3. Source and MRM parameters were optimized using Mass Hunter Source Optimizer software (version 1.1, Agilent Technologies Inc., Santa Clara, CA, USA). Final source parameters were as follows: drying gas temperature: 230 °C, drying gas flow: 20 L/min (nitrogen), nebulizer pressure: 40 psi (nitrogen), sheath gas temperature: 390 °C, sheath gas flow: 12 L/min (nitrogen), capillary voltage: +4,500 V, nozzle voltage: +300 V, high pressure radio frequency (HPRF): 210 V, low pressure radio frequency (LPRF): 160 V. MRM details are listed in Table 1. MassHunter (Quant) software (version B08, Agilent Technologies Inc., Santa Clara, CA, USA) was used for data acquisition and processing.

Table 1. Multiple reaction monitoring (MRM) transitions of docetaxel sodium adduct, used in method A.

Precursor Ion (*m/z*)	Product Ion (*m/z*)	Collision Energy	Cell Accelerator Voltage	Polarity
830.3	549.1	25	4	Positive
830.3	304.1	20	2	Positive

Method B: For identification of degradation products, an Agilent 1290 II HPLC connected to an Agilent 6550 iFunnel QTOF with Agilent Jet Stream source was used (Agilent Technologies Inc., Santa Clara, CA, USA). Separation of docetaxel and its metabolites was achieved on an Agilent Poroshell Phenyl Hexyl column (50 mm × 2.1 mm, 1.9 μm particle size) equipped with a corresponding guard column (5 mm × 2.1 mm, 1.9 μm particle size) using water (solvent A) and acetonitrile (solvent B) each containing 0.1% formic acid (*v/v*) as mobile phase. At a flow rate of 0.350 mL/min, a longer gradient was applied: 5% B for 0.5 min, to 37% B at 5 min, 50% B at 10 min, to 98% B at 15 min, 2 min hold, back to 5% B at 17.1 min, stop time 19 min. The column compartment was kept at 40 °C. The injection volume was 5 μL. A needle wash (acetonitrile, methanol, isopropanol, water) was applied for 20 s. The mass spectrometric parameters were as follows: drying gas temperature: 230 °C, drying gas flow 14 L/min (nitrogen), nebulizer pressure 40 psi (nitrogen), sheath gas temperature: 375 °C, sheath gas flow: 12 L/min (nitrogen), capillary voltage +4,500 V, nozzle voltage +300 V, high pressure radio frequency 200 V, low pressure radio frequency 100 V, fragmentor 365 V. Data acquisition was performed in auto MS/MS mode using a mass range of *m/z* 100–1000 at a scan rate of 1 spectrum/s for MS1 and *m/z* 50–1000 for MS2 experiments at 3 spectra/s. The collision energy was adjusted depending on the target *m/z* value (offset 4 eV, slope 3 eV/*m/z* 100).

2.7. Validation

Method A was used for automated real-time quantitation of docetaxel and validated in terms of selectivity, carry-over, lower limit of quantitation (LLOQ), calibration function, accuracy, and precision following the recommendations of the European Medicines Agency's (EMA) guideline on bioanalytical method validation [15]. All calibration (CAL) and quality control (QC) samples were freshly prepared in serum-free model differentiation medium as sample diluents.

Selectivity and carry-over: The guidelines require the analysis of matrix from four different lots. Since the matrix was artificial, no remarkable differences had to be considered. Thus, only one batch was used for assessing selectivity. Blank samples (serum-free model differentiation medium) were analyzed and compared with samples spiked with docetaxel at the LLOQ. Less than 20% detector response of the LLOQ is required for the blank samples. Carry-over was determined by analyzing blank samples after the injection of a high concentration QC (HQC) sample (7,500 ng/mL). Again, less than 20% detector response of the LLOQ is required to comply with the EMA guidelines.

Lower limit of quantitation and calibration: The LLOQ needs to be determined with sufficient accuracy and precision and with at least 5 times higher detector response than a blank sample. For evaluation, matrix-matched samples of 0.1, 0.25, 0.5, 1.0, 5.0 ng/mL were investigated. Additionally, the limit of detection (LOD) was determined based on calculations according to ICH guidelines [16]. Calibration samples in medium ranged from the LLOQ of 0.001 µg/mL to the upper limit of quantitation (ULOQ) of 10 µg/mL. In addition to an analyte free matrix sample, eight levels of calibration samples were prepared in triplicate and analyzed on two consecutive days.

Accuracy and precision: Accuracy and precision were assessed on serum-free medium samples spiked with docetaxel at 4 different QC levels with 5 replicates per level in a concentration range from the LLOQ to the ULOQ covering the calibration range. Samples were analyzed on two different days. Mean concentrations and the coefficient of variation (CV) of QC samples were required to be within ±15% in general, or ±20% at the LLOQ of the nominal concentrations, respectively. Within-run and between-run accuracy and precision were determined.

2.8. *Sample Preparation for the Identification of Degradation Products*

The degradation products of docetaxel were analyzed in the differentiation medium cultivated with the models (Table 2). To handle these samples, a protein precipitation procedure was performed. Aliquots of 100 µL of the samples were added to 400 µL of cold acetonitrile and centrifuged at 3328× *g* for 10 min. The serum-free supernatant was then transferred into LC-MS/MS vials for further analysis, according to method B.

Table 2. LC-MS data of docetaxel (highlighted gray) and postulated degradation products, acquired using method B.

Degradation Product	Formula	RT (min)	*m/z*	Exact Mass	Adduct	Mass Accuracy (ppm)
Carbamate	$C_{38}H_{45}NO_{12}$	4.30	708.3010	708.3015	$[M + H]^+$	0.65
10DABIII	$C_{29}H_{36}O_{10}$	4.55	545.2378	545.2381	$[M + H]^+$	0.60
Epi-carbamate	$C_{38}H_{45}NO_{12}$	4.72	708.3004	708.3015	$[M + H]^+$	1.47
Epi-10DABIII	$C_{29}H_{36}O_{10}$	5.31	567.2196	567.2201	$[M + Na]^+$	0.76
Oxo-10DABIII	$C_{29}H_{34}O_{10}$	5.40	565.2041	565.2044	$[M + Na]^+$	0.56
Epi-oxo-10DABIII	$C_{29}H_{34}O_{10}$	5.84	565.2040	565.2044	$[M + Na]^+$	0.67
1-7 **Docetaxel**	$C_{43}H_{53}NO_{14}$	7.95	830.3374	830.3358	$[M + Na]^+$	−1.9
Epi-Docetaxel	$C_{43}H_{53}NO_{14}$	9.08	830.3377	830.3358	$[M + Na]^+$	−2.26
Oxo-Docetaxel	$C_{43}H_{51}NO_{14}$	9.94	828.3200	828.3202	$[M + Na]^+$	0.19
Epi-oxo-Docetaxel	$C_{43}H_{51}NO_{14}$	11.07	828.3192	828.3202	$[M + Na]^+$	1.16

2.9. *Pharmacokinetic Analysis*

Pharmacokinetic analyses were conducted in R [17]. First, a non-compartmental analysis was performed. Assumptions were: (i) dose was calculated by concentration in the reservoir x volume (Figure 1a(3)); (ii) area under the concentration curve (AUC) 0–48 h lasted until 48 h and AUC 48–96 h until the end of the experiment; (iii) for the concentration between 48–96 h the unmeasured concentrations were not considered. Afterwards, interval AUCs were calculated. For 0–48 h, the AUC was calculated from 0.0001 h (start of the experiment) to the end of the 1st cycle; for 48–96 h, the AUC was calculated from the time "end of the 1st cycle" to "end of the 2nd cycle". However, the end of the 2nd cycle varied, since in some experiments, the last concentrations could not be measured. The maximum concentration (C_{max}) was determined based on the measured concentrations; time to maximum concentration (t_{max}) was the corresponding time to C_{max}.

3. Results

3.1. TOM Models with Sampling Port

The TOM models reproducibly showed an unstructured and hyperproliferative epithelial layer with pleomorphic tumor cells, also separating from the epithelial layer into the lamina propria. Neither the sampling port nor the cultivation within the autosampler of the UHPLC-MS/MS device influenced the tumor growth. The effects of docetaxel on the tumor size in TOM models by supplementing the differentiation medium with either two drug doses or the vehicle control were determined. Whereas the vehicle control did not change the tumor morphology (Figure 1b), docetaxel caused a dose-dependent reduction of tumor size with abundant epithelial cell death (Figure 1c). The average tumor size declined from 347 ± 72 µm (untreated) to 100 ± 45 µm (max docetaxel concentration, $n = 4$ each).

3.2. Docetaxel Epimerization and Degradation Products

During electrospray ionization, docetaxel mainly forms a sodium adduct ($[M + Na]^{+}_{theor}$=830.3358), which is used as precursor ion for all MS/MS experiments. As shown in Figure 2 (top), the product ion spectrum of docetaxel shows three major fragments at *m/z* 549.2095 (taxane nucleus (10-deacetylbaccatin III, 10DABIII), $[C_{29}H_{34}O_9 + Na]^+$, exact mass *m/z* 549.2095, mass error $\Delta m/z = 0$ ppm), *m/z* 304.1159 (phenylpropionic acid side chain, $[C_{14}H_{19}NO+Na]^+$, exact mass *m/z* 304.1155, $\Delta m/z = -1.17$ ppm), and *m/z* 248.0537 (side chain with loss of the tert-butyl moiety, $[C_{10}H_{11}NO_5 + Na]^+$, exact mass *m/z* 248.0529, $\Delta m/z = -3.05$ ppm). The two main fragments *m/z* 549. 1 and *m/z* 304.1 were later chosen for MRM transitions in real-time quantitation (method A).

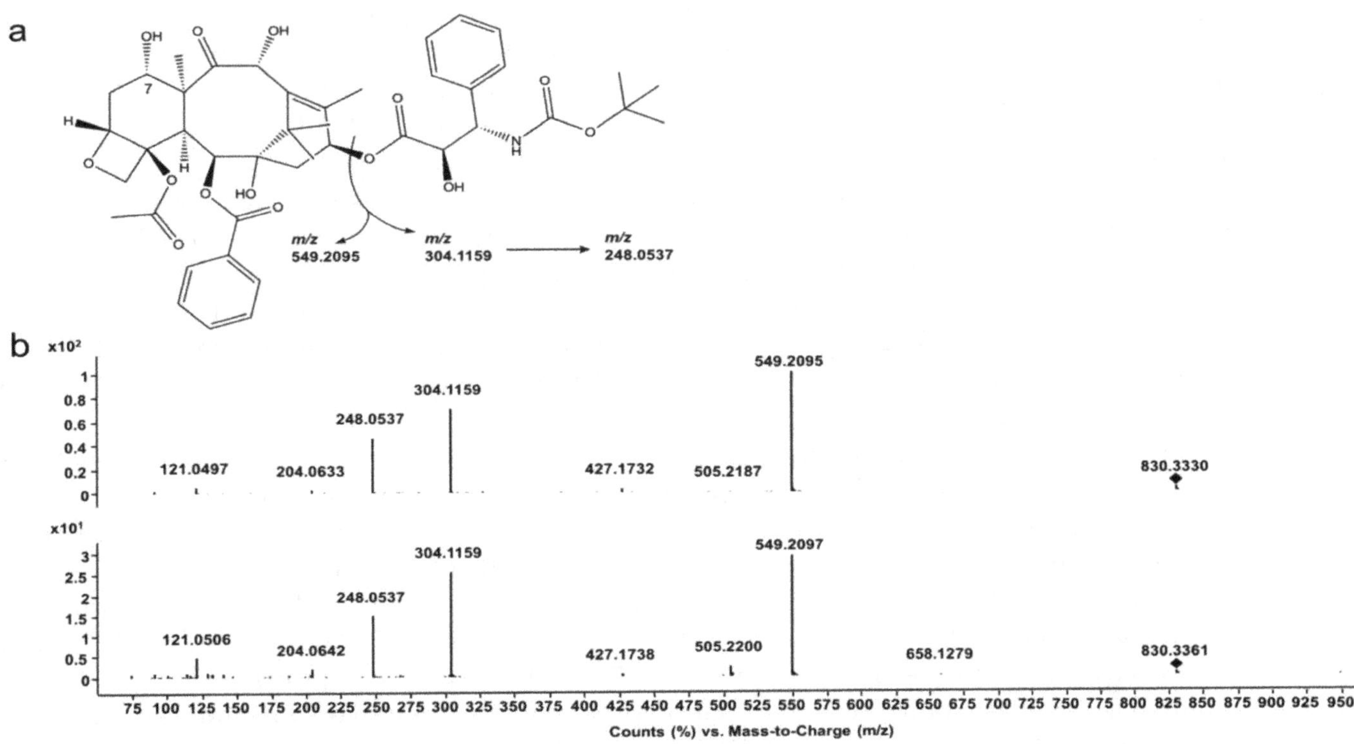

Figure 2. Docetaxel structure fragmentation. (**a**) Chemical structure of docetaxel and main fragmentation products. (**b**) Product ion spectra of docetaxel (top) and its potential 7-epimer (bottom), precursor $[M + Na]^{+}_{theor}$ = 830.3358 indicated with black rhombus.

Analyses of docetaxel reference substance as well as cell culture media without cells, and TOM models, revealed a second peak with almost identical MRM transitions (method A, chromatogram showing transitions in Figure S1) and product ions (method B, Figure 2 (bottom)). It already appeared only minutes after preparing the samples for analysis with serum-free medium as sample diluent. This degradation product is postulated to be the 7-epimer of docetaxel (epi-docetaxel), which is known to occur in basic and acidic conditions [18,19]. Since the epimerization could not be avoided in calibration or quality control samples as well, the combined peak areas of docetaxel and the 7-epimer were considered for all further quantitation experiments of docetaxel.

Based on accurate mass data, we postulated further degradation products beside the main degradant epi-docetaxel. Oxidized species of docetaxel and several hydrolysis products (ester and carbamate hydrolysis), as well as oxidation of the products of ester hydrolysis and their respective epimers (Table 2, Figures S3 and S4) are assigned. Two oxidized species of docetaxel show abundant sodium adducts in MS1 of *m/z* 828.3200 (oxo-docetaxel, RT: 9.94 min, $[C_{43}H_{51}NO_{14} + Na^+]^+$, exact mass *m/z* 828.3202, $\Delta m/z$ = 0.19 ppm) and *m/z* 828.3192 (epi-oxo-docetaxel, RT: 11.07 min, $[C_{43}H_{51}NO_{14} + Na^+]^+$, exact mass *m/z* 828.3192, $\Delta m/z$ = 1.16 ppm). Their MS/MS spectra show abundant fragments at $m/z_{\text{oxo-docetaxel}}$ 772.2534 and $m/z_{\text{epi-oxo-docetaxel}}$ 772.2584 ($[C_{39}H_{43}NO_{14} + Na]^+$, exact mass *m/z* 772.2576, $\Delta m/z_{\text{oxo-docetaxel}}$ =−1.07 ppm and $\Delta m/z_{\text{epi-oxo-docetaxel}}$ =5.41 ppm), which may originate from the loss of the tert-butyl residue. They both show a fragment corresponding to an oxidation at the taxane nucleus at $m/z_{\text{oxo-docetaxel}}$ 547.1927 and $m/z_{\text{epi-oxo-docetaxel}}$ 547.1955 ($[C_{29}H_{32}O_9 + Na]^+$, exact mass *m/z* 547.1939, $\Delta m/z_{\text{oxo-docetaxel}}$ = 2.11 ppm and $\Delta m/z_{\text{epi-oxo-docetaxel}}$ = −3.01 ppm). Analogously to docetaxel, the fragment *m/z* 304.1173 originated from the intact phenylpropionic acid side chain ($[C_{14}H_{19}NO_5 + Na]^+$, exact mass *m/z* 304.1155, $\Delta m/z_{\text{oxo-docetaxel}}$ = −5.77 ppm).

Further degradation products of docetaxel resulted from the ester hydrolysis of the taxane nucleus and the phenylpropionic acid side chain and are postulated here as 10DABIII (*m/z* 545.2378, RT: 4.55 min, $[C_{29}H_{36}O_{10} + H]^+$, exact mass *m/z* 545.2381, $\Delta m/z$ = 0.60 ppm) and epi-10DABIII (*m/z* 567.2196, RT: 5.31 min, $[C_{29}H_{36}O_{10} + Na]^+$, exact mass *m/z* 567.2201, $\Delta m/z$ = 0.83 ppm). A loss of benzoic acid, acetic acid and two losses of water from 10DABIII resulted in the fragment *m/z* 327.1587 ($[C_{20}H_{22}O_4 + H]^+$, exact mass *m/z* 327.1591, $\Delta m/z$ = 1.18 ppm). Epi-10DABIII showed a fragment at *m/z* 445.1791 ($[C_{22}H_{30}O_8 + Na]^+$, exact mass *m/z* 445.1833, $\Delta m/z$ = 9.41 ppm) which may correspond to the loss of the benzoic acid moiety and *m/z* 385.1615 ($[C_{20}H_{26}O_6 + Na]^+$, exact mass *m/z* 385.1622, $\Delta m/z$ = 1.71 ppm), which indicates a subsequent loss of acetic acid.

These two hydrolyzed esters most likely exist in an oxidized form as well, which are proposed as oxo-10DABIII (*m/z* 565.2041, RT: 5.40 min, $[C_{29}H_{34}O_{10} + Na]^+$, exact mass *m/z* 565.2044, $\Delta m/z$ = 0.56 ppm) and epi-oxo-10DABIII (*m/z* 565.2040, RT: 5.84 min, $[C_{29}H_{34}O_{10} + Na]^+$, exact mass *m/z* 565.2044, $\Delta m/z$ = 0.74 ppm) based on their accurate mass data. They both show a distinct fragment at $m/z_{\text{oxo-10DABIII}}$ 443.1661 and $m/z_{\text{epi-oxo-10DABIII}}$ 443.1680 ($[C_{22}H_{28}O_8 + Na]^+$, exact mass *m/z* 443.1676, $\Delta m/z_{\text{oxo-10DABIII}}$ = 3.47 ppm and $\Delta m/z_{\text{epi-oxo-10DABIII}}$ = −0.81 ppm), most likely originating from the loss of the benzoic acid moiety.

Furthermore, the hydrolysis of the carbamate function of docetaxel revealed two more products: 'Carbamate' showed an *m/z* 708.3010 in MS1 ($[C_{38}H_{45}NO_{12} + H]^+$, exact mass *m/z* 708.3015, $\Delta m/z$ = 0.64 ppm), and an abundant fragment of *m/z* 182.0818 in MS/MS which may originate from the cleavage of the remaining phenylpropionic acid side chain and the taxane nucleus ($[C_9H_{11}NO_3 + H]^+$, exact mass *m/z* 182.0812, $\Delta m/z$ = −3.46 ppm). 'Epi-carbamate' showed a similar product ion spectrum with the same base peak of *m/z* 182.0820 ($[C_9H_{11}NO_3 + H]^+$, exact mass *m/z* 182.0812, $\Delta m/z$ = −4.56 ppm) and *m/z* 708.3004 ($[C_{38}H_{45}NO_{12} + H]^+$, exact mass *m/z* 708.3015, $\Delta m/z$ = 1.47 ppm) in MS1.

An exemplary chromatogram of the degradation products following two applications of 70 μg/mL docetaxel for 48 h each is shown in Figure S2. We found only trace amounts of docetaxel degradation products in the TOM model media following the two applications of 7 μg/mL docetaxel for 48 h each. Therefore, we did not consider the degradation products in the real-time pharmacokinetic analyses.

3.3. Validation

As method A is used for quantitation in the online hyphenation of the tumor model with UHPLC based analysis, it was validated according to the guideline of the EMA [15].

Selectivity and carry-over: The method fulfilled the criteria for selectivity (<20% response in blank artificial matrix compared to response obtained at LLOQ) with a maximum of 7.45% detector response. Carry-over was a more critical parameter since the concentration range was very broad. Even after the optimization of the injector wash procedures, the detector response of analyte-free matrix samples exceeded the allowed 20% LLOQ detector response with a maximum of 29.42% after injection of HQC samples. Therefore, additional blank sample injections were included after samples of high concentrations resulted in successful prevention of carry-over.

Lower limit of quantitation and calibration: The concentration of 0.001 μg/mL showed acceptable accuracy (92.42–114.17%) and precision (6.58%CV) and was therefore chosen as the lowest point of the calibration. Based on the EMA guideline, the calculated LLOQ was 0.16 ng/mL and LOD 0.05 ng/mL, respectively.

For the calibration function, a quadratic fit after log-log transformation of the data provided the best results in terms of a combination of low residuals and best overall accuracy. All CAL samples met the requirements by EMA.

Accuracy and precision: The method (A) fulfilled the requirements given by EMA. Calculated concentrations of QC and CAL samples were within ±15% of the nominal values (Table 3), only 8.33% (within-day) and 15% (between-day) with only individual values outside.

Table 3. Accuracy and precision. c: docetaxel concentration, CV: coefficient of variation, RE: Relative error as measure of accuracy, LLOQ: lower limit of quantitation, LQC: lower quality control, MQC: middle quality control, HQC: higher quality control.

QC	Within-Day (n = 5)				Between-Day (n = 5)		
	Expected c (ng/mL)	Mean Calculated c (ng/mL)	CV (%)	RE (%)	Mean Calculated c (ng/mL)	CV (%)	RE (%)
LLOQ	1.00	1.06	7.26	5.71	1.01	11.40	1.62
LQC	3.00	2.76	2.27	−7.87	2.67	3.37	−10.94
MQC	3000	3027	7.83	0.89	3254	9.48	8.48
HQC	7500	6982	7.79	−6.91	7676	9.57	2.35

3.4. Docetaxel Pharmacokinetics in TOM Models

The area under the concentration curves (AUC), the maximum concentration (C_{max}), and the time to maximum concentration (t_{max}) as main pharmacokinetic parameters for the concentration versus time profiles of docetaxel within the sampling port are summarized in Table 4.

The course of the concentration versus time curves was comparable between the applied drug doses (Figure 3). Following the administration of docetaxel by supplementing the differentiation medium of TOM models in the reservoir at 0 h, the drug concentration increased until a plateau phase. The time to maximum concentration t_{max}, 39 ± 7.9 h was almost independent of the administered docetaxel dose, while the C_{max} depended on the administered docetaxel dose. Following the exchange of the differentiation medium, again supplemented with the same docetaxel doses, we detected 2.4- to 9.1-fold increased maximum concentrations and 2.4- to 8.8-fold increased AUCs in the sampling port compared to the respective values following the first docetaxel administration. Furthermore, we detected about 4- to 7-fold higher docetaxel concentrations in the sampling port compared to the applied docetaxel concentration (Figure 3b,c). This effect was not observed when applying 7 or 7000 ng/mL docetaxel (Figure 3a,d). Again, the t_{max} values were close to the end of the treatment cycle with values ranging between 82 and 89 h.

Table 4. Main pharmacokinetic parameters following 1st docetaxel application (0–48 h) and 2nd docetaxel application (48–96 h). c: docetaxel concentration, AUC: area under the curve.

c (ng/mL)	AUC (0–48 h) Mean (h × ng/mL)	CV (%)	C_{max} (0–48 h) Mean (ng/mL)	CV (%)	t_{max} (0–48 h) t_{max} (h)	CV (%)
7	66.3	44.6	1.9	194.5	43.9	14.5
70	444.4	12.5	14.4	25.3	39.5	20.7
700	13,324	26.0	461	29.0	41	9.9
7000	85,658	8.3	2492	10.4	32	21.4

c (ng/mL)	AUC (48–96 h) Mean (h × ng/mL)	CV (%)	C_{max} (48–96 h) Mean (ng/mL)	CV (%)	t_{max} (48–96 h) t_{max} (h)	CV (%)
7	151.4	84.4	6.0	65.1	82.8	16.2
70	3915.1	75.0	131.4	78.5	82.7	15.5
700	78,890	75.1	2850	66.3	83	16.6
7000	211,171	12.2	5920	7.3	90	13.7

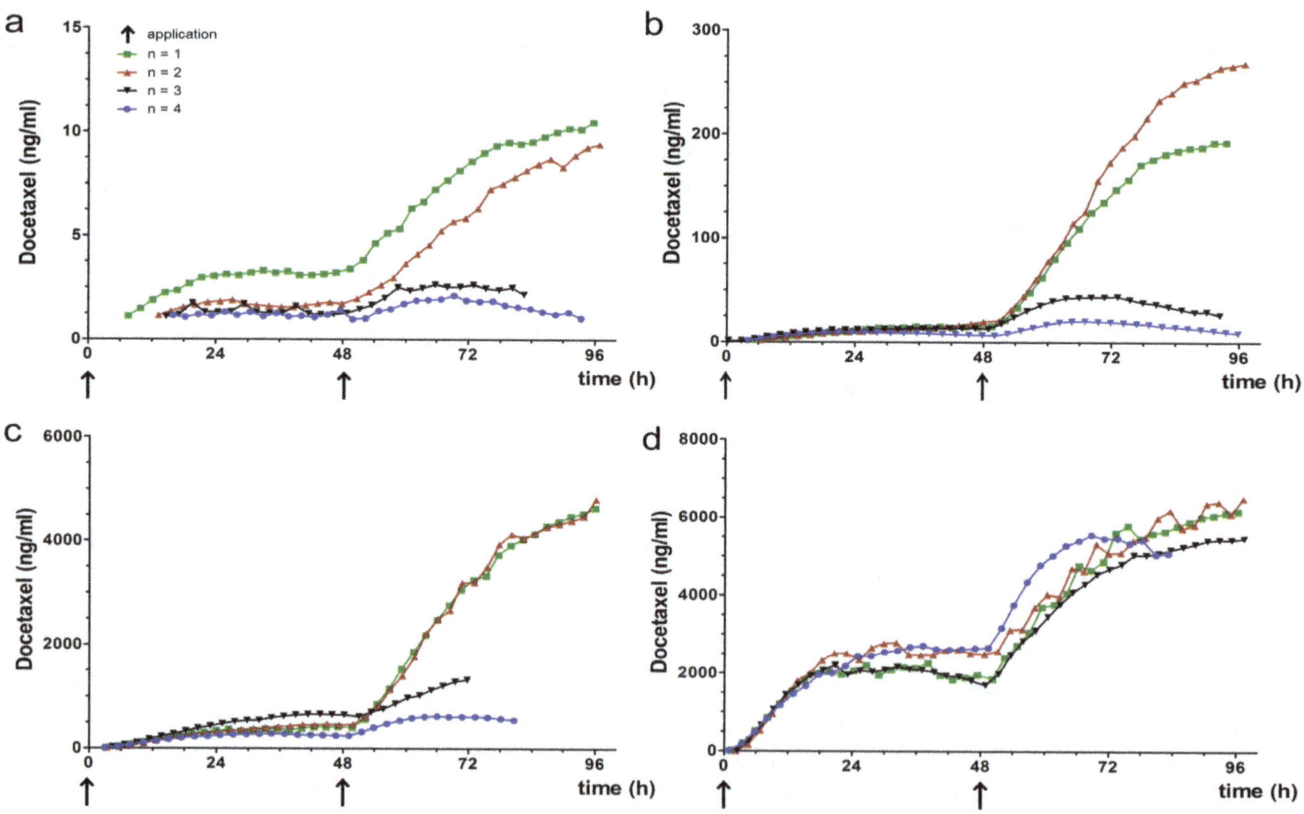

Figure 3. Concentration-time curves of docetaxel. Docetaxel concentrations in the sampling port of TOM models following the application of (**a**) 7, (**b**) 70, (**c**) 700 or (**d**) 7000 ng/mL docetaxel. Docetaxel was supplemented to the differentiation at 0 and 48 h (arrows), $n = 4$ for each concentration.

Moreover, the concentration versus time curves showed a different shape in two experiments (blue and black curve vs. red and green curve in Figure 3a–c). The slope of the blue and black curves markedly differed from the slope of the red and green curves after the second docetaxel administration. The relatively constant docetaxel concentrations within the sampling port could result from evaporation of medium from the reservoir (Figure 1a(3)), causing in loss of contact of the model with the reservoir.

Evaporation also affected the accessibility of the sample fluid for the autosampler needle, since we did not measure docetaxel from certain time points on (e.g., black curve in Figure 3c).

4. Discussion

An automated UHPLC-MS/MS method with online sampling in TOM models is presented here. This proof-of-concept study demonstrated the feasibility of real-time monitoring of drug levels in TOM models without any sample preparation. To achieve this, both the analytical method for docetaxel quantitation in human blood samples [20] and the culture of TOM models [14] needed to be adapted only slightly. Our approach was validated according to EMA guidelines [15] and is easily transferrable to other in vitro disease models.

In vitro studies frequently use drug doses far higher than the maximum tolerated dose in patients [21]. This overdosing causes effects in vitro that are not reproducible in vivo, contributing to the high attrition rate of investigational new drugs in clinical trials. Even if the patients tolerate such high doses, they will be prone to off-target effects. Aside from the bench-to-bedside extrapolation of drug doses, clinical data can be useful to conduct more relevant studies for investigation of personalized adaptations. Considering the maximum plasma concentration at the highest single dose recommended in the drug product of marketed drugs provides an upper limit for in vitro studies [22]. This concept is particularly useful to test potential new indications for approved drugs. We used docetaxel as a model drug to develop our analytical approach since both the efficacy and the pharmacokinetics of docetaxel are well-known [22]. After calculating a steady-state concentration of 74 ng/mL docetaxel in patients following an intravenous application of 75 mg/m^2 (for details, see [14]), we selected 7; 70; 700; and 7000 ng/mL as test concentrations in TOM models. The AUC within the TOM models ranged between 66.32 and 85,658.15 h × ng/mL following the first, and between 151 and 211,171 h×ng/mL following the second docetaxel application. Together with C_{max} values below 2492 and 5920 ng/mL, these in vitro results were in range of the clinical application of 100 mg/m^2, which results in an AUC of 4600 h × ng/mL and C_{max} of 3700 ng/mL [23].

Focusing on the nominal concentration of 70 ng/mL, we detected less docetaxel in the sampling port than has been found in human blood samples. This discrepancy supports the hypothesis of the poor uptake of anticancer drugs into solid tumors [6]. Likewise, paclitaxel penetrates only to the periphery of spheroids [5]. Nevertheless, docetaxel uptake into the TOM models increased following the second drug application. Since apoptosis results in enhanced drug uptake into inner cell layers of solid tumors [8], tumor cells dying after the first application should favor docetaxel uptake into TOM models.

Moreover, our method provides an in-depth insight into the formation of docetaxel degradation products. Since docetaxel epimerization is associated with a loss of potency and tumor resistance development in vivo [24], the considerable epimer formation will affect the efficacy of docetaxel. In contrast, the trace amounts of oxidation products and carbamates should not limit docetaxel effects in TOM models, although they are 10- to 40-fold less active [25]. The degradation products were identified by QTOF-MS and related to degradation products known from the literature [26]. Nevertheless, our approach allows for only limited insights into clinically relevant clearance due to the absence of hepatic metabolism and biliary excretion. If tumor cells metabolize the applied drugs, the quantitation of local metabolites will be feasible as well, but in the case at hand, we observed docetaxel epimerization and formation of degradation products as artifacts also in cell-free medium.

Differences between docetaxel concentrations in human patients and TOM models also arise from differences in protein binding. Whereas plasma protein binding of docetaxel is 97% in the patients [22], protein binding in medium containing fetal bovine serum is saturable. Paclitaxel, close in chemical structure to docetaxel, shows a protein binding between 79% at 500 ng/mL and 20% at 15,000 ng/mL [27]. Thus, we expect higher amounts of free drug available compared to the patients, especially following the application of 7000 ng/mL docetaxel. Nevertheless, we were not able to discriminate free against total docetaxel concentration, since the membrane of the sampling port has a pore size of 400 nm. Most protein sizes range between 1 and 100 nm, making protein diffusion into the sampling port likely. This might also explain higher C_{max} values in the sampling port than the administered concentration in the reservoir, since we quantified all docetaxel within the sampling port. The first docetaxel administration saturated the protein binding and intracellular fluids, the second application directly increased the concentration in the interstitial fluid of TOM models and the sampling port. However, we assume complete equilibration between the interstitial fluid of the TOM model and the sampling fluid within two hours, equal to the time interval we selected between two measurements. Thus, signals of the concentration over time curve earlier between zero and two hours might not recapitulate the concentration within the interstitial fluid of the TOM model, but provide an insight into the lag-time between docetaxel application and first appearance within the sampling port. As to be expected, the lag-time decreases with increasing docetaxel concentrations: 11.1 ± 3 h (7 ng/mL docetaxel application) compared to 1.82 ± 0.6 h (7000 ng/mL docetaxel application).

Since classical microdialysis already allowed insights into tissue-specific drug [28] and cytokine levels [29], the automated determination of pharmacokinetic profiles will enable patient-specific analyses in higher throughput. PK-PD modelling already improved dose selection and characterization of drug effects on tumor growth, overall survival and safety [30], but requires relevant data for the patient and his/her tumor. Nonclinical testing together with pharmacometrics may provide a more detailed insight by testing drugs in patient-specific models and extrapolating drug concentrations in tumors to adapt dose regimen for patients.

UHPLC-MS/MS again proved as the method of choice as it was already useful for a wide range of applications in pharmacology, toxicology, and forensics [31–33]. Despite first dilute and inject attempts to reduce the time-consuming sample preparation [34–39], UHPLC-MS/MS analyses still often utilizes extensive sample preparation to separate the molecule of interest from interfering proteins and potential enzymatic degradation processes [40]. Our method (A) used for quantitation of docetaxel was successfully validated in terms of selectivity, carry-over, lower limit of quantitation (LLOQ), calibration function, accuracy, and precision according to EMA guidelines for bioanalytical method validation. A very broad concentration range of 1–10,000 ng/mL was covered compared to already published methods [20,41], allowing the analysis of docetaxel administered ranging from 7 to 7000 ng/mL. The method proved to be accurate and precise, showed acceptable carry-over after including blank injections between high and low concentration samples, as well as fitness-for purpose in LLOQ. Furthermore, the method was fast, being able to separate docetaxel and 7-epi-docetaxel in less than 3.7 min (total run-time including cleaning of injector 9.75 min).

Future studies will compare differences between the patients' drug responses and drug delivery systems to optimize the dose regimen and application form. For increased efficacy, model size and sampling volume may be further optimized in the direction of high-throughput, and therefore, enhance personalized medicine.

5. Conclusions

We developed and evaluated a real-time approach to automatically measure docetaxel concentrations in TOM models. Partial epimerization and neglectable amounts of degradation products were detected instantaneously upon application of docetaxel to the medium. The courses of concentration versus time curves for 96 h were comparable among four different docetaxel concentrations. The first drug application resulted in an increase of docetaxel concentration, followed by a plateau phase, and exceeded after the second drug application. This proof-of-concept study paves the way for real-time pharmacokinetic and further online investigations in 3D tumor models and beyond, and thus, helps to improve preclinical drug development and personalized medicine.

Supplementary Materials:
Figure S1: Multiple reaction monitoring (MRM) chromatogram, Figure S2: Overlay of extracted ion chromatograms of docetaxel and degradation products, Figure S3: Product ion spectra of degradation products, Figure S4:

Suggested chemical structure of docetaxel and degradation products, structural differences in comparison to docetaxel are displayed in red color.

Author Contributions: Conceptualization, J.F.J., L.G., B.W., C.Z., and M.K.P.; methodology, J.F.J., L.G., B.W., C.Z., and M.K.P.; validation, J.F.J., L.G., and C.Z.; formal analysis, J.F.J., L.G. and C.Z.; investigation, J.F.J., L.G., J.G., L.M.C..; resources, C.Z., U.K., M.K.P.; data curation, J.F.J., L.G., J.G.-M., L.M.C.; writing—original draft preparation, J.F.J., L.G., C.Z.; writing—review and editing, J.F.J., L.G., U.K., C.Z., M.K.P.; visualization, J.F.J., L.G., J.G., C.Z.; supervision, C.Z., M.K.P.; project administration, U.K., C.Z., M.K.P.; funding acquisition, C.Z., U.K., M.K.P. All authors have read and agreed to the published version of the manuscript.

Acknowledgments: The authors thank Kathleen Sauvetre, Université Angers, France, for technical help with the sampling port and Luis Ilia, Freie Universität Berlin, Germany, for help with the pharmacokinetic analyses. The publication of this article was funded by Freie Universität Berlin.

References

1. Horvath, C.J.; Milton, M.N. The TeGenero incident and the Duff Report conclusions: A series of unfortunate events or an avoidable event? *Toxicol. Pathol.* **2009**, *37*, 372–383. [CrossRef] [PubMed]
2. Zou, P.; Yu, Y.; Zheng, N.; Yang, Y.; Paholak, H.J.; Yu, L.X.; Sun, D. Applications of Human Pharmacokinetic Prediction in First-in-Human Dose Estimation. *AAPS J.* **2012**, *14*, 262–281. [CrossRef] [PubMed]
3. Andrade, E.L.; Bento, A.F.; Cavalli, J.; Oliveira, S.K.; Schwanke, R.C.; Siqueira, J.M.; Freitas, C.S.; Marcon, R.; Calixto, J.B. Non-clinical studies in the process of new drug development—Part II: Good laboratory practice, metabolism, pharmacokinetics, safety and dose translation to clinical studies. *Braz. J. Med. Biol. Res.* **2016**, *49*, e5646. [CrossRef] [PubMed]
4. Nie, L.; Rubin, E.H.; Mehrotra, N.; Pinheiro, J.; Fernandes, L.L.; Roy, A.; Bailey, S.; de Alwis, D.P. Rendering the 3 + 3 Design to Rest: More Efficient Approaches to Oncology Dose-Finding Trials in the Era of Targeted Therapy. *Clin. Cancer Res.* **2016**, *22*, 2623–2629. [CrossRef]
5. Jang, S.H.; Wientjes, M.G.; Lu, D.; Au, J.L. Drug delivery and transport to solid tumors. *Pharm. Res.* **2003**, *20*, 1337–1350. [CrossRef]
6. Dewhirst, M.W.; Secomb, T.W. Transport of drugs from blood vessels to tumour tissue. *Nat. Rev. Cancer* **2017**, *17*, 738–750. [CrossRef]
7. Saleem, A.; Price, P.M. Early tumor drug pharmacokinetics is influenced by tumor perfusion but not plasma drug exposure. *Clin Cancer Res* **2008**, *14*, 8184–8190. [CrossRef]
8. Jang, S.H.; Wientjes, M.G.; Au, J.L. Determinants of paclitaxel uptake, accumulation and retention in solid tumors. *Invest. New Drugs* **2001**, *19*, 113–123. [CrossRef]
9. Fang, Y.; Eglen, R.M. Three-Dimensional Cell Cultures in Drug Discovery and Development. *SLAS Discov* **2017**, *22*, 456–472. [CrossRef]
10. Schütte, M.; Risch, T.; Abdavi-Azar, N.; Boehnke, K.; Schumacher, D.; Keil, M.; Yildiriman, R.; Jandrasits, C.; Borodina, T.; Amstislavskiy, V.; et al. Molecular dissection of colorectal cancer in pre-clinical models identifies biomarkers predicting sensitivity to EGFR inhibitors. *Nat. Commun.* **2017**, *8*, 14262. [CrossRef]
11. Wang, Q.; Zhang, J.; Pi, Z.; Zheng, Z.; Xing, J.; Song, F.; Liu, S.; Liu, Z. Application of online microdialysis coupled with liquid chromatography-tandem mass spectrometry method in assessing neuroprotective effect of Rhizoma coptidis on diabetic rats. *Anal. Methods* **2015**, *7*, 45–52. [CrossRef]
12. Graf, C.; Rühl, E. Imaging Techniques for Probing Nanoparticles in Cells and Skin. In *Biological Responses to Nanoscale Particles*; Springer: Berlin, Germany, 2019; pp. 213–239.
13. Rheinwald, J.G.; Beckett, M.A. Tumorigenic keratinocyte lines requiring anchorage and fibroblast support cultured from human squamous cell carcinomas. *Cancer Res* **1981**, *41*, 1657–1663. [PubMed]
14. Gronbach, L.; Wolff, C.; Klinghammer, K.; Stellmacherc, J.; Jurmeisterd, P.; Alexievc, U.; Schäfer-Kortinga, M.; Tinhofer, I.; Keilholz, U.; Zoschke, C. A multilayered epithelial mucosa model of head neck squamous cell carcinoma for analysis of tumor-microenvironment interactions and drug development. *Clin. Cancer Res.*. (in revision).
15. EMA. Guideline on Bioanalytical Method Validation. 2011. Available online: ema.europa.eu/en/documents/scientific-guideline/guideline-bioanalytical-method-validation_en.pdf (accessed on 2 February 2020).
16. EMA. ICH Topic Q 2 (R1) Validation of Analytical Procedures: Text and Methodology. 1995. Available online: ema.europa.eu/en/documents/scientific-guideline/ich-q-2-r1-validation-analytical-procedures-text-methodology-step-5_en.pdf (accessed on 2 February 2020).

17. R Development Core Team. *R: A Language and Environment for Statistical Computing*; R Foundation for Statistical Computing: Vienna, Austria, 2019.
18. Rao, B.M.; Chakraborty, A.; Srinivasu, M.K.; Devi, M.L.; Kumar, P.R.; Chandrasekhar, K.B.; Srinivasan, A.K.; Prasad, A.S.; Ramanatham, J. A stability-indicating HPLC assay method for docetaxel. *J. Pharm. Biomed. Anal.* **2006**, *41*, 676–681. [CrossRef]
19. Kumar, D.; Tomar, R.S.; Deolia, S.K.; Mitra, M.; Mukherjee, R.; Burman, A.C. Isolation and characterization of degradation impurities in docetaxel drug substance and its formulation. *J. Pharm. Biomed.* **2007**, *43*, 1228–1235. [CrossRef]
20. Yamaguchi, H.; Fujikawa, A.; Ito, H.; Tanaka, N.; Furugen, A.; Miyamori, K.; Takahashi, N.; Ogura, J.; Kobayashi, M.; Yamada, T.; et al. A rapid and sensitive LC/ESI–MS/MS method for quantitative analysis of docetaxel in human plasma and its application to a pharmacokinetic study. *J. Chromatogr. B Biomed. Appl.* **2012**, *893-894*, 157–161. [CrossRef]
21. Smith, M.A.; Houghton, P. A proposal regarding reporting of in vitro testing results. *Clin. Cancer Res.* **2013**, *19*, 2828–2833. [CrossRef]
22. Liston, D.R.; Davis, M. Clinically Relevant Concentrations of Anticancer Drugs: A Guide for Nonclinical Studies. *Clin. Cancer Res.* **2017**, *23*, 3489–3498. [CrossRef]
23. EMA. European Public Assessment Report "TAXOTERE", Annex I—Summary of Product. 2019. Available online: ema.europa.eu/documents/product-information/taxotere-epar-product-information_en.pdf (accessed on 2 February 2020).
24. Mohsin, S.; Arellano, I.H.; Choudhury, N.R.; Garg, S. Docetaxel epimerization in silicone films: A case of drug excipient incompatibility. *Drug Test. Anal.* **2014**, *6*, 1076–1084. [CrossRef]
25. Vuilhorgne, M.; Gaillard, C.; Sanderink, G.J.; Royer, I.; Monsarrat, B.; Dubois, J.; Wright, M. Metabolism of Taxoid Drugs. In *Taxane Anticancer Agents*; American Chemical Society: Washington, DC, USA, 1994; Volume 583, pp. 98–110.
26. Tian, J.; Stella, V.J. Degradation of paclitaxel and related compounds in aqueous solutions I: Epimerization. *J. Pharm. Sci.* **2008**, *97*, 1224–1235. [CrossRef]
27. Song, D.; Hsu, L.F.; Au, J.L. Binding of taxol to plastic and glass containers and protein under in vitro conditions. *J. Pharm. Sci.* **1996**, *85*, 29–31. [CrossRef] [PubMed]
28. Schuck, V.J.; Rinas, I.; Derendorf, H. In vitro microdialysis sampling of docetaxel. *J Pharm. Biomed. Anal.* **2004**, *36*, 807–813. [CrossRef] [PubMed]
29. Baumann, K.Y.; Church, M.K.; Clough, G.F.; Quist, S.R.; Schmelz, M.; Skov, P.S.; Anderson, C.D.; Tannert, L.K.; Giménez-Arnau, A.M.; Frischbutter, S.; et al. Skin microdialysis: methods, applications and future opportunities—An EAACI position paper. *Clin. Transl. Allergy* **2019**, *9*, 24. [CrossRef] [PubMed]
30. Pasqua, O.E.D. PKPD and Disease Modeling: Concepts and Applications to Oncology. In *Clinical Trial Simulations: Applications and Trends*; Kimko, H.H.C., Peck, C.C., Eds.; Springer: New York, NY, USA, 2011; pp. 281–306. [CrossRef]
31. Patteet, L.; Maudens, K.E.; Stove, C.P.; Lambert, W.E.; Morrens, M.; Sabbe, B.; Neels, H. The use of dried blood spots for quantification of 15 antipsychotics and 7 metabolites with ultra-high performance liquid chromatography - tandem mass spectrometry. *Drug Test. Anal.* **2015**, *7*, 502–511. [CrossRef]
32. Rodriguez-Aller, M.; Gurny, R.; Veuthey, J.L.; Guillarme, D. Coupling ultra high-pressure liquid chromatography with mass spectrometry: constraints and possible applications. *J. Chromatogr. A* **2013**, *1292*, 2–18. [CrossRef]
33. Novakova, L.; Pavlik, J.; Chrenkova, L.; Martinec, O.; Cerveny, L. Current antiviral drugs and their analysis in biological materials—Part II: Antivirals against hepatitis and HIV viruses. *J Pharm. Biomed. Anal.* **2018**, *147*, 378–399. [CrossRef]
34. Gorgens, C.; Guddat, S.; Schanzer, W.; Thevis, M. Screening and confirmation of myo-inositol trispyrophosphate (ITPP) in human urine by hydrophilic interaction liquid chromatography high resolution / high accuracy mass spectrometry for doping control purposes. *Drug Test. Anal.* **2014**, *6*, 1102–1107. [CrossRef]
35. Ambrosio, G.; Joseph, J.F.; Wuest, B.; Mazzarino, M.; de la Torre, X.; Diel, P.; Botre, F.; Parr, M.K. Detection and quantitation of ecdysterone in human serum by liquid chromatography coupled to tandem mass spectrometry. *Steroids* **2020**, *157*, 108603. [CrossRef]

36. Holder, B.R.; McNaney, C.A.; Luchetti, D.; Schaeffer, E.; Drexler, D.M. Bioanalysis of acetylcarnitine in cerebrospinal fluid by HILIC-mass spectrometry. *Biomed. Chromatogr.* **2015**, *29*, 1375–1379. [CrossRef]
37. Kong, T.Y.; Kim, J.H.; Kim, J.Y.; In, M.K.; Choi, K.H.; Kim, H.S.; Lee, H.S. Rapid analysis of drugs of abuse and their metabolites in human urine using dilute and shoot liquid chromatography-tandem mass spectrometry. *Arch. Pharm. Res.* **2017**, *40*, 180–196. [CrossRef]
38. Bourgogne, E.; Wagner, M. [Sample preparation and bioanalysis in mass spectrometry]. *Ann. Biol. Clin. (Paris)* **2015**, *73*, 11–23. [CrossRef] [PubMed]
39. Parr, M.K.; Ambrosio, G.; Wuest, B.; Mazzarino, M.; de la Torre, X.; Sibilia, F.; Joseph, J.F.; Diel, P.; Botrè, F. Targeting the Administration of Ecdysterone in Doping Control Samples. *bioRxiv* **2019**. [CrossRef]
40. Plock, N.; Kloft, C. Microdialysis–theoretical background and recent implementation in applied life-sciences. *Eur. J. Pharm. Sci.* **2005**, *25*, 1–24. [CrossRef] [PubMed]
41. Hendrikx, J.J.; Hillebrand, M.J.; Thijssen, B.; Rosing, H.; Schinkel, A.H.; Schellens, J.H.; Beijnen, J.H. A sensitive combined assay for the quantification of paclitaxel, docetaxel and ritonavir in human plasma using liquid chromatography coupled with tandem mass spectrometry. *J. Chromatogr. B Analyt. Technol. Biomed. Life Sci.* **2011**, *879*, 2984–2990. [CrossRef]

3

Quercetin is a Flavonoid Breast Cancer Resistance Protein Inhibitor with an Impact on the Oral Pharmacokinetics of Sulfasalazine in Rats

Yoo-Kyung Song [1,2,†], Jin-Ha Yoon [3,†], Jong Kyu Woo [3], Ju-Hee Kang [3], Kyeong-Ryoon Lee [2], Seung Hyun Oh [3], Suk-Jae Chung [1,*] and Han-Joo Maeng [3,*]

1 College of Pharmacy, Seoul National University, Seoul 08826, Korea; yksong777@gmail.com
2 Laboratory Animal Resource Center, Korea Research Institute of Bioscience and Biotechnology, Ochang 28116, Korea; Kyeongrlee@kribb.re.kr
3 College of Pharmacy, Gachon University, Incheon 21936, Korea; jinha89@daum.net (J.-H.Y.); apoptosis@snu.ac.kr (J.K.W.); applekjh0503@hanmail.net (J.-H.K.); eyeball@gachon.ac.kr (S.H.O.)
* Correspondence: sukjae@snu.ac.kr (S.-J.C.); hjmaeng@gachon.ac.kr (H.-J.M.)
† These authors contributed equally to this work.

Abstract: The potential inhibitory effect of quercetin, a major plant flavonol, on breast cancer resistance protein (BCRP) activity was investigated in this study. The presence of quercetin significantly increased the cellular accumulation and associated cytotoxicity of the BCRP substrate mitoxantrone in human cervical cancer cells (HeLa cells) in a concentration-dependent manner. The transcellular efflux of prazosin, a stereotypical BCRP substrate, was also significantly reduced in the presence of quercetin in a bidirectional transport assay using human BCRP-overexpressing cells; further kinetic analysis revealed IC_{50} and Ki values of 4.22 and 3.91 μM, respectively. Moreover, pretreatment with 10 mg/kg quercetin in rats led to a 1.8-fold and 1.5-fold increase in the AUC_{8h} (i.e., 44.5 ± 11.8 min·μg/mL vs. 25.7 ± 9.98 min·μg/mL, $p < 0.05$) and C_{max} (i.e., 179 ± 23.0 ng/mL vs. 122 ± 23.2 ng/mL, $p < 0.05$) of orally administered sulfasalazine, respectively. Collectively, these results provide evidence that quercetin acts as an in vivo as well as in vitro inhibitor of BCRP. Considering the high dietary intake of quercetin as well as its consumption as a dietary supplement, issuing a caution regarding its food–drug interactions should be considered.

Keywords: quercetin; breast cancer resistance protein; inhibitor; prazosin; sulfasalazine; kinetic analysis; pharmacokinetics; food–drug interactions

---

1. Introduction

Flavonoids are a large group of polyphenolic antioxidants present in various human foods, such as vegetables, fruits, and tea. Quercetin is a major plant flavonol, a subclass of flavonoids with a 3-hydroxyflavone structure; it is present in high levels in onions, kale, broccoli, and tea [1,2]. Quercetin is mostly present in foods in the form of glycosides, which are efficiently hydrolyzed in the small intestine to release quercetin aglycone when ingested [3]. Dietary consumption of quercetin is estimated to be between 25 and 50 mg per day, accounting for approximately 70% of the total dietary flavonol and flavonone intake [4–6]. Moreover, it is well recognized that quercetin has diverse biological effects, including antioxidative, antiviral, antiulcer, and anticancer activities [7–10]. These activities have led to its consumption in various dosages and forms (e.g., 200–1000 mg aglycone per capsule/tablet [11]) as dietary supplements.

However, a recent analysis reported that the increased demand and consumption of dietary supplements is likely associated with a risk of adverse events. Indeed, a high number of adverse events (i.e., 23,000 emergency department visits per year in the United States) are attributed to dietary supplements [12]. In particular, flavonoids can modulate the activity of major ATP-binding cassette (ABC) efflux transporters [13]. For example, several studies have consistently shown that quercetin interacts with both P-glycoprotein (P-gp) [14–16] and multidrug resistance-associated protein 1 (MRP1) [17], inhibiting the efflux of substrates in the specific transporter-overexpressing cells in vitro or increasing the bioavailability/brain accumulation of substrate drugs in vivo by affecting the transporters' activity. Moreover, our research group recently reported that repeated pretreatment with quercetin could upregulate the human multidrug resistance protein 1 (MDR1) gene via a vitamin D receptor-dependent pathway in Caco-2 cells [18]. Therefore, the increasing use of dietary supplements containing quercetin emphasizes the need to investigate the potential clinical interactions that can be induced by the flavonoid.

Among ABC transporters, breast cancer resistance protein (BCRP; encoded by the ABCG2 gene) is a major efflux transporter abundantly expressed at the apical membrane of intestinal/kidney epithelial cells and hepatocytes. The transporter functions as a physiological barrier against oral absorption as well as a determinant of the disposition of substrate drugs [19]. Recently, several studies have attempted to determine whether quercetin interacts with BCRP. Sesink et al. reported that the flavonoid can be transported by the mouse Bcrp1 transporter in MDCKII/mBcrp1 cells [20]; moreover, its presence was shown to inhibit the cellular accumulation of the BCRP substrates Hoechst 33342 and mitoxantrone in BCRP-overexpressing MCF-7 cells [21,22]. However, such observations in cell systems cannot be directly translated to substantial effects on efflux transporter activity in vivo. For example, a study reported that coadministration of topotecan (a BCRP substrate) with the flavonoids chrysin or 7,8-benzoflavone (potent inhibitors of the transporter in BCRP-overexpressing MCF-7 cells) resulted in no significant effects on the pharmacokinetics of the substrate in rats or P-gp-knockout mice [23]. Therefore, considering that no apparent in vitro to in vivo association regarding BCRP inhibition by flavonoids was found [23], a more pharmacokinetic-based understanding of the interaction of quercetin with BCRP is needed. To our knowledge, the in vivo pharmacokinetic inhibition of BCRP by quercetin has not been previously reported.

Therefore, the objective of this study was to conduct an integrated study including in vitro and in vivo pharmacokinetic assessments on the inhibition of BCRP by quercetin. Here, we showed that quercetin can increase the cellular accumulation and associated cytotoxicity of the BCRP substrate mitoxantrone in human cervical cancer HeLa cells. Importantly, the high inhibitory potency of quercetin in limiting transporter-mediated efflux was demonstrated using the kinetic parameters (e.g., IC_{50} and Ki) associated with the efflux. Finally, the in vivo pharmacokinetics of the possible inhibition were studied in rats using sulfasalazine, a selective BCRP probe that was previously proven to show increased absorption by impaired BCRP function [24–26].

2. Materials and Methods

2.1. Materials

Quercetin (Figure 1), mitoxantrone (MX), Ko143, and sulfasalazine were purchased from Sigma-Aldrich (St Louis, MO, USA). Prazosin was purchased from Tokyo Chemical Industry (Tokyo, Japan). High-performance liquid chromatography-grade methanol and formic acid were purchased from Fisher Scientific (Pittsburgh, PA, USA) and Fluka (Cambridge, MA, USA), respectively.

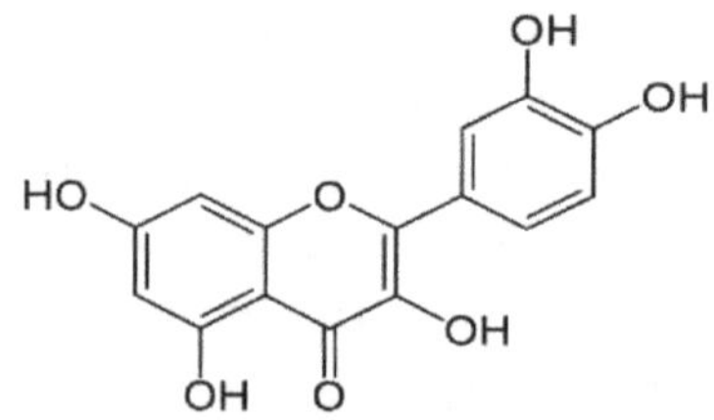

Figure 1. Chemical structure of quercetin.

2.2. Cell Culture

For the cellular accumulation and cytotoxicity studies, HeLa (human cervical cancer) cells were cultured in Dulbecco's modified Eagle's medium (DMEM; Welgene Inc., Daegu, Korea) supplemented with 10% fetal bovine serum (FBS; Welgene Inc., Daegu, Korea) and 100 U/mL penicillin–100 μg/mL streptomycin at 37 °C in a humidified incubator with 5% CO_2. For the bi-directional transport study, previously established human BCRP-overexpressing MDCKII cells [27] were used. Briefly, a plasmid construct containing cDNA for human BCRP was transfected into wildtype MDCKII cells to functionally express the transporter. MDCKII cells were grown in DMEM containing 10% FBS, 1% nonessential amino acid solution, 100 units/mL penicillin, and 0.1 mg/mL streptomycin under a humidified atmosphere containing 5% CO_2 at 37 °C.

2.3. RT-PCR Analysis

To measure the gene expression levels at the RNA level of BCRP, reverse-transcription polymerase chain reaction (RT-PCR) was performed. Total RNA was isolated from Hela, Caco-2, MCF-7, and SW620 cells using TRIzol reagent (Invitrogen, Carlsbad, CA, USA); complementary DNA (cDNA) was synthesized from 2 μg of the RNA extracted from cells, using the PrimeScript RT reagent Kit (TaKaRa, Shiga, Japan). cDNA was then amplified by PCR using human-specific primers: BCRP, 5′-TTC TCC ATT CAT CAG CCT CG-3′ (forward) and 5′-TGGTTGGTCGTCAGGAAGA-3′ (reverse); GAPDH 5′-GAA GGT GAA GGT CGG AGT C-3′ and 5′-GAAGATGGTGATGGGATTTC-3′ (reverse). Reverse transcription PCR (RT-PCR) was performed in a T-100TM thermal cycler (Bio-Rad, Hercules, CA, USA) using AccuPower PCR Premix (Bioneer, Daejeon, Korea), according to the manufacturer's protocol. The thermocycler conditions used for amplification were 95 °C for 5 min (hot start), 94 °C for 45 s, 55 °C for 30 s, and 72 °C for 30 s in 30 (BCRP) or 26 (GAPDH) cycles. Subsequently, the resultant products were analyzed by separation on a 1.5% agarose gel in tris-acetate/ethylenediaminetetraacetic acid (EDTA) buffer.

2.4. FACS-Cellular Accumulation Study

The cellular accumulation of quercetin was measured by FACSCalibur flow cytometry (Becton Dickinson, San Jose, CA, USA). For FACScan analysis, 2×10^5 HeLa cells/well were seeded into 6-well cell culture plates on the day before the experiment. On the following day, cells were treated with vehicle or quercetin and 1 μM MX. A time course experiment was conducted on HeLa cells following treatment with quercetin (1 and 100 μM) for 2, 4, and 6 h. After treatment, the cells were harvested by trypsinization and transferred to a fluorescence-activated cell sorting (FACS) tube, pelleted by centrifugation (1500 rpm, 5 min), and then resuspended in 200 μL of PBS. Flow cytometry analysis was performed using red fluorescence. A minimum of 10,000 cells were acquired per sample.

2.5. Cytotoxicity Assay

To determine the cytotoxic efficacy (i.e., the anticancer activity) of mitoxantrone associated with its intracellular accumulation, we performed the Cell Counting Kit-8 assay (CCK-8 assay kit; Dojindo Molecular Technologies, Kumamoto, Japan) following the manufacturer's instructions. HeLa cells (at a density of 1×10^4 cells per well) were seeded and cultured overnight in 96-well plates. Then, the medium was replaced with fresh medium containing the test drugs (mitoxantrone alone, mitoxantrone with 1 μM or 100 μM quercetin); the antiproliferation potential was examined at different drug concentrations after 24 h of incubation [28]. Additionally, 1 μM Ko143 was used as a positive control for BCRP inhibition. The absorbance was measured at a wavelength of 450 nm using a microplate reader (BioTeK, Highland Park, WI, USA).

2.6. Bi-Directional Transport Study

For the evaluation of the in vitro inhibitory potential of human BCRP by quercetin, the basolateral-to-apical (B-to-A) and apical-to-basolateral (A-to-B) permeability coefficients (P_{app}) of prazosin (the stereotypical substrate of BCRP) were determined in BCRP-overexpressing MDCKII cells in the presence of various concentrations of quercetin. Briefly, MDCKII cells were seeded on Transwell® filters (12 mm diameter, 0.4 μm pore size; Corning, NY, USA) at a density of 0.5×10^6 cells·mL^{-1} and then cultured for 5 days before being used in the transport assays. The confluence and integrity of the tight junctions were confirmed via microscopic observations as well as the measurement of transepithelial resistance [29]. The cells were washed twice and pre-incubated with transport buffer (9.7 g/L Hanks' balanced salt solution, 2.38 g/L HEPES, and 0.35 g/L sodium bicarbonate, pH adjusted to 7.4) for 30 min at 37 °C. Transport was initiated by adding transport buffer containing 10 μM prazosin in the presence or absence of quercetin (in a final concentration range of 0.1–300 μM) to the donor compartment (500 μL for the apical chamber or 1.5 mL for the basolateral chamber), followed by incubation at 37 °C for 120 min. At the end of the incubation, aliquots (300 μL for the apical chamber and 500 μL for the basolateral chamber) of the incubation mixture were collected from the donor and receiver chambers and subjected to LC-MS/MS assays.

2.7. Experimental Animals

Eight male Sprague-Dawley rats weighing 230–270 g (Orient Bio Inc., Seongnam, Korea) were used in the in vivo studies. The experimental protocols involving animals were reviewed and approved by the Seoul National University Institutional Animal Care and Use Committee, according to the National Institutes of Health Principles of Laboratory Animal Care (publication number 85-23, revised in 1985). The animal protocol number was SNU-180521-4; this protocol was approved on 9 October 2018.

2.8. Oral Pharmacokinetic Study in Rats

To determine whether quercetin affects the intestinal efflux mediated by BCRP, we divided the male rats into two groups: A sulfasalazine (a substrate of BCRP) control group and a quercetin pretreatment plus sulfasalazine group ($n = 4$, each). Considering the similar expression levels of intestinal BCRP between male and female rats, male rats were used in this study [30,31]. Briefly, overnight fasted male SD rats were anesthetized by intramuscular administration of 50 mg/kg tiletamine HCl/zolazepam HCl (Zoletil®) (Vibrac, TX, USA) and 10 mg/kg xylazine HCl (Rompun®, Bayer, Puteaux, France). While the rats were anesthetized, the femoral artery (for blood sampling) and vein (for supplementing body fluids) were catheterized using polyethylene tubing (PE 50; Clay Adams, Parsippany, NJ, USA). Upon recovery from anesthesia (i.e., after 4 h), quercetin was administered by oral gavage at 10 mg/kg (or 0 mg/kg in the case of the sulfasalazine control group; DMSO/polyethylene glycol 400/saline [1:4:5 (v/v/v)]). The pretreatment dose of quercetin was determined based on the compound solubility in the dosing vehicle and the likely daily dose of human dietary supplement. Fifteen minutes after the pretreatment, a dosing solution containing sulfasalazine at 2 mg/kg was administered by oral gavage. Blood samples (150 μL) were collected at 5, 15, 30, 60, 120, 240, 360, and 480 min after the sulfasalazine administration. Immediately after each blood collection, an identical volume of saline was intravenously provided to the animal to compensate for fluid loss. To prevent blood clotting during blood collection, the cannula was filled with 25 IU/mL heparinized saline. The plasma fraction was separated from the blood samples by centrifugation (16,100 × g for 5 min at 4 °C) and stored at −80 °C until the LC-MS/MS assay.

2.9. Quantification Using LC-MS/MS

Chromatographic quantification of sulfasalazine and prazosin was carried out using an LC-tandem mass spectrometry (LC-MS/MS) system equipped with a Waters e2695 high-performance liquid chromatography system (Milford, MA, USA) and an API 3200 QTRAP mass spectrometer (Applied Biosystems, Foster City, CA, USA). Briefly, an aliquot (50 μL) of a sample was vortex-mixed with an acetonitrile solution containing glipizide (300 ng/mL, internal standard); this was followed by centrifugation (16,100 × g for 5 min at 4 °C). An aliquot (5 μL) of the supernatant was directly injected into the LC-MS/MS system. Separations were carried out using a gradient of 0.1% formic acid in acetonitrile and 0.1% formic acid in water at a flow rate of 0.7 mL/min using a reversed-phase high-performance LC column (Agilent Poroshell 120, EC-C18 2.7 μm, 4.6 × 50 mm). The following transitions were used for analyte detection: *m/z* 399.0 → *m/z* 380.8 for sulfasalazine and *m/z* 384.1 → *m/z* 95.0 for prazosin. For the internal standard glipizide, the transition *m/z* 445.8 → *m/z* 320.9 was used. The limits of quantification were 10 ng/mL for sulfasalazine and 50 nM for prazosin.

2.10. Data Analysis

2.10.1. In Vitro Kinetic Analysis

The apparent permeability coefficient (P_{app}) of prazosin was estimated using the following equation (Equation (1)):

$$P_{app} = \frac{1}{A} \times \frac{1}{C_0} \times \frac{dQ}{dt} \quad (1)$$

where dQ/dt, A, and C_0 represent the transport rate, the surface area of the insert, and the initial concentration of the compound in the donor compartment, respectively. The efflux ratio (ER) was calculated by dividing the B-to-A apparent permeability coefficient ($P_{app,\ B\text{-to-}A}$) by the A-to-B apparent permeability coefficient ($P_{app,\ A\text{-to-}B}$). In the inhibition studies, the percentage of the control efflux ratio (%ER) was also calculated by dividing the value for ER in the presence of the inhibitor by that in the absence of the inhibitor (i.e., in the control). When necessary, the half maximal inhibitory concentration (IC_{50}) was determined by nonlinear regression analysis using WinNonlin Professional 5.0.1 software (Pharsight Corporation, Mountain View, CA, USA) and the following equation (Equation (2)):

$$V = V_{max} - (V_{max} - V_0) \times \left[\frac{[I]^n}{[I]^n + (IC_{50})^n}\right] \quad (2)$$

where V, V_{max}, V_0, [I], and n represent the rate of transport in the presence of the inhibitor, the maximal rate of transport, the basal rate of transport, the concentration of the inhibitor, and the Hill coefficient, respectively. When it was necessary to convert the IC_{50} to the inhibitory constant (Ki), the following equation (Equation (3)) [32] was used under the assumption that competitive inhibition existed between the substrate and the inhibitor:

$$K_i = \frac{IC_{50}}{1 + \frac{[S]}{K_m}} \quad (3)$$

where [S] is the concentration of the substrate and K_m represents the Michaelis–Menten constant.

2.10.2. Non-Compartmental Pharmacokinetic Analysis

Standard non-compartmental pharmacokinetic analysis was carried out using WinNonlin Professional 5.0.1 software (Pharsight, Cary, NC, USA) to calculate the pharmacokinetic parameters, including the peak concentration (C_{max}), time of the peak concentration (t_{max}), elimination half-life ($t_{1/2}$), area under the plasma concentration–time curve from time zero to the last sampling point, 8 h (AUC_{8h}), and elimination clearance (CL/F).

2.11. Statistical Analysis

For the comparison of means among the groups, one-way ANOVA (analysis of variance; for cytotoxicity and bi-directional transport studies) followed by Tukey's post hoc test were used. In these in vitro studies, a value of $p < 0.05$ was considered statistically significant. For the comparison of means between the groups for in vivo studies, the two-tailed/unpaired Student's t-test was used and a value of $p < 0.05$ with a statistical power more than 0.8 (Minitab 19.2, Minitab Inc., State College, PA, USA) was considered statistically significant.

3. Results

3.1. FACS-Cellular Accumulation Study

The expression of BCRP in Hela cells was confirmed by RT-PCR and compared with other cells, which were known to express high (Caco-2 and MCF-7) or low (SW620) levels of BCRP (Supplementary Figure S1) [33,34]. In the FACS-cellular accumulation study, the potential of quercetin to inhibit BCRP was first investigated by observing the cellular uptake of mitoxantrone (MX). The cellular uptake of MX with or without quercetin was analyzed by flow cytometry. The fluorescence intensity of a single cell measured by flow cytometry can be a good indication of the amount of MX internalized by each cell. As shown in Figure 2A, the peak fluorescence intensity of MX uptake was shifted to a higher level when MX was co-administered with quercetin, suggesting the promotion of MX internalization in HeLa cells. In the MX single treatment group, the percentage of cells with a significant uptake of MX was higher by 17.2% at 4 h of treatment and 27.1% at 6 h of treatment than at 2 h of treatment with MX alone as a control. In contrast, the cellular uptake of MX in the presence of quercetin was considerably higher by 30.2% at 4 h of treatment and 35.9% at 6 h of treatment (co-treatment with 1 μM quercetin) and by 45.3% at 4 h of treatment and 67.4% at 6 h of treatment (co-treatment with 100 μM quercetin) than at 2 h of treatment with MX alone. We also tested the internalization of MX when co-administered with 1 μM Ko143, a BCRP inhibitor. The results showed a considerably high number of cells that internalized MX when 1 μM Ko143 was co-administered with MX (Figure 2B). Thus, quercetin significantly promoted the cellular uptake of MX in HeLa cells likely via the inhibition of BCRP-mediated efflux.

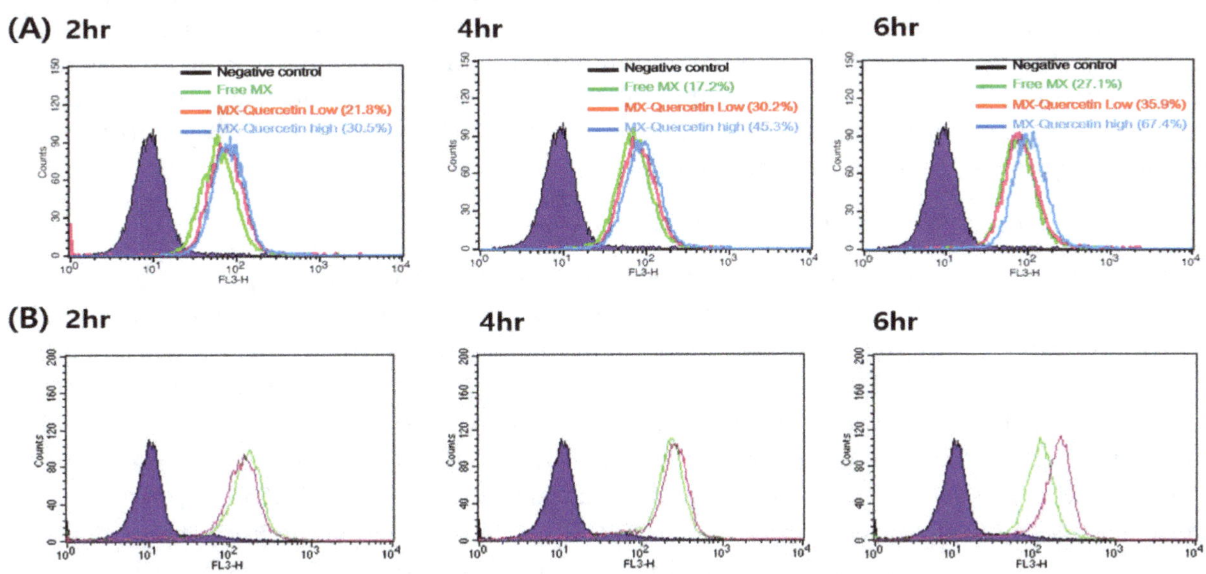

Figure 2. Representative histogram of mitoxantrone (MX) uptake in HeLa cells. (**A**) Flow cytometry measurement of MX fluorescence in HeLa cells incubated with MX alone (green line) or MX with 1 (red line) or 100 μM quercetin (blue line) for 2, 4, and 6 h. (**B**) Flow cytometry measurement of MX fluorescence in HeLa cells incubated with MX alone (green) or MX with 1 μM Ko143, a specific breast cancer resistance protein (BCRP) inhibitor (purple line), for 2, 4, and 6 h.

3.2. Cytotoxicity of Mitoxantrone in the Presence of Quercetin

To further confirm the effect of quercetin on the reversal of BCRP-mediated chemoresistance in HeLa cells, we examined the cytotoxicity (i.e., anticancer activity) of mitoxantrone in the absence and presence (1 or 100 μM) of quercetin. In this study, CCK-8 was used for the examination of mitoxantrone-associated cytotoxicity. As shown in Figure 3, mitoxantrone displayed concentration-dependent cytotoxicity in HeLa cells, which was further boosted in the presence of 1 μM Ko143, a stereotypical BCRP inhibitor. Likewise, the presence of 1 or 100 μM quercetin effectively enhanced the cytotoxicity associated with mitoxantrone as the IC_{50} decreased to 19.3% (1.13 μM) or 8.2% (0.478 μM), respectively, which differed from that observed with mitoxantrone alone (5.83 μM; Figure 3A). In addition, the cytotoxicity of quercetin alone without mitoxantrone was also examined. Treatment with 100 μM quercetin alone led to no significant changes in cell viability in comparison with the control (0.1% DMSO), demonstrating that the increased cytotoxicity observed in mitoxantrone-treated cells was not likely associated with the toxicity of quercetin (Supplementary Figure S2).

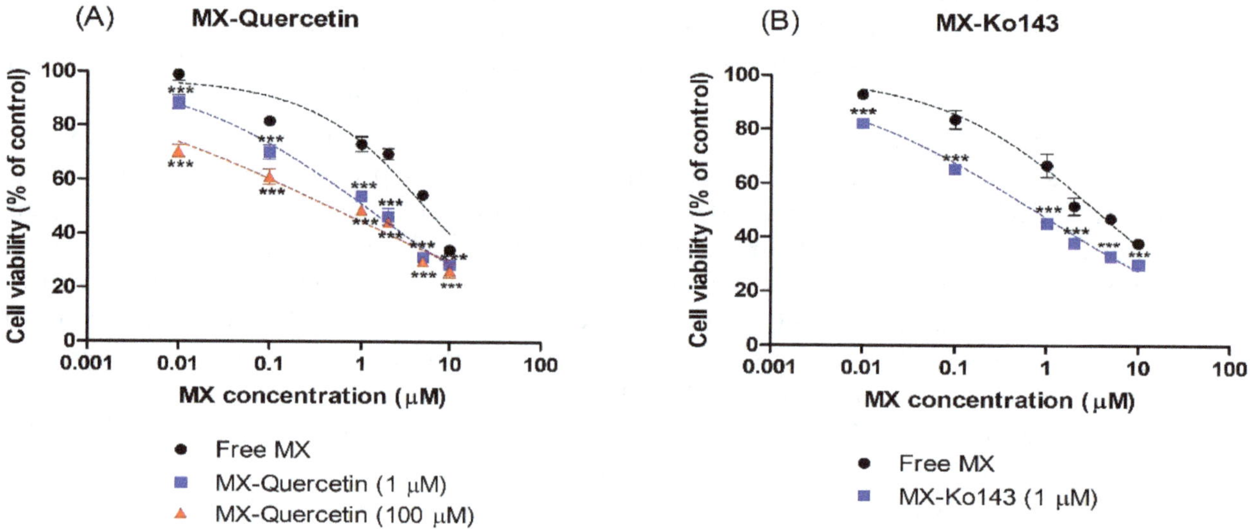

Figure 3. Effect of co-incubation of mitoxantrone (MX) with (**A**) quercetin (1 or 100 μM) and (**B**) Ko143 (1 μM) on the cell viability of HeLa cells. The Cell Counting Kit-8 (CCK-8) assay was used to determine the cytotoxicity associated with the cellular accumulation of MX after 24 h of incubation. Asterisks indicate statistical differences (* $p < 0.05$; ** $p < 0.01$; and *** $p < 0.001$) from the control group (i.e., without the quercetin or Ko143) according to one-way ANOVA, followed by Tukey's post hoc test. Data are presented as the mean ± SD of quintuplicate runs.

3.3. Bi-Directional Transport Study in MDCKII/BCRP Cells

We performed bi-directional transport studies in MDCKII cells expressing human BCRP (MDCKII/BCRP) to investigate the in vitro inhibitory potency of quercetin against BCRP in a concentration-dependent manner. Co-incubation with quercetin increased the $P_{app, A\text{-to-}B}$ of prazosin (Figure 4A) while simultaneously decreasing the $P_{app, B\text{-to-}A}$ (Figure 4B) with an increasing concentration of quercetin, leading to a concentration-dependent decrease in the overall ER (Figure 4C). Additionally, the functional expression of the efflux transporter in MDCKII/BCRP cells was also confirmed in this study, with an ER of 5.4 for prazosin (the stereotypical substrate of BCRP [27,35,36]), which decreased to 0.9 in the presence of the known inhibitor Ko143 (Figure 5C). Notably, the inhibitory effect of 10 μM quercetin on the B-to-A transport and efflux ratio was comparable to 1 μM Ko143 (Figure 5; $p > 0.05$). At quercetin concentrations higher than 10 μM, the ERs were less than 1.2, indicating the nearly complete inhibition of prazosin efflux (the complete inhibition of efflux would theoretically result in an ER of ~1, Figure 5). Kinetic analysis of the transport process yielded an estimated IC_{50} value of 4.22 μM for quercetin. Assuming the mechanism of inhibition to be competitive, the inhibitory constant (Ki) value was then estimated to be 3.91 μM using the K_m value of 128 μM [27] for prazosin.

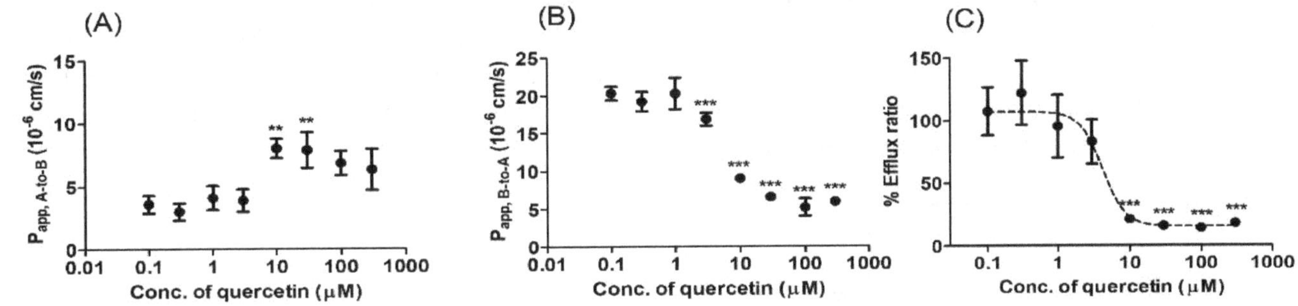

Figure 4. Bi-directional transport of prazosin in BCRP-overexpressing Madin-Darby Canine Kidney-II (MDCKII/BCRP) cells under various concentrations of quercetin (0.1–300 μM). (**A**) Apical-to-basolateral apparent permeability coefficient ($P_{app, A\text{-}to\text{-}B}$) and (**B**) basolateral-to-apical apparent permeability coefficient ($P_{app, B\text{-}to\text{-}A}$) of prazosin. (**C**) The percentage of the control efflux ratio (%ER, compared to the value without inhibitor) is shown together with the best-fit values generated from the nonlinear regression analysis based on Equation (2). Asterisks indicate statistical differences (* $p < 0.05$; ** $p < 0.01$; and *** $p < 0.001$) from the control (i.e., without quercetin) according to one-way ANOVA, followed by Tukey's post hoc test. Data are presented as the mean ± SD of triplicate runs. Data are presented as the mean ± SD of triplicate runs.

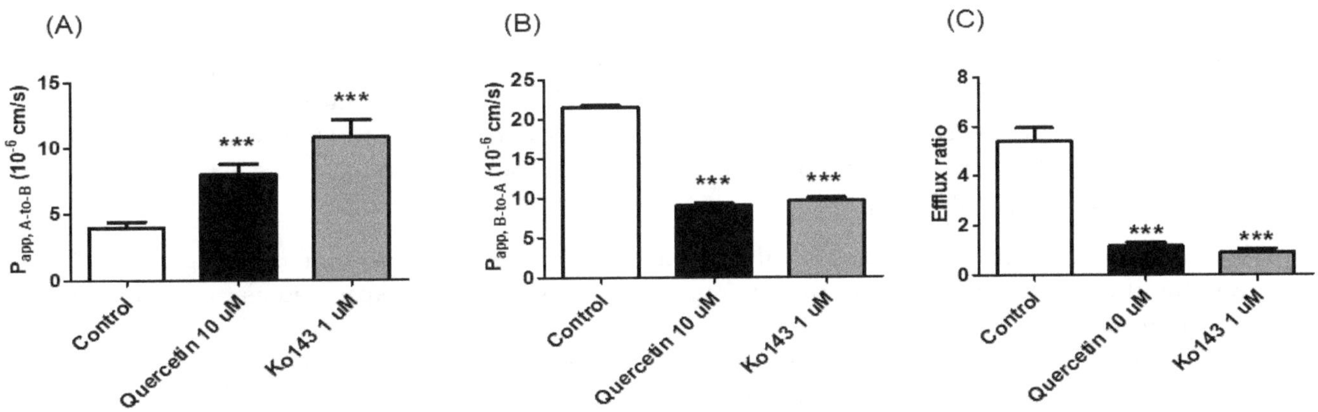

Figure 5. Effect of 10 μM quercetin or 1 μM Ko143 on the apparent permeability coefficient and efflux ratio of prazosin, a BCRP substrate, in MDCKII/BCRP cells. (**A**) Apical-to-basolateral apparent permeability coefficient ($P_{app, A\text{-}to\text{-}B}$), (**B**) basolateral-to-apical apparent permeability coefficient ($P_{app, B\text{-}to\text{-}A}$), and (**C**) efflux ratios of prazosin in the absence of inhibitor (i.e., the control) or in the presence of quercetin (10 μM) or Ko143 (the standard inhibitor of BCRP; 1 μM). Asterisks indicate statistical differences (* $p < 0.05$; ** $p < 0.01$; and *** $p < 0.001$) from the control group (i.e., without the inhibitor) according to one-way ANOVA, followed by Tukey's post hoc test. Data are presented as the mean ± SD of triplicate runs.

3.4. Oral Pharmacokinetic Study in Rats with or without Quercetin

To investigate the possible pharmacokinetic impact of quercetin as a BCRP inhibitor, we performed an oral pharmacokinetic study with sulfasalazine, a BCRP substrate, in rats. In this study, the change in the plasma concentration of sulfasalazine was used as an indicator of the in vivo interaction of BCRP with quercetin. To our knowledge, sulfasalazine has only limited interactions with other efflux transporters, including P-gp and MRP2 [34], whereas prazosin (the substrate used in the bi-directional transport study) is a dual substrate of P-gp and BCRP in vivo [37]. Thus, sulfasalazine is considered a relatively selective in vivo probe substrate of BCRP [25,26]. The mean plasma concentration–time profiles following the oral administration of 2 mg/kg sulfasalazine with or without pretreatment with 10 mg/kg quercetin in rats are shown in Figure 6. The pharmacokinetic parameters, as estimated using non-compartmental analysis, are summarized in Table 1. The plasma AUC_{8h} of sulfasalazine with or without quercetin pretreatment was 44.5 ± 11.8 min·μg/mL and 25.7 ± 9.98 min·μg/mL, respectively; this value was higher by 1.8-fold in the quercetin pretreatment group than in the control group, but it was not significantly different ($p < 0.05$, power < 0.8). More importantly, the C_{max} was significantly higher by 1.5-fold ($p < 0.05$, power > 0.8) in the quercetin pretreatment group (179 ± 23.0 ng/mL) than in the control group (i.e., 122 ± 23.2 ng/mL), whereas there was no significant change in the elimination half-life ($t_{1/2}$) of sulfasalazine. Collectively, these results suggest that pretreatment with quercetin led to the increased oral absorption of sulfasalazine in vivo.

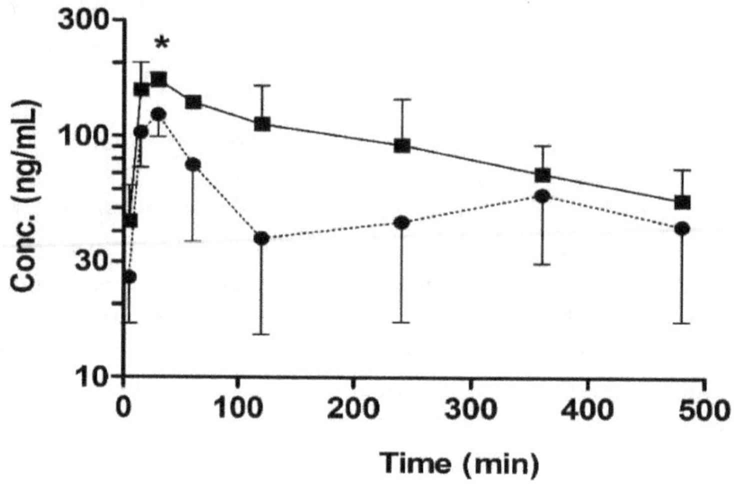

Figure 6. Temporal profiles of orally administered sulfasalazine (2 mg/kg) with or without the pre-administration of quercetin (10 mg/kg). Key: Control (•; without quercetin), quercetin pre-administration (■). Asterisks indicate statistical differences from the control (i.e., without quercetin) according to a two-tailed/unpaired Student's t-test (* $p < 0.05$, power > 0.8). Data are expressed as the mean ± SD of quadruplicate runs.

Table 1. Pharmacokinetic parameters of sulfasalazine after its oral administration (2 mg/kg dose) with and without pretreatment with quercetin (10 mg/kg) in rats. Data are expressed as the mean ± SD ($n = 4$ per group).

Parameter	Control	Pre-Administration Group (10 mg/kg Quercetin)
$t_{1/2}$ (min)	383 ± 111	242 ± 80.7
t_{max} (min)	30 ± 0	22.5 ± 8.70
C_{max} (ng/mL)	122 ± 23.2	179 ± 23.0 *
AUC_{8h}(min·ng/mL)	25700 ± 9980	44500 ± 11800
CL/F (mL/min/kg)	52.5 ± 33.5	33.2 ± 10.2

* significantly different from the control (i.e., without the pre-administration of quercetin) ($p < 0.05$, power > 0.8).

4. Discussion

Increasing lines of evidence from animal and human studies regarding food–drug interactions have indicated that a wide range of flavonoids can interact with ABC transporters, thereby leading to overexposure or underexposure of clinically important substrate drugs [13]. However, the accurate prediction of such interactions has been found to be difficult owing to limited in vitro data. The objective of this study was to investigate the inhibitory potential of quercetin against BCRP in vitro and in vivo. This study, which integrated the in vitro and in vivo effects of quercetin, was indeed necessary because a thorough understanding of the pharmacokinetic influence of this flavonoid is needed because of its high dietary intake as well as the lack of clear corresponding pharmacokinetic data.

Here, we demonstrated that the presence of quercetin can effectively enhance the cellular accumulation and associated cytotoxicity of mitoxantrone in HeLa cells (Figures 2 and 3), consistent with previous reports [38]. In the current study, the efficacy of quercetin as a BCRP inhibitor was quantitatively demonstrated via a significant reduction in the IC_{50} of mitoxantrone even in the presence of quercetin at a concentration as low as 1 μM (i.e., it decreased to 19.3% of the control value; from 5.83 to 1.13 μM). When the concentration of quercetin increased to 100 μM, the IC_{50} of mitoxantrone was further decreased (i.e., to 8.23% of the control value; 0.48 μM), similar to that in the presence of Ko143 (i.e., 0.62 μM), a stereotypical BCRP inhibitor. In addition, pharmacokinetically relevant parameters were obtained in a bi-directional transport study using MDCKII/BCRP cells, where the IC_{50} values of quercetin for the inhibition of BCRP-mediated efflux were estimated to be 4.22 μM. Assuming the mechanism of inhibition to be competitive, the IC_{50} value was further transformed to a Ki value of 3.91 μM, using the K_m value of 128 μM [27] for prazosin. The values obtained in the bi-directional transport studies were comparable to those previously observed in MCF-7/MX and MDCKII/BCRP cells using Hoechst 33342 accumulation (IC_{50} values of 7.6 and 6.9 μM, respectively) [21]. In both assays, it was shown that while quercetin is a less potent inhibitor compared to Ko143, it can show a similar inhibitory effect compared to 1 μM Ko143 in higher concentrations (Figures 3 and 5).

The US Food and Drug Administration recommends that orally administered compounds with an $[I_{gut}]$ value (the maximal gastrointestinal concentration; defined as the dose divided by 250 mL) divided by the Ki value greater than 10 be evaluated for potential in vivo interactions [36]. For quercetin, the estimated $[I_{gut}]$ value (662 μM, assuming a dietary quercetin intake of 50 mg/day) or even the estimated intestinal concentration (86.2 μM, when the intestinal fluid volume is assumed to be 1.92 L [39]) divided by the Ki (3.91 μM) value is far greater than 10. Thus, although the bioavailability of quercetin is somewhat low [40] and the daily dietary intake reportedly results in sub-micromolar concentrations in circulation [3], the substantially higher concentration in the gut is likely to result in the inhibition of intestinal BCRP and thereby an increase in the intestinal absorption of BCRP transporter substrates.

Consequently, the in vivo inhibitory potency of quercetin was further assessed to clarify its interaction with intestinal BCRP. In this study, the pharmacokinetic profile of orally administered sulfasalazine was used as an indicator of any alterations in intestinal BCRP activity. While sulfasalazine has been reported to be effluxed by P-gp and MRP2 to a low extent, previous studies have consistently demonstrated that the intestinal absorption of the compound following its oral administration was essentially unaffected in P-gp- or MRP2-knockout rats in contrast to the significantly higher AUC_{8h} and C_{max} values observed in BCRP-knockout rats [24], strongly suggesting that sulfasalazine is a good probe for observing intestinal BCRP activity. In this study, higher AUC_{8h} and C_{max} values of sulfasalazine (1.8-fold ($p < 0.05$, power < 0.8) and 1.5-fold ($p < 0.05$, power > 0.8), respectively) were observed in the presence of 10 mg/kg quercetin than in its absence (Table 1). The increased absorption in the presence of quercetin is clearly significant, but the degree is somewhat lower than that expected considering the approximately 20-fold increase observed in knockout rats [24] and, especially, the low Ki value of the flavonoid obtained in the current study. One possible reason for this discrepancy might be the rapid conjugation of quercetin to quercetin-3-glucuronide that occurs in the small intestine [20]. Once quercetin enters the intestinal cells by passive diffusion or uptake by the uptake transporters, it is subjected to glucuronidation by a UDP-glucuronosyltransferase present in both rat and human intestines [41–43], which results in the rapid clearance of quercetin from sites adjacent to the efflux transporter. Indeed, the oral bioavailability of quercetin was only 5.3% and the C_{max} value was the sub-micromolar range (i.e., 0.21 μg/mL) following 10 mg/kg oral administration to rats [44]. Another possibility that might result in relatively limited alterations in sulfasalazine absorption is the involvement of OATP2B1 in the intestinal absorption of sulfasalazine [25]. Sulfasalazine is a high-affinity substrate of OATP2B1 [25,45], whereas quercetin has been reported to be an inhibitor of OATP2B1 [46]. Therefore, the relatively low increase in sulfasalazine exposure in the presence of quercetin may be attributed to complex interactions between the simultaneous inhibition of the efflux by BCRP and the uptake by OATP2B1. In addition, considering that we only observed a single dosing of quercetin on the sulfasalazine pharmacokinetics, further studies regarding multiple dosing of quercetin are likely needed.

In a previous study by Zhang et al., an apparent discrepancy between the in vitro and in vivo inhibition of BCRP by the flavonoids chrysin and 7,8-benzoflavone was reported. In their investigation, the flavonoids were demonstrated to be potent inhibitors of human BCRP but weak inhibitors of mouse BCRP [23]; one possible explanation for this discrepancy may be species differences between the human and rodent transporters. Although a further study regarding food–drug interaction is required in humans, this may also be true for quercetin, in which case the clinical impact of the modulation of BCRP activity in humans may be much greater than that estimated from pharmacokinetic studies performed in rats.

5. Conclusions

The in vitro and in vivo inhibitory potencies of quercetin against BCRP were examined focusing on functional and/or kinetic aspects. Quercetin significantly increased the cellular accumulation and associated cytotoxicity of mitoxantrone in HeLa cells in a concentration-dependent manner. The transcellular efflux of prazosin was significantly reduced in the presence of quercetin as observed in a bi-directional transport assay using MDCKII/BCRP cells. These modulations in BCRP activity were consistent with the in vivo results, where pretreatment with quercetin led to not very dramatically different but still significantly higher intestinal absorption of sulfasalazine compared to that in the control group. Collectively, these results provide evidence that quercetin acts as a potent inhibitor of BCRP both in vitro and in vivo. Considering the high dietary intake of quercetin as well as its consumption as a dietary supplement, careful attention should be paid to potential flavonoid–drug interactions.

Supplementary Materials:
Figure S1: mRNA expression levels of BCRP in HeLa, Caco-2, MCF-7 and SW620 cell lines using RT-PCR, Figure S2: Effect of 100 μM quercetin alone on the cell viability of HeLa cells.

Author Contributions: Conceptualization, H.-J.M. and Y.-K.S.; methodology, investigation and formal analysis, Y.-K.S., J.-H.Y., J.K.W., J.-H.K., K.-R.L., S.H.O. and H.-J.M.; resources, S.-J.C. and H.-J.M.; writing—original draft preparation and visualization, Y.-K.S., J.K.W. and H.-J.M.; writing—review and editing, S.-J.C. and H.-J.M.; supervision, S.-J.C. and H.-J.M; project administration, H.-J.M.; funding acquisition, H.-J.M. All authors have read and agreed to the published version of the manuscript.

References

1. Hertog, M.; Hollman, P.; Katan, M. Flavonol and flavone content of vegetables and fruits. In *Flavonols and Flavones in Foods and Their Relation with Cancer and Coronary Heart Disease Risk*; CIP-Data Koninklijke Bibliotheek: The Hague, The Netherlands, 1994.
2. Hertog, M.G.L.; Hollman, P.C.H.; Van De Putte, B. Content of potentially anticarcinogenic flavonoids of tea infusions, wines, and fruit juices. *J. Agric. Food Chem.* **1993**, *41*, 1242–1246. [CrossRef]
3. Kelly, G.S. Quercetin. *Altern. Med. Rev.* **2011**, *16*, 172–195. [PubMed]
4. Sampson, L.; Rimm, E.; Hollman, P.C.; De Vries, J.H.; Katan, M.B. Flavonol and flavone intakes in US health professionals. *J. Am. Diet. Assoc.* **2002**, *102*, 1414–1420. [CrossRef]
5. De Vrie, J.H.; Janssen, P.; Hollman, P.C.; Van Staveren, W.A.; Katan, M.B. Consumption of quercetin and kaempferol in free-living subjects eating a variety of diets. *Cancer Lett.* **1997**, *114*, 141–144. [CrossRef]
6. Formica, J.; Regelson, W. Review of the biology of quercetin and related bioflavonoids. *Food Chem. Toxicol.* **1995**, *33*, 1061–1080. [CrossRef]
7. Takahama, U. Inhibition of lipoxygenase-dependent lipid peroxidation by quercetin: Mechanism of antioxidative function. *Phytochemistry* **1985**, *24*, 1443–1446. [CrossRef]
8. Lamson, D.W.; Brignall, M.S. Antioxidants and cancer, part 3: Quercetin. *Altern. Med. Rev. J. Clin. Ther.* **2000**, *5*, 196–208.
9. Ohnishi, E.; Bannai, H. Quercetin potentiates TNF-induced antiviral activity. *Antivir. Res.* **1993**, *22*, 327–331. [CrossRef]
10. De La Lastra, A.; Martin, M.; Motilva, V. Antiulcer and Gastroprotective Effects of Quercetin: A Gross and Histologic Study. *Pharmacology* **1994**, *48*, 56–62. [CrossRef] [PubMed]

11. Vida, R.G.; Fittler, A.; Somogyi-Végh, A.; Poór, M. Dietary quercetin supplements: Assessment of online product informations and quantitation of quercetin in the products by high-performance liquid chromatography. *Phytother. Res.* **2019**, *33*, 1912–1920. [CrossRef]
12. Geller, A.I.; Shehab, N.; Weidle, N.J.; Lovegrove, M.C.; Wolpert, B.J.; Timbo, B.B.; Mozersky, R.P.; Budnitz, D.S. Emergency Department Visits for Adverse Events Related to Dietary Supplements. *N. Engl. J. Med.* **2015**, *373*, 1531–1540. [CrossRef] [PubMed]
13. Alvarez, A.; Real, R.; Pérez, M.; Mendoza, G.; Prieto, J.G.; Merino, G. Modulation of the activity of ABC transporters (P-glycoprotein, MRP2, BCRP) by flavonoids and drug response. *J. Pharm. Sci.* **2010**, *99*, 598–617. [CrossRef] [PubMed]
14. Reddy, D.R.; Khurana, A.; Bale, S.; Ravirala, R.; Reddy, V.S.S.; Mohankumar, M.; Godugu, C. Natural flavonoids silymarin and quercetin improve the brain distribution of co-administered P-gp substrate drugs. *SpringerPlus* **2016**, *5*, 1618. [CrossRef] [PubMed]
15. Choi, J.-S.; Piao, Y.-J.; Kang, K.-W. Effects of quercetin on the bioavailability of doxorubicin in rats: Role of CYP3A4 and P-gp inhibition by quercetin. *Arch. Pharmacal Res.* **2011**, *34*, 607–613. [CrossRef]
16. Wang, Y.; Cao, J.; Zeng, S. Involvement of P-glycoprotein in regulating cellular levels of Ginkgo flavonols: Quercetin, kaempferol, and isorhamnetin. *J. Pharm. Pharmacol.* **2005**, *57*, 751–758. [CrossRef]
17. Van Zanden, J.J.; Wortelboer, H.M.; Bijlsma, S.; Punt, A.; Usta, M.; Van Bladeren, P.J.; Rietjens, I.M.C.M.; Cnubben, N.H. Quantitative structure activity relationship studies on the flavonoid mediated inhibition of multidrug resistance proteins 1 and 2. *Biochem. Pharmacol.* **2005**, *69*, 699–708. [CrossRef]
18. Chae, Y.-J.; Cho, K.H.; Yoon, I.-S.; Noh, C.-K.; Lee, H.-J.; Park, Y.; Ji, E.; Seo, M.-D.; Maeng, H.-J. Vitamin D Receptor-Mediated Upregulation of CYP3A4 and MDR1 by Quercetin in Caco-2 cells. *Planta Medica* **2015**, *82*, 121–130. [CrossRef]
19. Ni, Z.; Bikadi, Z.; Rosenberg, M.F.; Mao, Q. Structure and function of the human breast cancer resistance protein (BCRP/ABCG2). *Curr. Drug Metab.* **2010**, *11*, 603–617. [CrossRef]
20. Sesink, A.L.; Arts, I.C.; De Boer, V.C.; Breedveld, P.; Schellens, J.H.; Hollman, P.C.; Russel, F.G. Breast cancer resistance protein (Bcrp1/Abcg2) limits net intestinal uptake of quercetin in rats by facilitating apical efflux of glucuronides. *Mol. Pharmacol.* **2005**, *67*, 1999–2006. [CrossRef]
21. Pick, A.; Müller, H.; Mayer, R.; Haenisch, B.; Pajeva, I.; Weigt, M.; Bönisch, H.; Müller, C.E.; Wiese, M. Structure–activity relationships of flavonoids as inhibitors of breast cancer resistance protein (BCRP). *Bioorg. Med. Chem.* **2011**, *19*, 2090–2102. [CrossRef]
22. Zhang, S.; Yang, X.; Morris, M.E. Flavonoids Are Inhibitors of Breast Cancer Resistance Protein (ABCG2)-Mediated Transport. *Mol. Pharmacol.* **2004**, *65*, 1208–1216. [CrossRef] [PubMed]
23. Zhang, S.; Wang, X.; Sagawa, K.; Morris, M.E. Flavonoids chrysin and benzoflavone, potent breast cancer resistance protein inhibitors, have no significant effect on topotecan pharmacokinetics in rats or mdr1a/1b (–/–) mice. *Drug Metab. Dispos.* **2004**, *33*, 341–348. [CrossRef] [PubMed]
24. Zamek-Gliszczynski, M.J.; Bedwell, D.W.; Bao, J.Q.; Higgins, J.W. Characterization of SAGE Mdr1a (P-gp), Bcrp, and Mrp2 Knockout Rats Using Loperamide, Paclitaxel, Sulfasalazine, and Carboxydichlorofluorescein Pharmacokinetics. *Drug Metab. Dispos.* **2012**, *40*, 1825–1833. [CrossRef] [PubMed]
25. Kusuhara, H.; Furuie, H.; Inano, A.; Sunagawa, A.; Yamada, S.; Wu, C.; Fukizawa, S.; Morimoto, N.; Ieiri, I.; Morishita, M.; et al. Pharmacokinetic interaction study of sulphasalazine in healthy subjects and the impact of curcumin as an in vivo inhibitor of BCRP. *Br. J. Pharmacol.* **2012**, *166*, 1793–1803. [CrossRef] [PubMed]
26. Zaher, H.; Khan, A.A.; Palandra, J.; Brayman, T.G.; Yu, L.; Ware, J.A. Breast Cancer Resistance Protein (Bcrp/abcg2) Is a Major Determinant of Sulfasalazine Absorption and Elimination in the Mouse. *Mol. Pharm.* **2006**, *3*, 55–61. [CrossRef]
27. Song, Y.-K.; Park, J.E.; Oh, Y.; Hyung, S.; Jeong, Y.-S.; Kim, M.-S.; Lee, W.; Chung, S.-J. Suppression of Canine ATP Binding Cassette ABCB1 in Madin-Darby Canine Kidney Type II Cells Unmasks Human ABCG2-Mediated Efflux of Olaparib. *J. Pharmacol. Exp. Ther.* **2018**, *368*, 79–87. [CrossRef]
28. Kang, J.-W.; Cho, H.-J.; Lee, H.J.; Jin, H.-E.; Maeng, H.-J. Polyethylene glycol-decorated doxorubicin/carboxymethyl chitosan/gold nanocomplex for reducing drug efflux in cancer cells and extending circulation in blood stream. *Int. J. Boil. Macromol.* **2019**, *125*, 61–71. [CrossRef]
29. Irvine, J.D.; Takahashi, L.; Lockhart, K.; Cheong, J.; Tolan, J.W.; Selick, H.E.; Grove, J.R. MDCK (Madin-Darby Canine Kidney) Cells: A Tool for Membrane Permeability Screening. *J. Pharm. Sci.* **1999**, *88*, 28–33. [CrossRef]

30. Merino, G.; Van Herwaarden, A.E.; Wagenaar, E.; Jonker, J.W.; Schinkel, A.H. Sex-Dependent Expression and Activity of the ATP-Binding Cassette Transporter Breast Cancer Resistance Protein (BCRP/ABCG2) in Liver. *Mol. Pharmacol.* **2005**, *67*, 1765–1771. [CrossRef]
31. Tanaka, Y.; Slitt, A.L.; Leazer, T.M.; Maher, J.M.; Klaassen, C.D. Tissue distribution and hormonal regulation of the breast cancer resistance protein (Bcrp/Abcg2) in rats and mice. *Biochem. Biophys. Res. Commun.* **2004**, *326*, 181–187. [CrossRef]
32. Yung-Chi, C.; Prusoff, W.H. Relationship between the inhibition constant (KI) and the concentration of inhibitor which causes 50 per cent inhibition (I50) of an enzymatic reaction. *Biochem. Pharmacol.* **1973**, *22*, 3099–3108. [CrossRef]
33. To, K.K.; Robey, R.; Zhan, Z.; Bangiolo, L.; Bates, S.E. Upregulation of ABCG2 by romidepsin via the aryl hydrocarbon receptor pathway. *Mol. Cancer Res.* **2011**, *9*, 516–527. [CrossRef] [PubMed]
34. Ikai, A.; Watanabe, M.; Sowa, Y.; Kishimoto, M.; Yanagisawa, A.; Fujiwara, H.; Otsuji, E.; Sakai, A.T. Phosphorylated retinoblastoma protein is a potential predictive marker of irinotecan efficacy for colorectal cancer. *Int. J. Oncol.* **2016**, *48*, 1297–1304. [CrossRef] [PubMed]
35. Lepist, E.-I.; Phan, T.K.; Roy, A.; Tong, L.; MacLennan, K.; Murray, B.; Ray, A.S. Cobicistat Boosts the Intestinal Absorption of Transport Substrates, Including HIV Protease Inhibitors and GS-7340, In Vitro. *Antimicrob. Agents Chemother.* **2012**, *56*, 5409–5413. [CrossRef]
36. FDA. In Vitro Metabolism and Transporter Mediated Drug-Drug Interaction Studies: Guidance for Industry; US Department of Health and Human Services, Food and Drug Administration, Center for Drug Evaluation and Research (CDER). 2017. Available online: https://www.fda.gov/media/108130/download (accessed on 24 October 2017).
37. Zhou, L.; Schmidt, K.; Nelson, F.R.; Zelesky, V.; Troutman, M.D.; Feng, B. The effect of breast cancer resistance protein (Bcrp) and P-glycoprotein (Mdr1a/1b) on the brain penetration of flavopiridol, Gleevec, prazosin and PF-407288 in mice. *Drug Metab. Dispos.* **2009**, *37*, 946–955. [CrossRef]
38. Cooray, H.C.; Janvilisri, T.; Van Veen, H.W.; Hladky, S.B.; A Barrand, M. Interaction of the breast cancer resistance protein with plant polyphenols. *Biochem. Biophys. Res. Commun.* **2004**, *317*, 269–275. [CrossRef]
39. Tachibana, T.; Kato, M.; Watanabe, T.; Mitsui, T.; Sugiyama, Y. Method for predicting the risk of drug–drug interactions involving inhibition of intestinal CYP3A4 and P-glycoprotein. *Xenobiotica* **2009**, *39*, 430–443. [CrossRef]
40. Khaled, K.A.; El-Sayed, Y.M.; Al-Hadiya, B.M. Disposition of the Flavonoid Quercetin in Rats After Single Intravenous and Oral Doses. *Drug Dev. Ind. Pharm.* **2003**, *29*, 397–403. [CrossRef]
41. Murota, K.; Terao, J. Antioxidative flavonoid quercetin: Implication of its intestinal absorption and metabolism. *Arch. Biochem. Biophys.* **2003**, *417*, 12–17. [CrossRef]
42. Radominska-Pandya, A.; Little, J.M.; Pandya, J.T.; Tephly, T.R.; King, C.D.; Barone, G.W.; Raufman, J.-P. UDP-glucuronosyltransferases in human intestinal mucosa. *Biochim. Biophys. Acta (BBA)-Lipids Lipid Metab.* **1998**, *1394*, 199–208. [CrossRef]
43. Crespy, V.; Morand, C.; Manach, C.; Besson, C.; Demigne, C.; Remesy, C. Part of quercetin absorbed in the small intestine is conjugated and further secreted in the intestinal lumen. *Am. J. Physiol. Content* **1999**, *277*, G120–G126. [CrossRef] [PubMed]
44. Chen, X.; Yin, O.Q.P.; Zuo, Z.; Chow, M.S. Pharmacokinetics and Modeling of Quercetin and Metabolites. *Pharm. Res.* **2005**, *22*, 892–901. [CrossRef] [PubMed]
45. Tomaru, A.; Morimoto, N.; Morishita, M.; Takayama, K.; Fujita, T.; Maeda, K.; Kusuhara, H.; Sugiyama, Y. Studies on the intestinal absorption characteristics of sulfasalazine, a breast cancer resistance protein (BCRP) substrate. *Drug Metab. Pharmacokinet.* **2012**, *28*, 71–74. [CrossRef] [PubMed]
46. Mandery, K.; Bujok, K.; Schmidt, I.; Keiser, M.; Siegmund, W.; Balk, B.; Koenig, J.; Fromm, M.F.; Glaeser, H. Influence of the flavonoids apigenin, kaempferol, and quercetin on the function of organic anion transporting polypeptides 1A2 and 2B1. *Biochem. Pharmacol.* **2010**, *80*, 1746–1753. [CrossRef]

4

Modeling of Body Weight Metrics for Effective and Cost-Efficient Conventional Factor VIII Dosing in Hemophilia A Prophylaxis

Alanna McEneny-King [1], Pierre Chelle [1], Severine Henrard [2], Cedric Hermans [3], Alfonso Iorio [4,5] and Andrea N. Edginton [1,*]

1 School of Pharmacy, University of Waterloo, Waterloo, ON N2L 3G1, Canada; amceneny@uwaterloo.ca (A.M.-K.); pierre.chelle@uwaterloo.ca (P.C.)

2 Louvain Drug Research Institute, Clinical Pharmacy Research Group and Institute of Health and Society (IRSS), Université catholique de Louvain, 1348 Brussels, Belgium; severine.henrard@uclouvain.be

3 Haemostasis and Thrombosis Unit, Division of Haematology, Cliniques universitaires Saint-Luc, Université catholique de Louvain, 1348 Brussels, Belgium; cedric.hermans@uclouvain.be

4 Department of Health Evidence, Research Methods and Impact, McMaster University, Hamilton, ON L8S 4L8, Canada; iorioa@mcmaster.ca

5 Department of Medicine, McMaster University, Hamilton, ON L8S 4L8, Canada

* Correspondence: aedginto@uwaterloo.ca

Abstract: The total body weight-based dosing strategy currently used in the prophylactic treatment of hemophilia A may not be appropriate for all populations. The assumptions that guide weight-based dosing are not valid in overweight and obese populations, resulting in overdosing and ineffective resource utilization. We explored different weight metrics including lean body weight, ideal body weight, and adjusted body weight to determine an alternative dosing strategy that is both safe and resource-efficient in normal and overweight/obese adult patients. Using a validated population pharmacokinetic model, we simulated a variety of dosing regimens using different doses, weight metrics, and frequencies; we also investigated the implications of assuming various levels of endogenous factor production. Ideal body weight performed the best across all of the regimens explored, maintaining safety while moderating resource consumption for overweight and obese patients.

Keywords: hemophilia A; conventional factor VIII; dose metrics; obesity; population pharmacokinetics

---

1. Introduction

Hemophilia A is an inherited bleeding disorder resulting from a deficiency in clotting factor VIII (FVIII), causing spontaneous and recurring joint bleeds, eventually leading to arthropathy and premature death if left untreated. The mainstay of severe hemophilia treatment is prophylactic replacement of the missing factor. The typical aim of prophylaxis is to maintain a clotting factor level of at least 1 IU dL^{-1}, based on the observation that patients with moderate hemophilia (i.e., those with baseline factor levels >1 IU dL^{-1}) are less prone to the spontaneous bleeds and subsequent arthropathy seen in more severe cases [1]. In a study of 65 boys with severe hemophilia A, only regular prophylactic infusions were shown to prevent joint damage as compared to on-demand treatment [2]. While there is global unanimity that prophylaxis should be initiated before joint disease is sustained [3,4], the implementation of this approach is quite variable [5]. No optimal dosing regimen has been identified; instead, an individualized approach that accounts for the patient's physical activity, current (and accepted future) musculoskeletal condition, and the availability of resources has been suggested [6,7]. Ideally, the patient's pharmacokinetic (PK) profile is taken into account to define a truly individualized regimen that optimizes both safety and resource utilization [8]. To facilitate the adoption of PK-based dosing regimens, tools such as the Web Accessible Population Pharmacokinetics Service—Hemophilia (WAPPS-Hemo [9,10]) provide estimates of individual PK parameters from a minimal number of samples by leveraging population PK data. Despite the development of these platforms, the majority of hemophilia patients are still dosed according to total body weight, as initially proposed by Ingram in 1981 [11]. For instance, hemophilic children in Canada are started on a once-weekly regimen (50 IU kg^{-1}), then step up to either twice weekly (30 IU kg^{-1}) or every 48 h (25 IU kg^{-1}) as required; prophylaxis regimens in the Netherlands (Utrecht protocol: 15–30 IU kg^{-1} three times per week) and Sweden (Malmö protocol: 25–40 IU kg^{-1} three times per week), though proposing different intensities and targeting different levels, are based on the same principle [12].

The normalization of life expectancy of individuals with hemophilia brings new challenges to hemophilia care. Overweight and obesity rates amongst hemophiliacs now match the epidemic proportions that are seen in the general population [13]. A 2011 study conducted in Ontario found 28.8% of enrolled hemophiliacs were overweight or obese, compared to 26% of healthy controls [14]. Obesity also comes with a higher risk for hemophilic arthropathy; joint range of motion has been shown to negatively correlate with body mass index (BMI) [15]. Furthermore, the total body weight-based dosing regimen currently used in hemophilia treatment may not be appropriate for overweight and obese populations. Calculations for weight-adjusted dosing are based on the following formula:

$$\text{Dose (IU)} = \frac{\text{total body weight (kg)} \times \text{desired increase in FVIII level (\%)}}{\text{IVR}} \tag{1}$$

In vivo recovery (IVR) is a parameter used to describe clotting factor pharmacokinetics, and reflects the rise in factor activity (in this case, FVIII) after a dose is administered. Although it has been suggested that an individual IVR value be determined for each patient [16], typically an IVR of 2 IU $dL^{-1}/IU\ kg^{-1}$ is assumed. For example, a desired increase to normal FVIII levels (100%) would lead to a 50 IU kg^{-1} dose being administered. However, the assumption that IVR equals 2 for all is not always valid. A study by Henrard et al. found that overweight patients (BMI > 29.6 $kg{\cdot}m^{-2}$) had a median IVR of 2.70, while underweight patients (BMI < 20.3 $kg{\cdot}m^{-2}$) had a median IVR of 1.60 [17].

The emerging proportion of overweight and obesity in the general population has prompted research efforts aimed at identifying pharmacokinetic differences (and the corresponding dose adjustments) in this population. The relationship between body size and clearance is well established; a 2012 systematic review of this topic found that more than half of all identified models for clearance included a covariate for body size, most commonly as a power function [18]. Obesity specifically influences several factors affecting drug disposition, including body composition, metabolism by CYP450 enzymes, and plasma protein levels [19]. The most striking differences are observed for highly lipophilic drugs, where volume of distribution changes dramatically in the obese population [20]. However, this is not the case for clotting factor concentrates. FVIII concentrates are typically confined to the vascular space, with volumes of distribution approximating plasma volume (48 $mL{\cdot}kg^{-1}$) [21]. Since vasculature represents a very small fraction (0.005–0.010) of adipose tissue volume [22], an excess (or scarcity) of fat does not significantly alter the volume of distribution of FVIII. As a result, overweight and obese patients are likely overdosed when dose is calculated using total body weight [23]. A similar issue has been noted for dosing of unfractionated heparin, another compound whose volume of distribution is approximately equal to the plasma volume; obese children achieved comparable anticoagulation at a lower weight-based dose [24]. Hemophilia treatment is expensive, with annual costs in the hundreds of thousands for those on prophylaxis [2], and while prophylaxis does achieve better health outcomes, these come at a significant cost that is not automatically offset by prevention of other expenses [25]. As the clotting factor itself represents the majority of the cost of prophylaxis [26], overdosing can introduce a significant waste of resources [27]. This study will explore alternative dosing regimens that optimize both safety and resource utilization in overweight and obese hemophiliacs.

2. Methods

Population generation, simulation, and data analysis were all conducted in Matlab R2009.

2.1. Population Generation

The generated population of virtual individuals consists of two equal sized bins classified by BMI using the cut-offs defined by Henrard et al. [17] The first group consists of average weight subjects (BMI between 20.3 and 29.6 kg·m^{-2}); the second group represents an overweight and obese population with BMI between 29.6 kg·m^{-2} and 40.0 kg·m^{-2}. These cut-off values for BMI were found to be the strongest predictors of FVIII IVR. Each group contains 1000 simulated subjects with a uniform BMI distribution. Heights were derived from the distribution provided by the NHANES database [28]. A uniform distribution of BMI's was simulated and the total body weights were calculated as the product of BMI and the square of height.

2.2. Definitions of Weight Metrics

The following weight metrics were defined for each virtual patient from their simulated total body weight (TBW, kg), height (HT, cm) and BMI (kg·m^{-2}):

1. Lean body weight (LBW) [29]

$$\mathrm{LBW} = \frac{9270 \times \mathrm{TBW}}{6680 + 216 \times \mathrm{BMI}}, \tag{2}$$

2. Ideal body weight (IBW—Lorentz formula)

$$\mathrm{IBW} = \mathrm{HT} - 100 - \left(\frac{\mathrm{HT} - 150}{4}\right), \tag{3}$$

3. Adjusted body weight (ABW)

$$\mathrm{ABW}_{25} = \mathrm{IBW} + 0.25 \times (\mathrm{TBW} - \mathrm{BW}), \tag{4}$$

$$\mathrm{ABW}_{40} = \mathrm{IBW} + 0.4 \times (\mathrm{TBW} - \mathrm{IBW}). \tag{5}$$

We used the semi-mechanistic model for LBW developed by Janmahasatian et al. [30] as it has been found to better describe the full range of adult heights and weights [20]. IBW was calculated using Lorentz's formula, which takes into account the patient's height and sex but not total body weight. ABW was the first weight metric intended for use in pharmacokinetic studies; it involves adding a proportion of the excess weight above IBW [30]. This proportion is variable, ranging from 25–50%, with 40% being used most commonly; in this study, we examined both 25% (ABW_{25}) and 40% (ABW_{40}) correction factors. Correlation plots for all body size metrics are presented in Supplementary Figures S1 and S2 for normal and overweight/obese individuals, respectively.

2.3. Population Pharmacokinetic Model

Simulations were performed using the 2-compartment structure described by Garmann et al. [31] for BAY 81-8973 (Kovaltry®, Bayer, Leverkusen, Germany), built on 183 subjects. Of the 109 patients above 18 years of age, the BMI range was 15.0–38.3 kg·m^{-2}. The details of the model structure are presented in Table 1. For each simulated individual, PK parameters were calculated. Each virtual individual was then dosed based on various weight metrics and their PK was simulated.

Table 1. Details of the model developed by Garmann et al. [31]. CL: clearance; Q: intercompartmental clearance; V_1: volume of the central compartment; V_2: volume of the peripheral compartment; RUV: residual unexplained variability; BSV: between subject variability; LBW: lean body weight.

Parameter	Estimate	Covariate Effect	BSV (%CV)
CL ($dL{\cdot}h^{-1}$)	1.88	$\theta_{CL}\left(\frac{LBW}{51.1}\right)^{0.610}$	37.0
Q ($dL{\cdot}h^{-1}$)	1.90		
V_1 (dL)	30.0	$\theta_{V_1}\left(\frac{LBW}{51.1}\right)^{0.950}$	11.2
V_2 (dL)	6.37		
Proportional RUV (%CV)	26.7		
Additive RUV (IU dL^{-1})	1.10		

2.4. Simulation and Assessment of Treatment Regimens

For each virtual individual, FVIII levels and individual PK parameters were simulated assuming a baseline factor level of 0.5 IU dL^{-1}. FVIII levels were simulated using time steps of 0.2 h following dosing regimens for four weeks to ensure that steady state was reached, and results from the 5th week were used in subsequent analysis steps. In a first instance, we analyzed a typical dosing strategy (20 IU kg^{-1} TBW every 48 h) to evaluate its appropriateness.

We then simulated various regimens wherein equal doses were given at regular intervals (i.e., 48 h). Each patient was dosed from 10 IU kg^{-1} for each weight metric (10 IU kg^{-1} of TBW, 10 IU kg^{-1} of LBW, etc.) up to 210 IU kg^{-1}. Initially, the dose step was 2 IU kg^{-1} for doses up to 100 IU kg^{-1} and 10 IU kg^{-1} for doses between 100 and 210 IU kg^{-1}. After reviewing the results, the dose step was reduced to 0.1 IU kg^{-1} between 20 and 30 IU kg^{-1}, as this was the range of most interest. A regimen was considered to be safe for a BMI group if 95% of the simulated population within that group had factor levels above 1 IU dL^{-1} at all times ($C_{min} \geq 1$ IU dL^{-1}). The lowest dose per weight metric that met this safety criterion was identified and considered to be the optimal regimen for that particular metric and BMI group. A secondary measure of safety was the 95th quantile for time spent below 1 IU dL^{-1}; in other words, the amount of time per week spent below trough for the 5% of the population not meeting the safety criteria. To evaluate economic differences between regimens, we calculated the mean weekly consumption on each optimal regimen to determine which dosing regimen met safety requirements while minimizing resource expenditure. This process was then repeated for a Monday-Wednesday-Friday (M-W-F) dosing schedule. For these simulations, the optimal dose for each metric (determined in the previous simulations) was administered on Monday and Wednesday, and the Friday dose was increased until the safety criterion was reached. To evaluate the importance of the earlier assumption of 0.5 IU dL^{-1} baseline, we repeated the above simulations assuming a baseline of 0 IU dL^{-1} to observe if similar trends emerged.

3. Results

Simulations of the typical regimen of 20 IU kg^{-1} TBW every 48 h were completed and the results are summarized in Table 2. We then investigated the hypothesis that a TBW-based dosing regimen results in overdosing in overweight and obese patients by determining the TBW-based dose required to meet the 1 IU dL^{-1} safety criterion in 95% of these patients. At a dose of 20 IU kg^{-1} TBW, the median minimum concentration (C_{min}) throughout the week for these patients was 5.4 IU dL^{-1}; the average consumption associated with this dosing regimen was 7.25×10^3 IU per person per week. However, this population requires only 14 IU kg^{-1} TBW to meet the 95% safety criterion, which corresponds to an average weekly consumption of 5.07×10^3 IU per person.

Table 2. Comparison of the typical 20 IU kg^{-1} total body weight (TBW) dose and the lowest dose meeting the safety threshold (i.e., 14 IU kg^{-1} TBW) in overweight and obese patients. Results are presented as median (90% confidence interval).

Measure	Regimen	
	20 IU kg^{-1} TBW, Q48 h	**14 IU kg^{-1} TBW, Q48 h**
C_{min} (IU dL^{-1})	5.4 (1.2–17.3)	3.9 (1.0–12.3)
Consumption (IU per person per week)	7260 (5730–8780)	5080 (4010–6140)

Following this initial investigation, we explored dosing regimens using alternative weight metrics. The correlation between each weight metric and BMI is shown in Figure 1. We began by administering a dose of 10 IU kg^{-1} of each weight metric on a Q48 h dosing schedule. Once steady state was reached, the percentage of patients with $C_{min} \geq 1.0$ IU dL^{-1} was calculated. If this percentage was below 95%, the dose was incrementally increased until this threshold was reached. We then calculated the mean weekly consumption associated with the minimum dose required to reach the safety criterion for each metric to assess cost-effectiveness. Since a Monday-Wednesday-Friday dosing schedule is commonly used in hemophilia A prophylaxis, we performed analogous simulations using this schedule instead of a regular 48 h interval. We used the optimal doses found in the previous study on Monday and Wednesday, and then increased the dose on Fridays to compensate for the longer interval until the safety criterion was met.

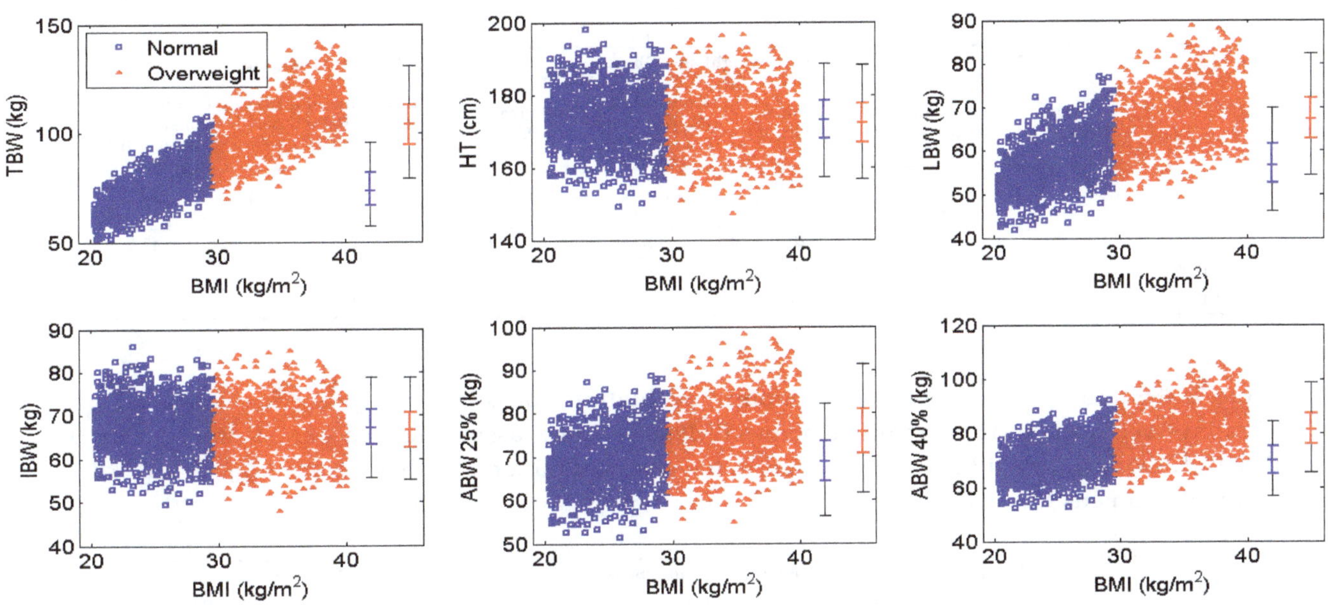

Figure 1. Correlation of body weight metrics with body mass index (BMI) for each BMI subgroup (blue = normal weight, red = overweight and obese). TBW: total body weight; HT: height; LBW: lean body weight; IBW: ideal body weight; ABW: adjusted body weight.

Tables 3 and 4 summarize the doses per kg of each weight metric required to reach the 95% safety criterion (when infused every 48 h or Monday-Wednesday-Friday, respectively) and the associated weekly consumption in each of the BMI categories and in the merged population, assuming a baseline factor level of 0.5 IU dL^{-1}. The most appropriate regimen is the one that meets the safety requirements while consuming the least amount of factor concentrate. For patients within the normal BMI range, LBW produced the optimal regimen for both dosing schedules; for the overweight and obese cohort, an IBW-based dosing regimen was found to be most cost-effective. Furthermore, the range of mean weekly consumption across the various weight metrics was much tighter for the normal BMI subgroup (125 IU per person per week) as compared to the overweight/obese subgroup (483 IU per person per week). When the two subgroups were combined, ABW with a 25% correction factor proved to be ideal for the Q48 h regimen, with IBW a very close second with a difference of just 5 IU per person per week. Both ABW_{25} and IBW perform almost identically in terms of safety for both BMI subgroups for the Q48 h regimen (Figure 2). However, IBW performed better than all other weight metrics when a Monday-Wednesday-Friday schedule was adopted, with a difference in consumption of over 100 IU per person per week when compared to the next best metric (LBW). Nevertheless, the amount of time spent below 1 IU dL^{-1} is significantly greater when following a Monday-Wednesday-Friday regimen as compared to the Q48 h dosing schedule (Figure 3b); additionally, an extremely high Friday dose (>125 IU kg^{-1} TBW) is required to meet the 95% safety requirement, whereas a dose of 18 IU kg^{-1} TBW is successful for the Q48 h regimen (Figure 3a).

Table 3. Summary of safety and economic evaluations of different weight metrics used in a Q48 h regimen across BMI subgroups, assuming a baseline factor level of 0.5 IU dL^{-1}. Dose is the dose required to have 95% of patients with a steady state C_{min} over 1 IU dL^{-1}. Optimal regimens for each subgroup and the overall population are bolded. IBW: ideal body weight, ABW: adjusted body weight.

Metric	Normal		Overweight and Obese		All BMI Categories		
	Dose ($IU\ kg^{-1}$)	**Mean Consumption (IU per Person per Week)**	**Dose ($IU\ kg^{-1}$)**	**Consumption (IU per Person per Week)**	**Dose ($IU\ kg^{-1}$)**	**Mean Consumption (IU per Person per Week)**	**Difference in Consumption from TBW**
TBW	20.0	5202	14.0	5074	18.0	5603	-
LBW	**25.6**	**5114**	21.3	5028	23.8	5186	−417
IBW	22.2	5222	**20.7**	**4828**	22.1	5176	−427
ABW_{25}	21.7	5239	20.0	5311	**20.4**	**5171**	**−432**
ABW_{40}	21.1	5173	18.0	5129	20.0	5301	−302

Table 4. Summary of safety and economic evaluations of different weight metrics used in a Monday-Wednesday-Friday regimen across BMI subgroups, assuming a baseline factor level of 0.5 IU dL^{-1}. Dose is the Friday dose required to have 90% of patients with a weekly $C_{min} \geq 1$ IU dL^{-1}. Optimal regimens for each subgroup and the overall population are bolded.

Metric	Normal		Overweight and Obese		All BMI Categories		
	Dose ($IU\ kg^{-1}$)	**Consumption (IU per Person per Week)**	**Dose ($IU\ kg^{-1}$)**	**Consumption (IU per Person per Week)**	**Dose ($IU\ kg^{-1}$)**	**Consumption (IU per Person per Week)**	**Difference in Consumption from TBW**
TBW	74	8174	54	9320	62	8716	-
LBW	**94**	**8082**	82	8740	88	8442	−274
IBW	78	8213	**84**	**8543**	**80**	**8312**	**−404**
ABW_{25}	78	8195	72	8558	76	8459	−258
ABW_{40}	76	8126	68	8792	72	8481	−235

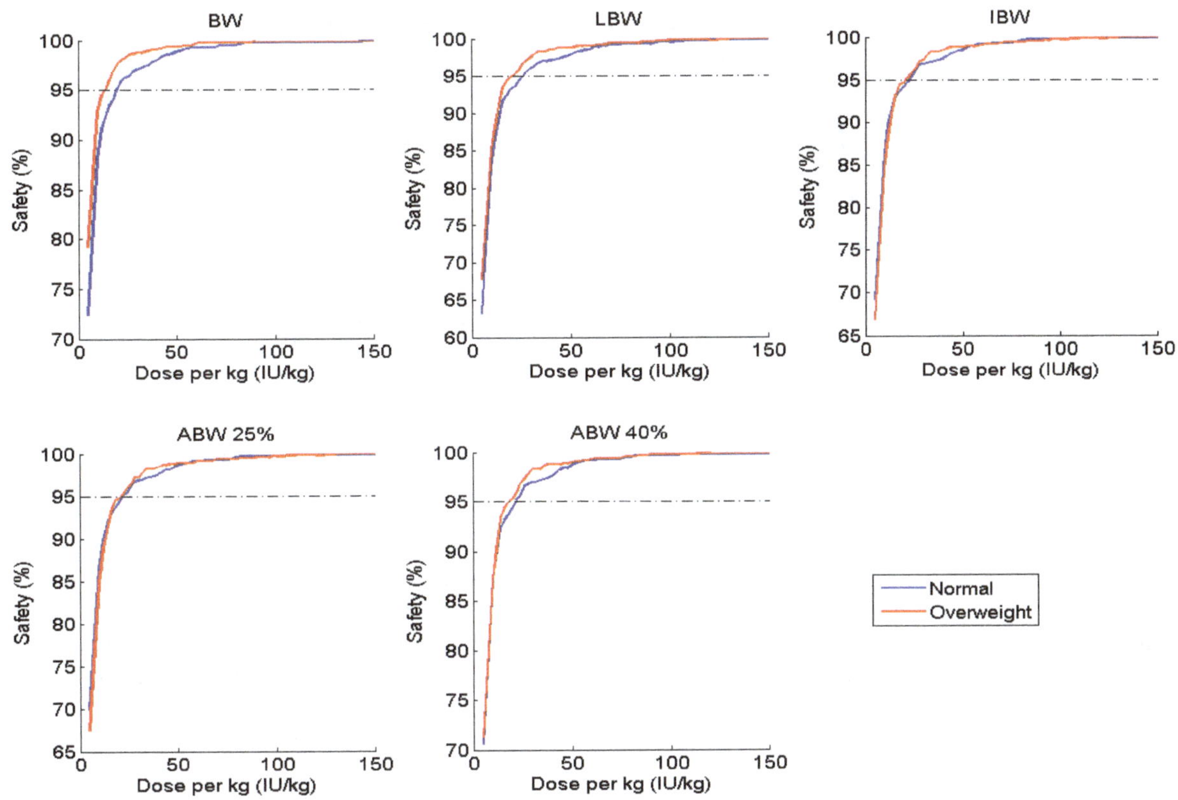

Figure 2. Percentage of patients with $C_{min} \geq 1$ IU dL^{-1} (safety) at various doses per kg of various weight metrics, stratified by BMI subgroup, administered at 48-h intervals.

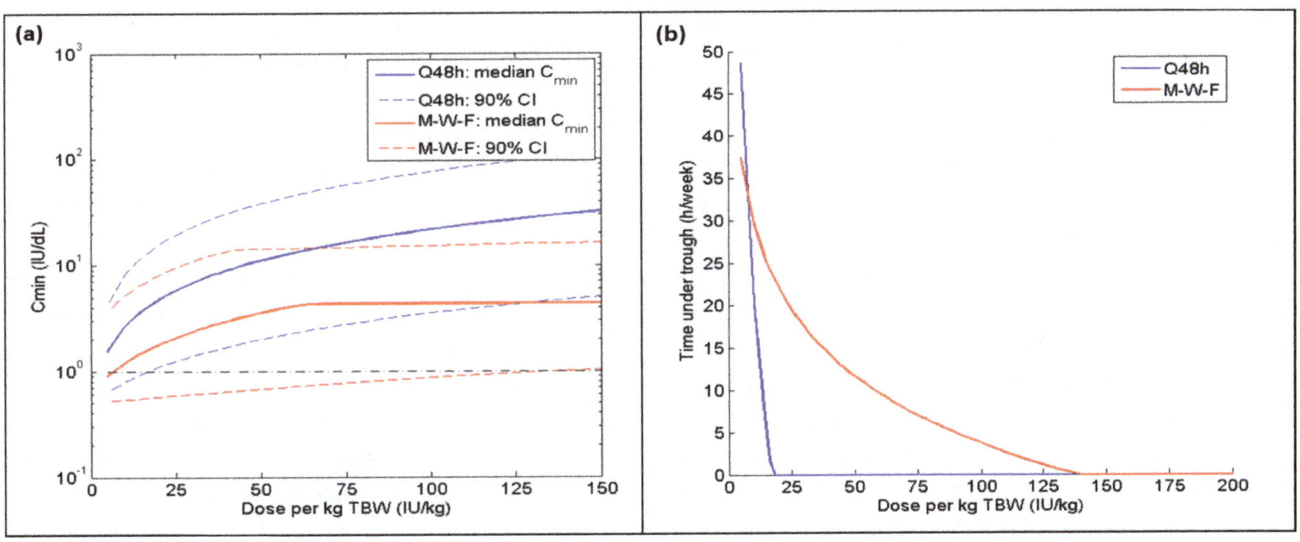

Figure 3. (**a**) Median and 90% confidence intervals for C_{min} and (**b**) 95th quantile for time spent below 1 IU dL^{-1} (hours per week) for TBW-based dosing regimen administered at different intervals for the combined group (normal + overweight/obese) for both Q48 h (blue) and Monday-Wednesday-Friday (red) dosing schedules. For the Q48 h regimen, all doses are increasing along the *X*-axis; for the Monday-Wednesday-Friday schedule, only the Friday dose is changing (Monday and Wednesday doses are fixed at 20 IU per kg TBW).

Ideal body weight continued to perform well in simulations with an assumed baseline of 0 IU dL^{-1}. The safety ratio versus dose curves are once again nearly identical for both BMI subgroups (Figure 4), although consumption was approximately doubled as compared to the Q48 h regimen.

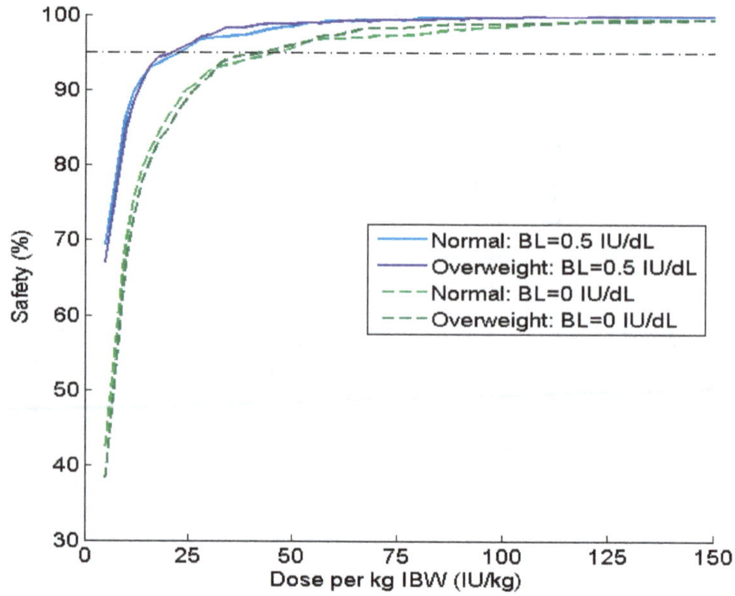

Figure 4. Comparison of safety profiles for patients simulated with baseline 0.5 IU dL^{-1} and 0 IU dL^{-1} for a Q48 h regimen. Safety (%) is the percentage of patients with $C_{min} \geq 1$ IU dL^{-1} at various doses per kg of IBW.

4. Discussion

We began by assessing the safety and cost-effectiveness of a typical 20 IU kg^{-1} TBW, Q48 h regimen in an overweight and obese patient population. For comparison, we determined the TBW-based dose required to meet the safety criterion. At a dose of 14 IU kg^{-1} TBW, 95% of patients had FVIII levels of at least 1 IU dL^{-1} at all times; the median C_{min} was 3.9 IU dL^{-1} and the mean consumption was just over 5000 IU per person per week. By contrast, the 20 IU kg^{-1} TBW regimen produced a median C_{min} of 5.4 IU dL^{-1} with a mean consumption of 7250 IU per person per week. Hence, the standard TBW-based dosing protocol results in over 40% higher consumption than required in the overweight and obese population; assuming a cost of $1 US per unit of concentrate, this amounts to over $100,000 US in excess spending per person annually. From this evaluation, it is clear that TBW does not represent the optimal body weight metric to guide FVIII dosing.

Simulations using dosing regimens based on alternative weight metrics (LBW, IBW, ABW_{25}, and ABW_{40}) were carried out using the two most common dosing schedules in hemophilia A prophylaxis: a regular 48 h regimen and a Monday-Wednesday-Friday regimen. Adapting a Monday-Wednesday-Friday timetable made it extremely difficult to meet the safety requirement, regardless of which weight metric was used to define the dose. While patients are often advised to increase their FVIII dose on Friday, a simple doubling of the dose is not sufficient. A potentially harmful Friday dose of 140 IU kg^{-1} TBW was required for 95% of patients to have a $C_{min} \geq 1$ IU dL^{-1}, compared to 18 IU kg^{-1} TBW to meet this safety minimum when infused every 48 h. Furthermore, the time spent below 1 IU dL^{-1} (and, consequently, the risk of bleeding events [32]) is significantly greater when following a Monday-Wednesday-Friday regimen, even if the Friday dose is twice or three times greater than the Monday and Wednesday doses (Figure 3b). In fact, a 2010 study in which FVIII was administered three times per week found that over 80% of bleeds occurred 48–72 h post-infusion [33]. The Monday-Wednesday-Friday treatment schedule, while more convenient, is no longer considered to be optimal therapy due to this increased vulnerability to bleeds during the weekend, with alternate day dosing representing the ideal regimen [34,35].

Due to analytical limitations, it can be difficult to obtain an exact measure of a patient's baseline factor level. Many assays have a lower limit of quantification of 1 IU dL^{-1} [36,37], which is greater than endogenous levels for severe hemophilia patients. To balance both safety and resource utilization, we ran initial simulations with an assumed baseline of 0.5 IU dL^{-1}. However, it is known that many severe hemophilia patients possess a genetic mutation such that no functional FVIII is produced endogenously. For this reason, the simulations were performed again using a baseline of 0 IU dL^{-1} to ensure similar trends were observed within this sub-population. Notably, a 95% safe ratio can be achieved in a population with no endogenous FVIII production at a reasonable dose (34 IU kg^{-1} TBW) if administered every 48 h. However, it is not possible to meet that safety threshold in this population if a Monday-Wednesday-Friday dosing schedule is employed. If the safety criteria is lowered to 90%, it can be met, but only with extremely high Friday doses (between 130 and 180 IU kg^{-1} for the various weight metrics) and associated weekly consumption (>16,000 IU per person per week); a study by Collins et al. found similarly high doses (>100 IU kg^{-1} for patients with average half-lives, and up to 400 IU kg^{-1} in extreme cases) were required to maintain FVIII levels above 1 IU dL^{-1} throughout the week when following this dosing schedule [38]. These results suggest that a regular dosing interval of 48 h offers significant advantages over the weekly Monday-Wednesday-Friday schedule in terms of both safety and cost-effectiveness.

After exploring all combinations of dosing schedule and baseline factor level, we determined that IBW-based dosing provides a safe and cost-effective regimen in the majority of scenarios, with ABW_{25} producing fairly similar results. Ideal body weight performed almost exactly the same in terms of safety between the normal and overweight groups across all of the doses and regardless of baseline, as evidenced by the closeness of the curves shown in Figures 2 and 4. Further, IBW was the most cost-effective in three out of four simulations; in the fourth, it differed by only 5 IU per person per week from the optimal regimen (ABW_{25}). If we compare the optimal regimen for a Q48 h schedule with a baseline of 0.5 IU dL^{-1} (i.e., 20.7 IU kg^{-1} IBW) to a 20 IU kg^{-1} TBW, this alterative regimen offers a savings of over 2000 IU per person per week (or nearly $110,000 US annually) for overweight and obese patients. Thus, IBW-based dosing offers a similar safety profile to the currently used TBW strategy while moderating the economic burden of clotting factor prophylaxis.

This exercise was limited by the constraints of the data. The model used herein was built on PK data from a specific brand of FVIII concentrate, although brand has not generally been found to significantly influence PK. A second limitation to the applicability of this approach is that the source data is largely from older (10+ years of age) patients, and the opinions on use of prophylaxis in adults are varied [39–41]. Obesity rates are also increasing rapidly amongst pediatric patients and similar dosing adjustments are likely appropriate in this population, but cannot be confirmed in this study. Further study of pediatric populations (and validated pediatric population PK models) is required in order to determine a dosing regimen that applies not only to all BMI's but also to all ages.

As the prevalence of obesity has risen in the general population, a number of studies have been conducted to investigate the frequency of overweight and obesity among hemophilia patients, complications such as co-morbidities and decreased quality of life, and recommendations for management strategies. Many pharmacokinetic studies exploring the relationship between excess body weight and plasma volume (and, by extension, in vivo recovery) have postulated that dosing according to body weight results in overdosing and an ineffective use of resources, suggesting instead that dosing be guided by LBW or IBW [42,43]. This study compared several weight metrics and confirmed that an IBW-based regimen is both safe and cost-effective across a range of BMI's. Ideal body weight produced slightly better results than other weight metrics because it is calculated based solely on height; as shown in Figure 1, there is no correlation between IBW and BMI as observed with the other metrics investigated.

Although we were able to identify a weight metric that is more suitable for a variable population, the high inter-individual variability in PK handling of factor concentrates precludes the definition of a single, "one dose fits all" strategy. In order to optimize prophylaxis, regimens should be tailored to the individual PK profile. This process has been facilitated by the development of the WAPPS-Hemo service (www.wapps-hemo.org), a Canadian-based user-friendly and industry-independent platform that produces estimates of individual PK parameters through a Bayesian iterative approach.

The WAPPS-Hemo service also includes a module for dosing regimen development, wherein clinicians can predict the effects of changing dose, frequency, or targeted trough for a specific patient before implementing these changes in practice. While PK-tailored dosing regimens may offer the best results, weight-based strategies are still the norm, but these can be optimized by adapting a different weight metric (i.e., IBW) to guide safe and cost-effective dosing at a population level.

5. Conclusions

In summary, we conducted simulations based on a previously published model of a conventional FVIII to explore the appropriateness of different weight metric-based dosing regimens for hemophilia A prophylaxis for overweight and obese patients. Regimens were required to produce a $C_{min} \geq 1$ IU dL^{-1} in 95% of the population, and then the average consumption for each regimen was calculated to evaluate resource-effectiveness. From this study, we conclude that ideal body weight performs the best, maintaining safety while tempering factor consumption for overweight and obese patients.

Supplementary Materials:
Figure S1: Correlation plots for all body size metrics used in simulations for the normal BMI subgroup. Diagonal elements contain histograms. Figure S2: Correlation plots for all body size metrics used in simulations for the overweight/obese subgroup. Diagonal elements contain histograms.

Acknowledgments: We thank Dirk Garmann for helpful comments. This work was funded by the Canadian Institute of Health Research (CIHR) as a doctoral award to AMK.

Author Contributions: Severine Henrard, Alanna McEneny-King, Andrea N. Edginton and Cedric Hermans conceived of the project. Alanna McEneny-King and Pierre Chelle completed the data analysis and all authors participated in manuscript preparation.

References

1. Den Uijl, I.E.; Mauser Bunschoten, E.P.; Roosendaal, G.; Schutgens, R.E.; Biesma, D.H.; Grobbee, D.E.; Fischer, K. Clinical severity of haemophilia A: Does the classification of the 1950s still stand? *Haemophilia* **2011**, *17*, 849–853. [CrossRef] [PubMed]
2. Manco-Johnson, M.J.; Abshire, T.C.; Shapiro, A.D.; Riske, B.; Hacker, M.R.; Kilcoyne, R.; Ingram, J.D.; Manco-Johnson, M.L.; Funk, S.; Jacobson, L.; et al. Prophylaxis versus episodic treatment to prevent joint disease in boys with severe hemophilia. *N. Engl. J. Med.* **2007**, *357*, 535–544. [CrossRef] [PubMed]
3. Fischer, K.; Collins, P.W.; Ozelo, M.C.; Srivastava, A.; Young, G.; Blanchette, V.S. When and how to start prophylaxis in boys with severe hemophilia without inhibitors: Communication from the SSC of the ISTH. *J. Thromb. Haemost.* **2016**, *14*, 1105–1109. [CrossRef] [PubMed]
4. Berntorp, E.; Spotts, G.; Patrone, L.; Ewenstein, B.M. Advancing personalized care in hemophilia A: Ten years' experience with an advanced category antihemophilic factor prepared using a plasma/albumin-free method. *Biologics* **2014**, *8*, 115–127. [CrossRef] [PubMed]
5. Petrini, P. Identifying and overcoming barriers to prophylaxis in the management of haemophilia. *Haemophilia* **2007**, *13* (Suppl. 2), 16–22. [CrossRef] [PubMed]
6. Oldenburg, J. Optimal treatment strategies for hemophilia: Achievements and limitations of current prophylactic regimens. *Blood* **2015**, *125*, 2038–2044. [CrossRef] [PubMed]
7. Bjorkman, S.; Folkesson, A.; Jonsson, S. Pharmacokinetics and dose requirements of factor VIII over the age range 3–74 years: A population analysis based on 50 patients with long-term prophylactic treatment for haemophilia A. *Eur. J. Clin. Pharmacol.* **2009**, *65*, 989–998. [CrossRef] [PubMed]
8. Carlsson, M.; Berntorp, E.; Bjorkman, S.; Lethagen, S.; Ljung, R. Improved cost-effectiveness by pharmacokinetic dosing of factor VIII in prophylactic treatment of haemophilia A. *Haemophilia* **1997**, *3*, 96–101. [CrossRef] [PubMed]
9. Iorio, A.; Keepanasseril, A.; Foster, G.; Navarro-Ruan, T.; McEneny-King, A.; Edginton, A.N.; Thabane, L. WAPPS-Hemo co-investigator network Development of a Web-Accessible Population Pharmacokinetic Service-Hemophilia (WAPPS-Hemo): Study Protocol. *JMIR Res. Protoc.* **2016**, *5*, e239. [CrossRef] [PubMed]

10. McEneny-King, A.; Foster, G.; Iorio, A.; Edginton, A.N. Data Analysis Protocol for the Development and Evaluation of Population Pharmacokinetic Models for Incorporation into the Web-Accessible Population Pharmacokinetic Service—Hemophilia (WAPPS-Hemo). *JMIR Res. Protoc.* **2016**, *5*, e232. [CrossRef] [PubMed]
11. Ingram, G.I. Calculating the dose of factor VIII in the management of haemophilia. *Br. J. Haematol.* **1981**, *48*, 351–354. [CrossRef] [PubMed]
12. Poon, M.C.; Lee, A. Individualized prophylaxis for optimizing hemophilia care: Can we apply this to both developed and developing nations? *Thromb. J.* **2016**, *14*, 32. [CrossRef] [PubMed]
13. Ullman, M.; Zhang, Q.C.; Brown, D.; Grant, A.; Soucie, J.M. Hemophilia Treatment Center Network Investigators Association of overweight and obesity with the use of self and home-based infusion therapy among haemophilic men. *Haemophilia* **2014**, *20*, 340–348. [CrossRef] [PubMed]
14. Revel-Vilk, S.; Komvilaisak, P.; Blanchette, V.; Stain, A.M.; Floros, G.; Cochrane, A.; Blanchette, C.; Hang, M.; Roberts, E.A.; Ling, S.C. The changing face of hepatitis in boys with haemophilia associated with increased prevalence of obesity. *Haemophilia* **2011**, *17*, 689–694. [CrossRef] [PubMed]
15. Young, G. New challenges in hemophilia: Long-term outcomes and complications. *Hematol. Am. Soc. Hematol. Educ. Program.* **2012**, *2012*, 362–368.
16. Shapiro, A.D.; Korth-Bradley, J.; Poon, M.C. Use of pharmacokinetics in the coagulation factor treatment of patients with haemophilia. *Haemophilia* **2005**, *11*, 571–582. [CrossRef] [PubMed]
17. Henrard, S.; Speybroeck, N.; Hermans, C. Impact of being underweight or overweight on factor VIII dosing in hemophilia A patients. *Haematologica* **2013**, *98*, 1481–1486. [CrossRef] [PubMed]
18. McLeay, S.C.; Morrish, G.A.; Kirkpatrick, C.M.; Green, B. The relationship between drug clearance and body size: Systematic review and meta-analysis of the literature published from 2000 to 2007. *Clin. Pharmacokinet.* **2012**, *51*, 319–330. [CrossRef] [PubMed]
19. Cheymol, G. Effects of obesity on pharmacokinetics implications for drug therapy. *Clin. Pharmacokinet.* **2000**, *39*, 215–231. [CrossRef] [PubMed]
20. Hanley, M.J.; Abernethy, D.R.; Greenblatt, D.J. Effect of obesity on the pharmacokinetics of drugs in humans. *Clin. Pharmacokinet.* **2010**, *49*, 71–87. [CrossRef] [PubMed]
21. Bjorkman, S.; Oh, M.; Spotts, G.; Schroth, P.; Fritsch, S.; Ewenstein, B.M.; Casey, K.; Fischer, K.; Blanchette, V.S.; Collins, P.W. Population pharmacokinetics of recombinant factor VIII: The relationships of pharmacokinetics to age and body weight. *Blood* **2012**, *119*, 612–618. [CrossRef] [PubMed]
22. Kawai, R.; Lemaire, M.; Steimer, J.L.; Bruelisauer, A.; Niederberger, W.; Rowland, M. Physiologically based pharmacokinetic study on a cyclosporin derivative, SDZ IMM 125. *J. Pharmacokinet. Biopharm.* **1994**, *22*, 327–365. [CrossRef] [PubMed]
23. Tuinenburg, A.; Biere-Rafi, S.; Peters, M.; Verhamme, P.; Peerlinck, K.; Kruip, M.J.; Laros-Van Gorkom, B.A.; Roest, M.; Meijers, J.C.; Kamphuisen, P.W.; et al. Obesity in haemophilia patients: Effect on bleeding frequency, clotting factor concentrate usage, and haemostatic and fibrinolytic parameters. *Haemophilia* **2013**, *19*, 744–752. [CrossRef] [PubMed]
24. Taylor, B.N.; Bork, S.J.; Kim, S.; Moffett, B.S.; Yee, D.L. Evaluation of weight-based dosing of unfractionated heparin in obese children. *J. Pediatr.* **2013**, *163*, 150–153. [CrossRef] [PubMed]
25. Risebrough, N.; Oh, P.; Blanchette, V.; Curtin, J.; Hitzler, J.; Feldman, B.M. Cost-utility analysis of Canadian tailored prophylaxis, primary prophylaxis and on-demand therapy in young children with severe haemophilia A. *Haemophilia* **2008**, *14*, 743–752. [CrossRef] [PubMed]
26. Johnson, K.A.; Zhou, Z.Y. Costs of Care in Hemophilia and Possible Implications of Health Care Reform. *Hematol. Am. Soc. Hematol. Educ. Program.* **2011**, *1*, 413. [CrossRef] [PubMed]
27. Majumdar, S.; Ostrenga, A.; Latzman, R.D.; Payne, C.; Hunt, Q.; Morris, A.; Iyer, R. Pharmacoeconomic impact of obesity in severe haemophilia children on clotting factor prophylaxis in a single institution. *Haemophilia* **2011**, *17*, 717–718. [CrossRef] [PubMed]
28. Fryar, C.D.; Gu, Q.; Ogden, C.L.; Flegal, K.M. Anthropometric Reference Data for Children and Adults: United States, 2011–2014. *Vital Health Stat. 3* **2016**, *39*, 1–46.
29. Janmahasatian, S.; Duffull, S.B.; Ash, S.; Ward, L.C.; Byrne, N.M.; Green, B. Quantification of lean bodyweight. *Clin. Pharmacokinet.* **2005**, *44*, 1051–1065. [CrossRef] [PubMed]
30. Green, B.; Duffull, S.B. What is the best size descriptor to use for pharmacokinetic studies in the obese? *Br. J. Clin. Pharmacol.* **2004**, *58*, 119–133. [CrossRef] [PubMed]

31. Garmann, D.; McLeay, S.; Shah, A.; Vis, P.; Maas Enriquez, M.; Ploeger, B.A. Population pharmacokinetic characterization of BAY 81–8973, a full-length recombinant factor VIII: Lessons learned—Importance of including samples with factor VIII levels below the quantitation limit. *Haemophilia* **2017**, *23*, 528–537. [CrossRef] [PubMed]
32. Collins, P.W.; Blanchette, V.S.; Fischer, K.; Bjorkman, S.; Oh, M.; Fritsch, S.; Schroth, P.; Spotts, G.; Astermark, J.; Ewenstein, B. Break-through bleeding in relation to predicted factor VIII levels in patients receiving prophylactic treatment for severe hemophilia A. *J. Thromb. Haemost.* **2009**, *7*, 413–420. [CrossRef] [PubMed]
33. Collins, P.; Faradji, A.; Morfini, M.; Enriquez, M.M.; Schwartz, L. Efficacy and safety of secondary prophylactic vs. on-demand sucrose-formulated recombinant factor VIII treatment in adults with severe hemophilia A: Results from a 13-month crossover study. *J. Thromb. Haemost.* **2010**, *8*, 83–89. [CrossRef] [PubMed]
34. Collins, P.W.; Fischer, K.; Morfini, M.; Blanchette, V.S.; Bjorkman, S.; International Prophylaxis Study Group Pharmacokinetics Expert Working Group. Implications of coagulation factor VIII and IX pharmacokinetics in the prophylactic treatment of haemophilia. *Haemophilia* **2011**, *17*, 2–10. [CrossRef] [PubMed]
35. Richards, M.; Williams, M.; Chalmers, E.; Liesner, R.; Collins, P.; Vidler, V.; Hanley, J. Paediatric Working Party of the United Kingdom Haemophilia Doctors' Organisation A United Kingdom Haemophilia Centre Doctors' Organization guideline approved by the British Committee for Standards in Haematology: Guideline on the use of prophylactic factor VIII concentrate in children and adults with severe haemophilia A. *Br. J. Haematol.* **2010**, *149*, 498–507. [PubMed]
36. Shapiro, A.D. Long-lasting recombinant factor VIII proteins for hemophilia A. *Hematol. Am. Soc. Hematol. Educ. Program.* **2013**, *2013*, 37–43. [CrossRef] [PubMed]
37. Barrowcliffe, T.W. Monitoring haemophilia severity and treatment: New or old laboratory tests? *Haemophilia* **2004**, *10* (Suppl. 4), 109–114. [CrossRef] [PubMed]
38. Collins, P.W.; Bjorkman, S.; Fischer, K.; Blanchette, V.; Oh, M.; Schroth, P.; Fritsch, S.; Casey, K.; Spotts, G.; Ewenstein, B.M. Factor VIII requirement to maintain a target plasma level in the prophylactic treatment of severe hemophilia A: Influences of variance in pharmacokinetics and treatment regimens. *J. Thromb. Haemost.* **2010**, *8*, 269–275. [CrossRef] [PubMed]
39. Ljung, R. Aspects of prophylactic treatment of hemophilia. *Thromb. J.* **2016**, *14*, 30. [CrossRef] [PubMed]
40. Jackson, S.C.; Yang, M.; Minuk, L.; Sholzberg, M.; St-Louis, J.; Iorio, A.; Card, R.; Poon, M.C. Prophylaxis in older Canadian adults with hemophilia A: Lessons and more questions. *BMC Hematol.* **2015**, *15*. [CrossRef] [PubMed]
41. Oldenburg, J.; Brackmann, H.H. Prophylaxis in adult patients with severe haemophilia A. *Thromb. Res.* **2014**, *134* (Suppl. 1), S33–S37. [CrossRef] [PubMed]
42. Graham, A.; Jaworski, K. Pharmacokinetic analysis of anti-hemophilic factor in the obese patient. *Haemophilia* **2014**, *20*, 226–229. [CrossRef] [PubMed]
43. Komwilaisak, P.; Blanchette, V. Pharmacokinetic studies of coagulation factors: Relevance of plasma and extracellular volume and body weight. *Haemophilia* **2006**, *12* (Suppl. 4), 33. [CrossRef]

5

Tissue Specific Modulation of cyp2c and cyp3a mRNA Levels and Activities by Diet-Induced Obesity in Mice: The Impact of Type 2 Diabetes on Drug Metabolizing Enzymes in Liver and Extra-Hepatic Tissues

Sarah Maximos [1,2], Michel Chamoun [3], Sophie Gravel [1,3], Jacques Turgeon [1,2,3] and Veronique Michaud [1,2,3,*]

1 Centre de recherche du Centre hospitalier de l'Université de Montréal (CRCHUM), Montreal, QC H2X 0A9, Canada; sarah.maximos@umontreal.ca (S.M.); sophie.gravel.3@umontreal.ca (S.G.); turgeoja@gmail.com (J.T.)
2 Faculty of Medicine, Université de Montréal, Montreal, QC H3T 1J4, Canada
3 Faculty of Pharmacy, Université de Montréal, Montreal, QC H3T 1J4, Canada; michel_chamoun94@hotmail.com
* Correspondence: v.michaud@umontreal.ca

Abstract: Various diseases such as type 2 diabetes (T2D) may alter drug clearance. The objective of this study was to evaluate the effects of T2D on CYP450 expressions and activities using high-fat diet (HFD) as a model of obesity-dependent diabetes in C57BL6 mice. The cyp450 mRNA expression levels for 15 different isoforms were determined in the liver and extra-hepatic tissues (kidneys, lungs and heart) of HFD-treated animals (n = 45). Modulation of cyp450 metabolic activities by HFD was assessed using eight known substrates for specific human ortholog CYP450 isoforms: in vitro incubations were conducted with liver and extra-hepatic microsomes. Expression levels of cyp3a11 and cyp3a25 mRNA were decreased in the liver (>2–14-fold) and kidneys (>2-fold) of HFD groups which correlated with a significant reduction in midazolam metabolism (by 21- and 5-fold in hepatic and kidney microsomes, respectively, $p < 0.001$). HFD was associated with decreased activities of cyp2b and cyp2c subfamilies in all organs tested except in the kidneys (for tolbutamide). Other cyp450 hepatic activities were minimally or not affected by HFD. Taken together, our data suggest that substrate-dependent and tissue-dependent modulation of cyp450 metabolic capacities by early phases of T2D are observed, which could modulate drug disposition and pharmacological effects in various tissues.

Keywords: cytochromes P450; drug metabolism; mRNA; diet induced obesity; diabetes

---

1. Introduction

Type 2 diabetes (T2D) has become a worldwide public health concern as prevalence of the disease continues to rise [1]. In 2014, the American Diabetes Association reported that 29.1 million Americans, or 9.3% of the population, had T2D [2]. In addition to anti-diabetic drugs, T2D patients commonly require multiple drug therapies to treat a wide range of comorbidities such as hypertension, stroke, dyslipidemia, atherosclerosis and coronary artery disease [3]. Clinical practice reveals that T2D patients show highly variable pharmacokinetics and responses to several drugs used to treat T2D and its related comorbidities [4–7]. For instance, variable drug dosages and effects are observed for drugs such as clopidogrel, warfarin, cyclosporine and tacrolimus, as well as for anti-hypertensive and cholesterol lowering drugs [8–14]. Hence, the treatment of co-morbidities in T2D is associated with variable drug response and unexpected toxicities [4,15–17].

Currently, information available on the underlying mechanisms responsible for this variability is uncertain. Patients with T2D have a high prevalence of metabolic syndrome (85% vs. 24% in general population), which is associated with a chronic low-grade inflammatory state [18–20]. Several reports showed that some inflammatory mediators may modulate expression levels and activities of numerous proteins including some isoenzymes of the cytochrome P450 (CYP450) superfamily [21–24]. In fact, interleukin-B (IL-1B), interleukin-6 (IL-6) and interferon-γ (INF-γ) have been associated with decreased expressions and activities of CYP450s, especially of CYP3A, in cultured human hepatocytes [25–27]. It is also known that pathophysiological changes resulting from obesity affect drug-metabolizing enzyme expressions and activities [28–30].

In humans, some studies have reported a decrease in CYP3A4 and an increase in CYP2E1 activities with obesity, while its effects on other isozymes remain uncertain [31–34]. For instance, Woolsey et al. have reported that CYP3A activity and CYP3A4 mRNA expression were reduced in humans and mice with nonalcoholic fatty liver disease [35]. However, results from animal studies are inconsistent from one study to the other [30,36–42]. These discrepancies could be explained by the type of diabetes being studied (i.e., T1D vs. T2D), and the strategy used to induce diabetes (i.e., genetically-modified animals vs. chemicals vs. diet). For instance, down-regulation of CYP1A2 and CYP3A1, and up-regulation of CYP3A2 are observed in Goto–Kakizaki rats (genetic model of non-obese T2D) [43]. Conversely, alloxan or streptozocin were associated with an increase expression of hepatic CYP1A2, CYP2B1/2, CYP3A1/23 and CYP2E1 in diabetic rats compared to controls [44–49]. No alteration in hepatic levels of cyp1a2 and cyp2e1 has been found in streptozocin-induced diabetic mice [41]. A study from Ghose et al. revealed a decrease of cyp3a activity, but unaffected cyp1a2 and cyp2e1 activities in high-fat diet (HFD) fed mice [38]. Finally, no difference was observed for cyp3a11 expression or activity in db/db mice (a genetic T2D mouse model) [37].

Several organs express various combinations of CYP450s and, thus, different patterns of CYP450 expression in tissues may be a key determinant of variability observed for drug response. Although extra-hepatic CYP450 activity is manifested to a lower magnitude compared to the liver [50], variability in tissue-specific metabolizing CYP450 enzymes may lead to variation in drug effects due to local metabolism in target organs. To date, there is a paucity of information on the influence of pathophysiological conditions such as T2D on the activity and expression of extra-hepatic CYP450s.

In this study, we sought to determine the effects of T2D on the expression and activities of hepatic and extra-hepatic CYP450 enzymes using the high fat-diet (HFD) diet-induced obesity (DIO) C57BL6 mouse as a T2D model [51]. DIO mice were stratified into two groups according to the effect of HFD on their body weight at the end of the treatment period: low-diet responders and high-diet responders. These two groups have been well characterized and correspond to the early diabetes situation observed in obese humans [51]. An extensive phenotyping characterization was conducted in many organs (liver, kidneys, lungs and heart) to assess the tissue-specific modulation of cyp450 expressions and activities.

2. Materials and Methods

2.1. Chemicals

Ebastine, hydroxyebastine, carboxyebastine, desalkylebastine, hydroxyebastine-d5, carebastine-d5, desalkylebastine-d5, bufuralol, hydroxybufuralol, hydroxybufuralol-d9, repaglinide, 2-despiperidyl-2-amino repaglinide (M1), 3′-hydroxyrepaglinide (M4), bupropion, hydroxubupropion, hydroxybupropion-d5, hydroxytolbutamide, carboxytolbutamide, 1′-hydroxytolbutaminde-d9, 4′-carboxytolbutamide-d9, 4-hydroxymidazolam, 4-hydroxymidazolam-d5, 6-hydroxychlorzoxazone and 12-hydroxydodecanoic-d20 acid were purchased from Toronto Research Chemicals (Toronto, ON, Canada). Hydroxychlorzoxazone-d2 was obtained from TLC PharmaChem (Mississauga, ON, Canada). Midazolam and 1′-hydroxymidazolam-d4 were purchased from Cerilliant (Round Road,

TX, USA). Chlorzoxazone, tolbutamide, dodecanoic acid, β-Nicotinamide-Adenine Dinucleotide Phosphate (NADP), glucose-6-phosphate (G6P), glucose-6-phosphate dehydrogenase (G6PD), dimethyl sulfoxide (DMSO), trishydroxymethylaminomethame (TRIS), and phenylmethanesulfonyl (PMSF) were purchased from Sigma-Aldrich (St. Louis, MO, USA). Ethynediaminetetraacetic acid (EDTA) and dithiothreitol were obtained from Bishop (Burlington, ON, Canada) and from Gibco®, Life Technologies Ltd. (Eugene, OR, USA), respectively. All other chemicals used were commercially available and were of analytical grade.

2.2. *Animals*

Five-week-old male C57BL/6 mice (n = 45) were purchased from Charles River Laboratories (Montreal, QC, Canada). Animals were housed in a temperature-, light-, and humidity-controlled environment, they were housed 2 per cage and were maintained at an ambient temperature of 21 °C on a 12-h light/dark cycle with free access to water and food ad libitum. The obese diabetic mice were developed according to the experimental protocol described previously [51]. Briefly, one week after their arrival, mice (mean weight 20.0 $\pm$ 1.0 g) were fed with a high-fat diet (HFD) (Bio-Serv Diet #F3282, Frenchtown, NJ, USA, 60% fat by energy) or the standard normal diet (ND) (Teklad Global 18% protein diet; Harlan Teklad, Madison, WI, USA, 15% fat by energy) for 8 weeks. Body weight was measured weekly while blood glucose and insulin were determined at Week 8. After 8 weeks of diet, HFD mice were stratified according to their body weight and two groups were formed as follows; low responders to HFD (LDR) (<39.9 g) and high responders to HFD (HDR) (39.9–45 g). Peyot et al. have demonstrated that the LDR are less obese, develop intermediate severity of insulin resistance and have mild impairment in glycemia, while the HDR are more obese, insulin resistant, hyperinsulinemic and hyperglycemic [51]. Animals were sacrificed by cervical dislocation, and organs including heart, lungs, kidneys and liver were quickly excised, washed with cold TRIS 100 mM buffer (pH 7.4) and immersed in liquid nitrogen (−80 °C). Experimental protocols were approved by the institutional committee of animal protection and were carried out in accordance with the Guide for the Care and Use of Experimental Animals of the Canadian Council on Animal Care.

2.3. *CYP450 mRNA Levels*

2.3.1. Isolation of RNA and Preparation of cDNA

For each organ tested (using a pool of 3 mice/organ), about 100 mg of tissue was homogenized in 1 mL of Trizol and incubated for 5 min at room temperature. Chloroform (200 μL) was added, the mixture shaken for 15 s and then, centrifuged at 16,000× g for 30 min at 4 °C. The aqueous supernatant (500 μL) was transferred and ethanol 70% was added (1:1 v/v). RNA was extracted using the Qiagen kit (RNeasy Mini kit; Qiagen Sciences, MD, USA) according to the manufacturer's recommendations. RNA concentration and quality was assessed by spectrometry. Total RNA (2 μg) from each sample was used for reverse transcription. RNA, random primers (6 μg) and dNTP (25 mM) were preheated for 5 min at 65 °C. Then, 5X-first strand buffer, 80 units of RNAse inhibitor, DTT (0.01 M) and 400 units of Superscript II (Invitrogen, Carlsbad, CA, USA) were added to a final volume of 40 μL. Reverse transcription was carried out for 50 min at 42 °C and stopped by heating to 70 °C for 15 min (final RNA concentration 50 ng/μL). The resulting cDNA was frozen at −80 °C until analyzed.

2.3.2. RT-qPCR Analysis

Real-time quantitative PCR was performed using TaqMan® probe and primer sets from Applied Biosystem (Foster, CA, USA). The assay IDs for selected cyp450s were: cyp2b9 (Mm00657910_m1), cyp2b10 (Mm01972453_s1), cyp2c29 (Mm00725580_s1), cyp2c37 (Mm00833845_m1), cyp2c39 (Mm04207909_g1), cyp2c40 (Mm04204172_mH), cyp2d9 (Mm00651731_m1), cyp2d10 (Mm00731648_m1), cyp2d22 (Mm00530542_m1), cyp2e1 (Mm00491127_m1), cyp2j5 (Mm00487292_m1), cyp2j6 (Mm01268197_m1), cyp3a11 (Mm00731567_m1), cyp3a13 (Mm00484110_m1), cyp3a25

(Mm01209536_m1) and cyp4a10 (Mm01622743_g1). As reference genes, gapdh (Mm99999915_g1) and b2m (Mm00437762_m1) were used as housekeeping genes. cDNA was diluted to 10 ng/reaction, mixed with TaqMan® PCR Master Mix (10 μL) and amplified using cycling conditions as follows: 45 cycles consisting of 10 s at 95 °C and 45 s at 60 °C. Reactions were run in a QuantStudio 6 Flex System (Life Technologies Inc., Burlington, ON, Canada).

The relative quantification of various gene expressions was calculated to the comparative CT method using the formula $2^{-\Delta CT}$ [52,53]. Only CT values ≤ 35 were included in the analyses. Since CT values > 35 were not reliable and considered below the detection level of the assay, a CT value of 35 to 38 was defined not quantifiable (NQ) while a value of CT > 38 as not detectable (ND). For their part, mRNA levels associated with the expression of each isoenzyme under a specific diet condition (ND, LDR, HDR) were determined using a calibrator and the following formula $2^{-\Delta\Delta CT}$ [52]. The calibrator was prepared at the same mRNA concentration using a pool of RNA obtained for each tissue (Clontech A Takara, Bio Company, Mountain View, CA, USA). Determination of mRNA levels was performed in triplicate for each sample, and three independent experiments were repeated to confirm results.

2.4. In Vitro CYP450 Metabolism in Liver and Extra-Hepatic Organs

2.4.1. Preparation of Microsomes

Microsomes from liver, kidneys, lungs and heart were prepared according to our previously described methods with slight modifications [54]. Briefly, tissue (pools of organs from 3 mice) was homogenized in an ice-cold buffer consisting of 50 mM-150 mM-1 mM TRIS-KCL-EDTA buffer (liver and kidneys) or 100 mM-150 mM-1 mM PO_4-KCL-EDTA buffer (lungs and heart) and both buffers containing protease inhibitors namely, PMFS (0.01 mM) and DTT (0.5 mM). Microsomal subcellular fraction was prepared by centrifugation (10,000 $g \times 20$ min, at 4 °C) followed by ultra-centrifugation (100,000 $g \times 90$ min, at 4 °C). The microsomal pellets were resuspended in the same buffer (without PMSF and DTT), and frozen at −80 °C until in vitro metabolism experiments were performed. The protein concentration of the microsomes was determined by the Bradford method using bovine serum albumin as the standard.

2.4.2. Effects of the HFD on Hepatic and Extra-Hepatic cyp450 Activities

In order to investigate the effects of the HFD as a representative model of type 2 diabetes on cyp450 activities, in vitro incubations were performed in presence of various microsomes with several probe drugs of CYP450s including bupropion, repaglinide, tolbutamide, bufuralol, chlorzoxazone, ebastine, midazolam and dodecanoic acid, which were used as markers of the functional orthologs of human CYP2B6, CYP2C8, CYP2C9, CYP2D6, CYP2J2, CYP2E1, CYP3A4/5 and CYP4A11, respectively. This study employed cocktails of probe substrates already accepted and validated to investigate the impact of diabetes on specific cyp450 activities. The production of each specific metabolite was quantified from substrate probes and variations of in vitro probes reactions can be inferred to affect all substrates metabolized by the same enzymes.

Assay conditions were previously optimized by standard incubations with probes (buffer, incubation period, protein contents and drug concentrations). All incubations were performed in triplicate. The incubation mixture containing microsomes [5 μL for liver (~20 mg proteins/mL) and 50 μL for kidney, lungs and heart microsomes (~7–14 mg proteins/mL)], NADPH-regenerating system solution (NADP 6.5 mM, G6P 16.5mM, $MgCl_2$ 5 mM and 0.2 U G6PD) and 100 mM phosphate buffer PO_4 (pH 7.4) or 100 mM TRIS buffer (pH 7.4, for tolbutamide and dodecanoic acid) were pre-incubated in a shaking bath for 10 min at 37 °C. Reaction was initiated by the addition of substrates (bupropion, tolbutamide, bufuralol, chlorzoxazone, midazolam, ebastine, dodecanoic acid or repaglinide) to the incubation mixture (total final volume of 500 μL). Bupropion, chlorzoxazone, ebastine and midazolam were incubated together as a cocktail as previously described whereas the other probe substrates were tested separately. The substrate concentrations used span a range from 38–620 μM for bupropion,

2.5–40 μM for bufuralol, 50–800 μM for chlorzoxazone, 0.125–2 μM for ebastine, 1.25–20 μM for dodecanoic acid, 0.25–4 μM for midazolam, 0.85–14 μM for repaglinide and 25–400 μM for tolbutamide (5 different concentrations were used with liver microsomes while one concentration (>2 km) to ensure saturation was selected to investigate cyp450 activities in extra-hepatic microsomes). After 30 min, the reaction was stopped using 1000 μL of ice-cold internal methanol containing isotope-labeled internal standard probe metabolite(s). Reaction mixtures were put on ice for 10 min, and following a centrifugation at 13,000 rpm for 10 min, and then the supernatant was transferred for analysis. For dodecanoic acid metabolite analysis, the solution was evaporated to dryness at 50 °C under a gentle stream of nitrogen, reconstituted with 200 μL of methanol and transferred to an injection vial for analysis.

2.5. High Performance Chromatography–Mass Spectrometry Analytical Methods

2.5.1. Chromatographic Conditions for the Metabolites of Bupropion, Midazolam and Ebastine

This analysis was performed on a Thermo Scientific Acclaim RSLC Polar Advantage C16 column (75 mm × 3.0 mm, 3 μm) and Phenomenex Security Guard Cartridge (C12, 4 mm × 2 mm) operating at 50 °C. The mobile phase was a gradient elution consisting of (A) 0.1% formic acid in acetonitrile and (B) 10 mM ammonium formate in water adjusted to pH 3; ratio A:B varied from 25:75 to 60:40 (*v*/*v*), at a flow rate 500 μL/min (a total run time of 10 min). A 10 μL aliquot of the extract was injected into LC-MSMS system.

A Thermo Scientific TSQ Quantiva Triple Quadrupole mass spectrometer (San Jose, CA, USA) was interfaced with a Thermo Scientific Ultimate 3000 XRS UHPLC system (San Jose, CA, USA) using a pneumatic assisted heated electrospray ion source. MS detection was performed in positive ion mode using selected reaction monitoring (SRM). Selection of optimal transitions and collision energy and tube lens voltage conditions for the metabolites and their respective internal standard are listed in Table S1.

2.5.2. Chromatographic Conditions for the Metabolites of Chlorzoxazone, Tolbutamide, Dodecanoic Acid, Bufuralol and Repaglinide

These analyses were carried out on a Phenomenex Luna PFP (2) column (150 mm × 3.0 mm I.D., 3 μm) with a Phenomenex PFP security guard cartridge operating at 40 °C. A mobile phase in isocratic mode was composed of acetonitrile and 0.01% formic acid having a fixed ratio of 40:60 (*v*/*v*) for chlorzoxazone, tolbutamide and dodecanoic acid, while a ratio of 50:50 was used for bufuralol and repaglinide. The flow rate was 0.30 mL/min (total run time 10 min). A 10 μL aliquot of the extract was injected into the LC-MSMS system.

The HPLC system consisted of a Shimadzu Prominence series UFLC pump and auto sampler (Kyoto, Japan). The tandem MS system used was a Thermo TSQ Quantum Ultra (San Jose, CA, USA). The mass spectrometer was interfaced with the HPLC system using a pneumatic assisted heated electrospray ion source. MS detection was performed in negative ion mode for chlorzoxazone, tolbutamide, and dodecanoic acid metabolites, and in positive ion mode for bufuralol and repaglinide metabolites using selected reaction monitoring (SRM). Selection of optimal transitions and collision energy and tube lens voltage conditions for the metabolites and their respective internal standard are shown in Table S2.

2.6. Statistical Analysis

Calibration curves were calculated from the equation $y = ax + b$, as determined by weighted $1/x$ and $1/x^2$ linear regressions of the calibration lines constructed from the peak-area ratios of metabolites to the internal standard (XCalibur software, Thermo Fisher, San Jose, CA, USA). Relative expression levels of CYP450s mRNAs were analyzed by one-way analysis of variance followed by the Dunnett post-hoc test. A difference with $p < 0.05$ was considered statistically significant. Enzyme kinetic parameters were determined by non-linear regression analysis using Michaelis–Menten equation and Lineweaver–Burk double reciprocal plot and data points were expressed as the mean ± S.D., K_m and V_{max} values and the 95% confidence interval for the intrinsic clearance. Data were analyzed using GraphPad Prism 5 (GraphPad Software, La Jolla, CA, USA) and SAS statistical software (Version 9.4 of the SAS System for Windows, Copyright©, SAS Institute Inc., Cary, NC, USA).

3. Results

3.1. Animal Model

Although no animal model exactly reflects human T2D, some have similar features. Human T2D is a heterogeneous disorder with a complex interplay between genetic, epigenetic and environmental factors. On one hand, diabetic animal models including chemically-induced or surgically-provoked develop hyperglycemia primarily by cytotoxic actions on beta cells rather than through insulin resistance. On the other hand, transgenic/knockout model are more useful to investigate the role of a specific candidate gene unlike heterogeneity as seen in humans. Moreover, the observed diabetes conditions are less stable; chemicals can produce toxic actions and development of digestive problems can be observed which could also affect CYP450 activities. Consequently, a validated nutritionally (high-fat diet; HFD) obese mouse model has been selected to characterize the effects of obesity-induced diabetes on CYP450 activities [51].

Weight, glycemia and insulinemia measured at week 8 were as follow; 29.2 ± 1.1 g, 9.7 ± 0.3 mmol/L and 1.37 ± 0.35 ng/mL in the chow-fed control group (n = 12); 36.4 ± 0.9 g, 9.4 ± 0.5 mmol/L and 2.59 ± 0.44 ng/mL for the LDR group (n = 12) and 43.1 ± 0.6 g, 10.5 ± 0.4 mmol/L and 6.82 ± 1.32 ng/mL, for the HDR group (n = 16), respectively. Weight, glycemia and insulinemia parameters were significantly higher for HFD groups compared to the control group ($p < 0.05$). Five mice were considered as extreme responders (outliers) since their weight was over 45.0 g and were excluded from our analysis.

3.2. Effects of HFD on cyp450 mRNA Expression Levels

3.2.1. General Pattern of cyp450 Expression

The relative expression of total cyp450 mRNA levels for 15 cyp450 isoforms found in hepatic and extra-hepatic tissues are illustrated for chow-fed control group (ND) and HFD groups in Figure 1 (and Table S3). Major differences were observed in the expression pattern of various cyp450s among tissues. On the other hand, the pattern of cyp450 expression was rather similar among the different diet group: hence, the HFD did not change the pattern of relative cyp450 expression levels in a specific organ. The highest relative levels of mRNAs were cyp2e1 in the liver, cyp2j5/cyp2e1 in kidneys, and cyp2d22 in both heart and lung tissues. The cyp2d, cyp2e and cyp2j subfamilies were expressed in all organs tested (i.e., liver, kidneys, heart and lungs). Moreover, high levels of cyp2b10 (representing approximately 20% of cyp450 mRNA expression) were also observed in the lungs.

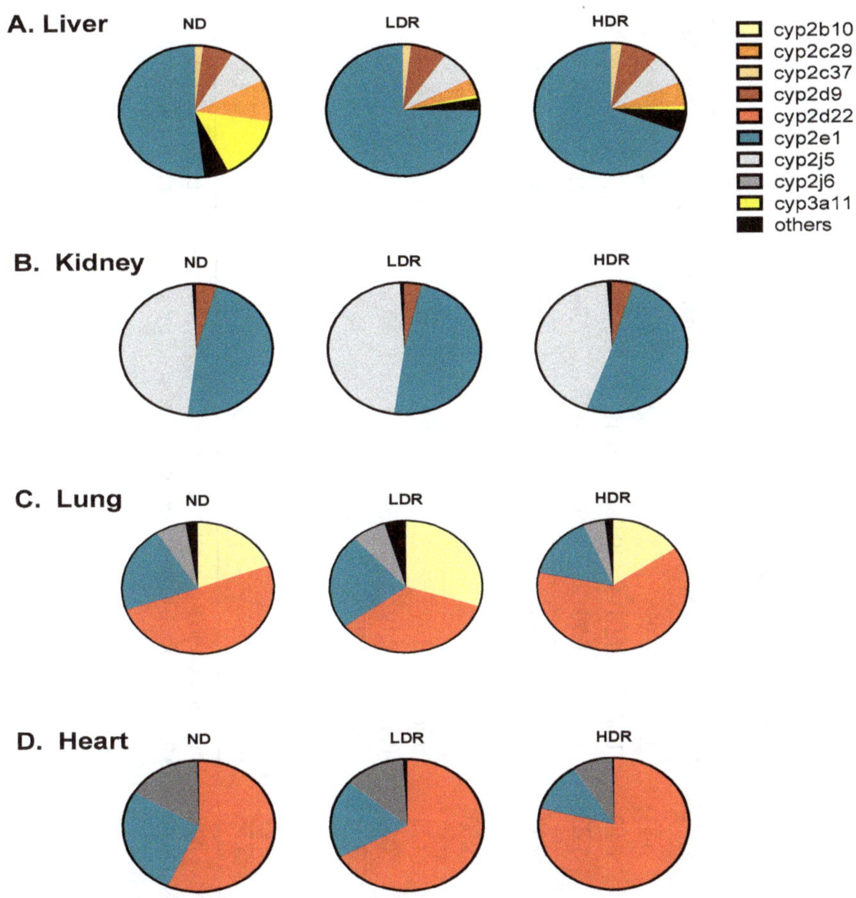

Figure 1. Cyp450 mRNA pie charts. Total mRNA transcripts for each isoenzyme are displayed as expressed in C57BL6 mouse microsomes according to diet group: (**A**) Liver; (**B**) Kidney; (**C**) Lung; and (**D**) Heart. ND, Normal diet; LDR, low-diet responders; and HDR, high-diet responders. Cyp450 mRNA transcript with a relative contribution >1% are illustrated, and "others" have a relative contribution <1%. Others include the following isoforms: Liver, cyp2b10, cyp2b29, cyp2c39, cyp2c40, cyp2d22, cyp2j6, cyp3a13, cyp3a25, and cyp4a10; Kidneys, cyp2b10, cyp2b29, cyp2c29, cyp2c37, cyp2c39, cyp2c40, cyp2d22, cyp2j6, cyp3a11, cyp3a13, cyp3a25, and cyp4a10; and Lungs, cyp2b29, cyp2c29, cyp2c37, cyp2c39, cyp2c40, cyp2d9, cyp2j5, cyp3a11, cyp3a13, cyp3a25, and cyp4a10.

3.2.2. Modulation of cyp450 mRNA Expression by HFD

Table 1 presents the relative mRNA transcripts for each cyp450 isoform found in each individual organ under HFD (LRD and HRD) vs. normal chow-diet (ND). Overall, our results showed that HFD altered the profile of mRNA expression in an isoenzyme-specific manner. Moreover, HFD altered the expression profile of cyp450 mRNAs in a tissue-specific fashion. Our major findings were: (1) mRNA levels of cyp3a11 were significantly decreased (approximately 14-fold) in the liver of both HFD groups (LRD and HRD) compared to ND ($p < 0.001$); (2) in contrast, a two-fold increase of hepatic mRNA levels of cyp2b9 ($p < 0.001$), cyp2c39 ($p < 0.01$) and cyp4a10 ($p < 0.05$) were observed in HDR compared to ND; and (3) cyp2b10 ($p < 0.01$) was also increased by two folds in the lungs.

Table 1. Relative mRNA transcripts for each cyp isoform in C57B/6 mice microsomes according to diet group.

Tissue	Diet	cyp2b9	cyp2b10	cyp2c29	cyp2c37	cyp2c39	cyp2c40	cyp2d9	cyp2d22	cyp2e1	cyp2j5	cyp2j6	cyp3a11	cyp3a13	cyp3a25	cyp4a10
Liver	ND	0.01	0.02	0.49	1.31	0.01	0.44	0.55	0.53	0.56	0.98	1.08	0.58	2.40	0.44	1.25
	LDR	4.89 *	NQ	0.25 *	1.77	0.01	0.20	0.81	0.59	1.02	1.05	0.88	0.04 ‡	3.07	0.17	1.22
	HDR	8.51 ‡	0.03	0.30	2.15	0.02 **	0.37	0.71	1.03	0.79	0.90	1.09	0.04 ‡	2.96	0.21	3.72
Kidney	ND	ND	0.54	2.35	ND	ND	8.62	1.65	1.32	1.28	4.89	4.56	1.41	1.37	2.00	1.42
	LDR	ND	0.46	3.08	ND	ND	3.08	1.35	1.38	1.29	4.68	4.62	0.57	2.12	1.79	1.13
	HDR	ND	0.42	1.59	ND	ND	5.92	1.65	1.50	1.29	4.18	4.03	0.72	2.41	0.95	2.43
Heart	ND	ND	1.21	0.26	ND	ND	ND	0.05	3.24	0.96	0.09	2.19	ND	NQ	ND	1.09
	LDR	ND	2.16	0.49	ND	ND	ND	0.07	3.40	0.62	0.19	1.85	ND	NQ	ND	2.15
	HDR	ND	1.68	0.30	ND	ND	ND	0.07	5.03	0.51 *	0.19	1.67	ND	NQ	NQ	1.47
Lung	ND	ND	0.73	1.11	ND	ND	ND	0.07	2.06	0.21	0.13	1.20	ND	3.26	0.06	3.28
	LDR	ND	1.66 ‡	2.96	ND	ND	ND	0.08	2.05	0.33 **	0.47	1.88	ND	8.15 **	0.07	9.90 *
	HDR	ND	1.17 **	1.00	ND	ND	ND	ND	5.76	0.32 *	0.83	1.69	ND	5.39	0.11	3.43

Results are expressed as mean N-fold differences in cyp gene relative to the average expression of housekeeping genes and a calibrator ($2^{-\Delta\Delta Ct\ sample}$). ND, Normal diet; LDR, low-diet responders; and HDR, high-diet responders. NQ = Not Quantifiable ($35 < Ct < 38$), ND = Not Detectable ($Ct > 38$). Each experiment was performed three times and in triplicates. One-way ANOVA was performed with Dunnett post-hoc test. LDR or HDR versus ND; * $p < 0.05$, ** $p < 0.01$, ‡ $p < 0.001$.

3.3. Modulation of cyp450 Hepatic Activities by DIO Mouse as a Model of T2D

3.3.1. Hepatic Activities

As shown in Figure 2 (Table 2), HFD induced variations in hepatic cyp450 activities in an isoform-dependent manner. A significant decrease in midazolam metabolism, a marker of cyp3a subfamily, was observed following HFD treatment; the intrinsic clearance of 1-hydroxymidazolam was reduced in LDR and HDR (23 and 40 µL/min/mg prot) groups compared to ND (107 µL/min/mg prot) ($p < 0.001$) (Table S4). This was mostly explained by a decrease in V_{max}; formation of 1-hydroxymidazolam decreased from 0.32 (ND) to 0.06 nmol/mg protein/min (LDR and HDR, $p < 0.001$) (Table 2). HFD treatment was also associated with a diminished hepatic activity of cyp2c subfamilies compared to ND group. The intrinsic clearance of tolbutamide (used as a probe of CYP2C9 in human) was significantly reduced from 0.80 to 0.54 and 0.57 µL/min/mg prot in ND, LDR and HDR groups, respectively ($p < 0.05$) (Table S4). Similarly, HFD affected also the repaglinide hydroxylation (CL_{int} to M1-hydroxyrepaglinide) from 10.6 µL/min/mg prot in ND compared to 1.0–1.4 µL/min/mg prot in HFD groups) (Table S4). Cyp2b activity as measured by bupropion hydroxylation tended to be slightly decreased in HDR group (CL_{int} in HDR vs. ND reduced by 22%). In contrast, no significant effect was observed on the hepatic hydroxylation of bufuralol (cyp2d), dodecanoic acid (cyp4a), chlorzoxazone (cyp2e1) and ebastine (cyp2j) as demonstrated by comparable pharmacokinetics values (Table 2).

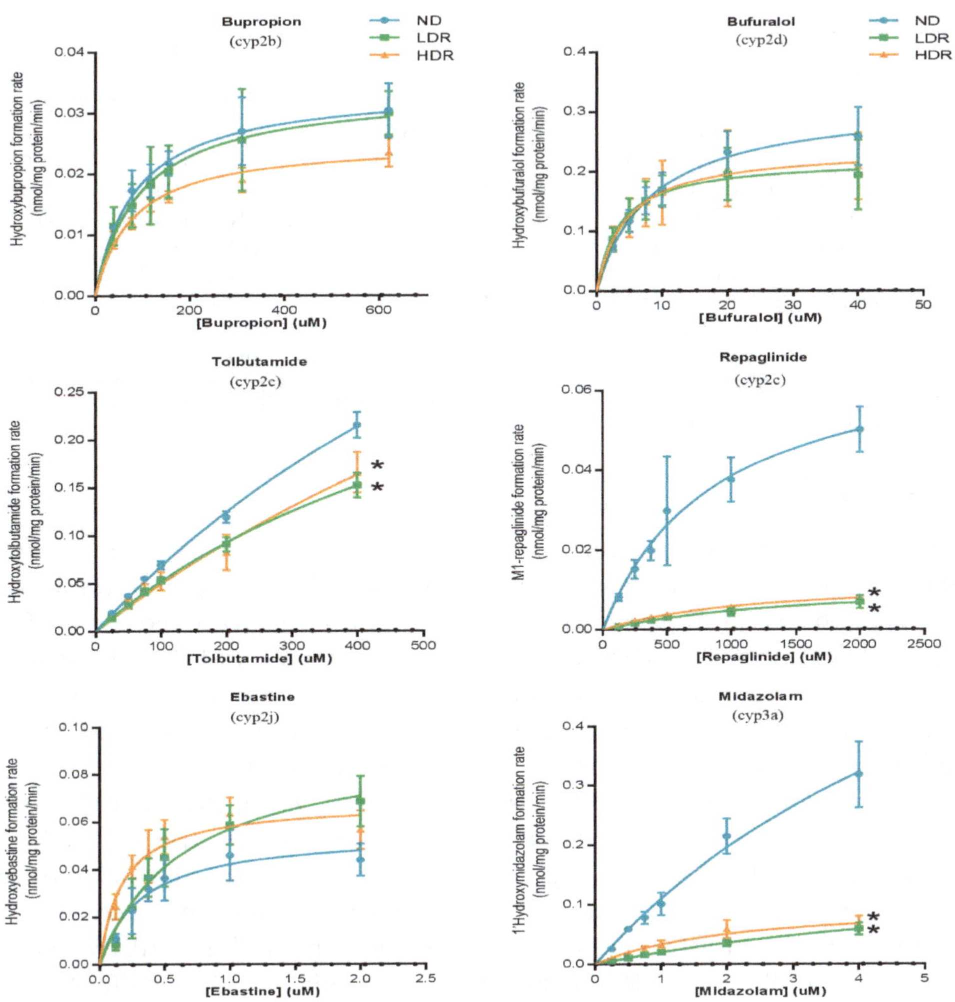

Figure 2. *Cont.*

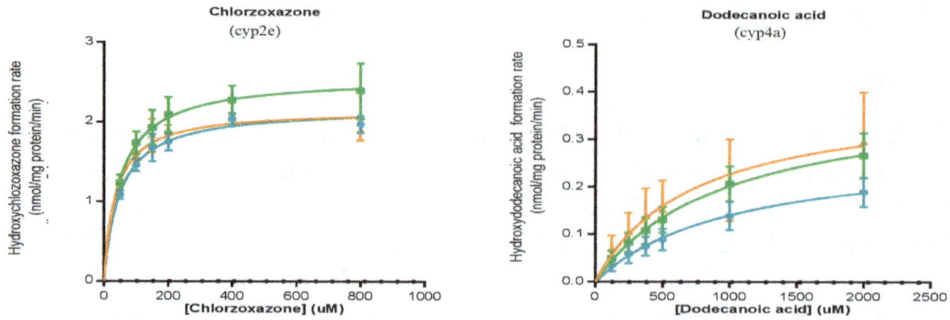

Figure 2. Hepatic cyp450 activities of cyp2b (bupropion), cyp2c (tolbutamide and repaglinide), cyp2d (bufuralol), cyp2e (chlorzoxazone), cyp2j (ebastine), cyp3a (midazolam) and cyp4a (dodecanoic acid) in C57BL6 mice fed a normal diet (ND) or a HFD (LDR, low-diet responders; and HDR, high-diet responders after an eight-week period of treatment). Data were expressed as the mean ± S.D. LDR or HDR vs. ND; * $p < 0.05$. N/F; activity not found, N/A; Not Available (in vitro incubation could not be determined) and dotted line represents the limit of quantification.

Table 2. Hepatic microsome activities for cyp2b (bupropion), cyp2c (tolbutamide and repaglinide), cyp2d (bufuralol), cyp2e (chlorzoxazone), cyp2j (ebastine), cyp3a (midazolam) and cyp4a (dodecanoic acid) in C57BL6 mice fed a normal diet (ND) or a HFD (LDR, low-diet responders; and HDR, high-diet responders after an eight-week period).

Liver	ND	LDR	HDR
	(nmol/mg protein/min)		
Bupropion → Hydroxybupropion	0.030 ± 0.004	0.030 ± 0.004	0.023 ± 0.002 **
Tolbutamide → Hydroxytolbutamide	0.22 ± 0.01	0.15 ± 0.01 ‡	0.17 ± 0.02 ‡
Repaglinide → M1-repaglinide	0.050 ± 0.006	0.007 ± 0.002 ‡	0.0081 ± 0.0003 ‡
Repaglinide → Hydroxyrepaglinide	0.0020 ± 0.0001	0.0010 ± 0.0002 ‡	0.0013 ± 0.0004 **
Bufuralol → Hydroxybufuralol	0.26 ± 0.05	0.19 ± 0.06	0.21 ± 0.06
Chlorzoxazone → Hydroxychlorzoxazone	2.0 ± 0.1	2.4 ± 0.3 **	1.9 ± 0.1
Ebastine → Hydroxyebastine and carebastine	0.044 ± 0.007	0.07 ± 0.01 ‡	0.057 ± 0.008 *
Midazolam → 1′-hydroxymidazolam	0.32 ± 0.06	0.06 ± 0.01 ‡	0.06 ± 0.01 ‡
Dodecanoic acid → 12-hydroxydecanoic acid	0.19 ± 0.03	0.27 ± 0.05	0.3 ± 0.1 *

Cyp450 activities are reported as the rate of metabolite formation in nmol/mg protein/min ± SD (* $p < 0.05$, ** $p < 0.01$, ‡ $p < 0.001$ compared to ND).

3.3.2. Extra-Hepatic Activities

Figure 3 (Table 3) illustrates the effects of diabetes induced by HFD on the formation rate of cyp450 probe metabolites measured in extra-hepatic tissues. A tissue-dependent modulation of cyp450 activities by HFD was observed. In the kidneys, HFD treatment produced a significant decrease in cyp3a activity; formation rate of 1-hydroxymidazolam was three- and five-times lower in LDR and HDR groups, respectively, compared to ND group ($p < 0.001$) (Table 3(A)). In contrast, the cyp3a activity measured in the lung was not affected by the HFD indicating a tissue-dependent modulation of cyp450 by HFD. No cyp3a activity was detectable in mouse hearts.

Our data showed that the formation of hydroxybupropion was approximately 20–50-times greater in the lungs compared to the liver and kidneys (regardless of the diet groups, $p < 0.0001$) (Table 3(B)). Renal and lung microsomes displayed a slight decrease in the hydroxylation of bupropion in HDR group vs. control diet group ($p < 0.01$) (Figure 3). Although the magnitude of activity was low, a similar observation was made for the hydroxylation of bupropion in the heart (0.150 vs. 0.037 and 0.025 pmol/mg protein/min in ND vs. LDR and HDR, respectively, $p < 0.001$) (Table 3(C)). In addition, ebastine (cyp2j) and dodecanoic acid (cyp4a) metabolisms were reduced by HFD, particularly in HDR, in renal and lung tissues. Ebastine hydroxylation in heart microsomes was not affected by HFD, whereas cyp4a activity could not be detected. In contrast, our results showed that DIO mouse were associated with an increase in tolbutamide (~20–50%) and bufuralol (~90–110%) metabolic activities in kidneys, while in lung microsomes, the hydroxylation of tolbutamide and bufuralol tended to decrease ($p < 0.01$ and $p < 0.001$, respectively, in HDR group). Overall, cyp450 activities tended to be reduced in HFD group with greater effects being observed in HDR.

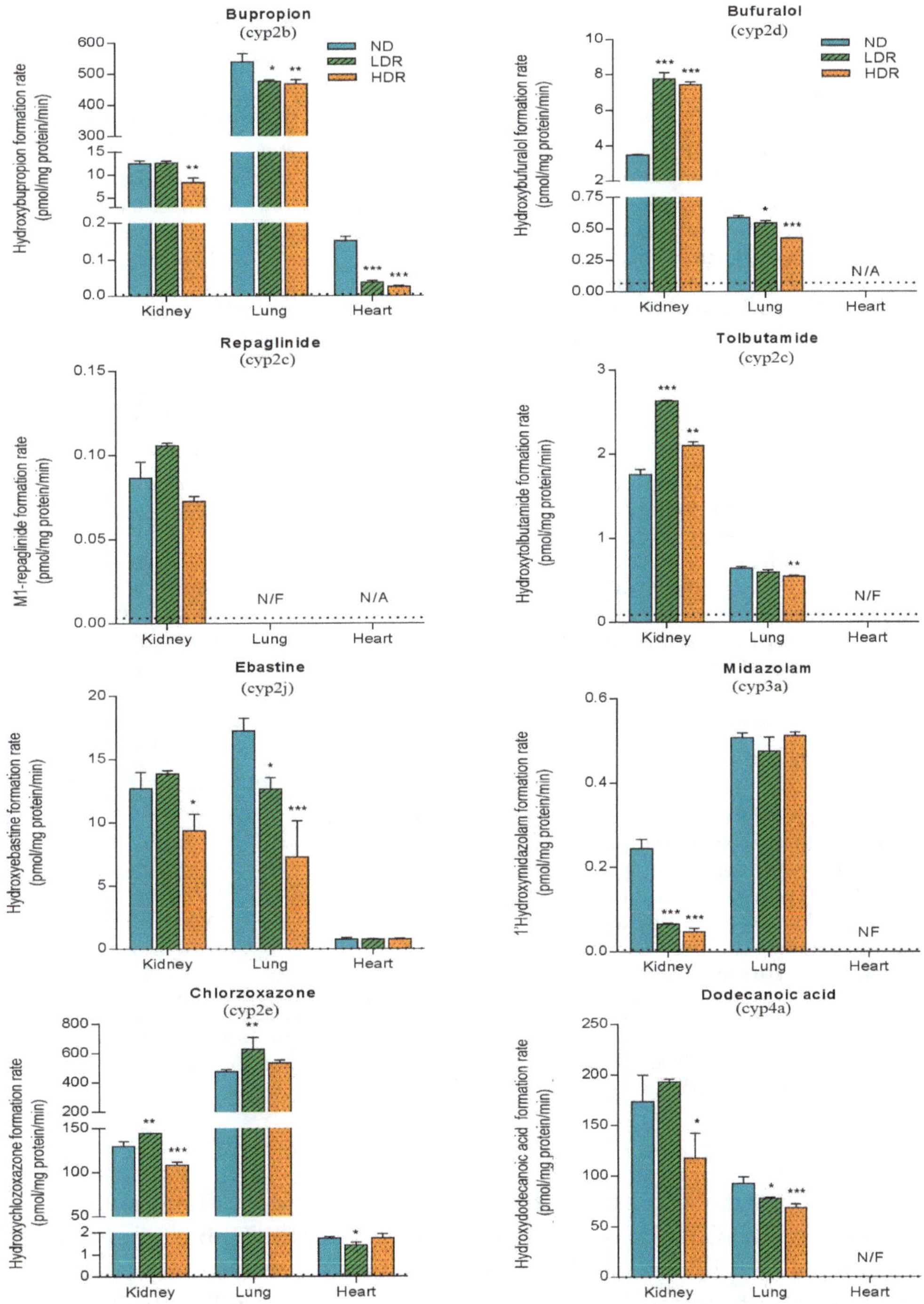

Figure 3. Extrahepatic cyp450 microsomal activities for cyp2b (bupropion), cyp2c (tolbutamide and repaglinide), cyp2d (bufuralol), cyp2e (chlorzoxazone), cyp2j (ebastine), cyp3a (midazolam) and cyp4a (dodecanoic acid) measured in the kidneys, lungs and heart in C57BL6 mice fed a normal diet (ND) or a HFD (LDR, low-diet responders; and HDR, high-diet responders after an eight-week period). Bars and error bars represent the mean ± SD, respectively. LDR or HDR vs. ND; * $p < 0.05$, ** $p < 0.01$, *** $p < 0.001$. N/F; activity not found, N/A; Not Available (in vitro incubation could not be determined) and dotted line represents the limit of quantification.

Table 3. Extra-hepatic microsome activities for cyp2b (bupropion), cyp2c (tolbutamide and repaglinide), cyp2d (bufuralol), cyp2e (chlorzoxazone), cyp2j (ebastine), cyp3a (midazolam) and cyp4a (dodecanoic acid) in C57BL6 mice fed a normal diet (ND) or a HFD (LDR, low-diet responders; and HDR, high-diet responders after an eight-week period): (**A**) renal microsomes; (**B**) lung microsomes; and (**C**) heart microsomes.

(A)

Kidney	ND	LDR	HDR
	(pmol/mg protein/min)		
Bupropion → Hydroxybupropion	12.5 ± 0.6	12.6 ± 0.4	8 ± 1 **
Tolbutamide → Hydroxytolbutamide	1.76 ± 0.06	2.63 ± 0.01 ‡	2.10 ± 0.04 **
Repaglinide → M1-repaglinide	0.09 ± 0.01	0.105 ± 0.002	0.073 ± 0.003
Bufuralol → Hydroxybufuralol	3.50 ± 0.03	7.7 ± 0.4 ‡	7.4 ± 0.2 ‡
Chlorzoxazone → Hydroxychlorzoxazone	130 ± 6	144.6 ± 0.2 **	108 ± 3 **
Ebastine → Hydroxyebastine and carebastine	13 ± 1	13.9 ± 0.3	9 ± 1 *
Midazolam → 1′-hydroxymidazolam	0.24 ± 0.02	0.065 ± 0.002 ‡	0.047 ± 0.008 ‡
Dodecanoic acid → 12-hydroxydecanoic acid	173 ± 27	193 ± 3	118 ± 24 *

(B)

Lung	ND	LDR	HDR
	(pmol/mg protein/min)		
Bupropion → Hydroxybupropion	538 ± 26	476 ± 4 *	467 ± 14 **
Tolbutamide → Hydroxytolbutamide	0.64 ± 0.02	0.59 ± 0.03	0.54 ± 0.01 **
Repaglinide → M1-repaglinide	N/F	N/F	N/F
Bufuralol → Hydroxybufuralol	0.59 ± 0.02	0.55 ± 0.02 *	0.425 ± 0.001 ‡
Chlorzoxazone → Hydroxychlorzoxazone	477 ± 16	629 ± 79 **	535 ± 19
Ebastine → Hydroxyebastine and carebastine	17 ± 1	12.6 ± 0.9 *	7 ± 3 ‡
Midazolam → 1′-hydroxymidazolam	0.51 ± 0.01	0.47 ± 0.04	0.51 ± 0.01
Dodecanoic acid → 12-hydroxydecanoic acid	93 ± 6	78 ± 1 *	68 ± 4 ‡

(C)

Heart	ND	LDR	HDR
	(pmol/mg protein/min)		
Bupropion → Hydroxybupropion	0.15 ± 0.01	0.037 ± 0.004 ‡	0.025 ± 0.003 ‡
Tolbutamide → Hydroxytolbutamide	N/F	N/F	N/F
Repaglinide → M1-repaglinide	N/A	N/A	N/A
Bufuralol → Hydroxybufuralol	N/A	N/A	N/A
Chlorzoxazone → Hydroxychlorzoxazone	1.7 ± 0.1	1.2 ± 0.1 *	1.7 ± 0.2
Ebastine → Hydroxyebastine and carebastine	0.8 ± 0.1	0.76 ± 0.06	0.78 ± 0.06
Midazolam → 1′-hydroxymidazolam	N/F	N/F	N/F
Dodecanoic acid → 12-hydroxydecanoic acid	N/F	N/F	N/F

Cyp450 activities determined at 3 km are reported as the rate of metabolite formation in pmol/mg prot/min ± SD (* $p < 0.05$, ** $p < 0.01$ and ‡ $p < 0.001$ compared to ND). N/F, activity not found; N/A, Not Available (in vitro incubation could not be determined).

4. Discussion

This study demonstrated that expression and activities of major cyp450s involved in the metabolism of drugs were modulated in DIO C57BL6 mice used as a model of T2D (Table S5). First, we demonstrated that cyp3a expression and activities were decreased by HFD. Second, cyp2c activities were reduced in all organs tested (except for tolbutamide in the kidneys). Finally, cyp2b activity, largely expressed in the lungs, was also decreased by HFD.

C57BL/6 mice were divided into three groups: ND, LDR and HDR. LDR were less obese and developed intermediate severity of insulin resistance, while HDR were more obese and developed severe insulin resistance. The extent of changes in cyp450 activities by HFD tended to be gradually decreased in LDR compared to HDR and some effects being only observed in HDR group. This observation suggests that modulation of some cyp450 activities happens at early stage of pre-diabetes and similar pathways of regulation involved in pre-diabetes development can also intervene on cyp450 activities in an isoform-dependent manner.

Obesity and diabetes have been shown to alter the expression and activity of hepatic CYP450s [14,28,29,35–38,40–42,55–57]. Clinical studies and animal experiments report mostly on hepatic CYP3A since it is the most important isoenzyme involved in the metabolism of prescribed drugs [58,59]. In humans, a significant decrease in CYP3A activity has been reported in diabetic human liver microsomes compared to healthy subjects [56], while a significant increase in CYP2E1 activity has been reported in obese T2D human liver microsomes [33]. In our study, we observed a significant decrease in hepatic cyp3a mRNA expression levels in HFD groups compared to normal diet group. Similarly, decreased levels of cyp3a11 mRNA expression have been reported in DIO mice [38,59,60]. Preliminary results from our clinical study using oral CYP450 probe cocktail demonstrate that oral clearance of midazolam was significantly reduced in subjects with T2D compared to subjects without T2D [61]. Our results on RNA transcripts are also consistent with phenotypic findings showing that cyp3a activity determined via hydroxylation of midazolam was significantly reduced in the two HFD groups compared to control group. In agreement with our finding, CYP3A activity has been reported to be also decreased in Zucker diabetic fatty (ZDF) rats using midazolam and testosterone as probes [40].

There are no or very limited data pertaining to the effects of T2D on cyp2c and cyp2b families. We observed that cyp2c and cyp2b subfamilies mRNA expression levels were not changed in the liver by HFD compared to normal group, except for cyp2b9 which was increased in HFD groups. Our results are in agreement with those reported by Yoshinari et al. and Guo et al. who demonstrated unchanged relative mRNA levels of cyp2c and cyp2b subfamilies in the liver [59,60]. In contrast, it has been reported a decrease of cyp2b10 mRNA levels in CD1 mice fed with HFD [38]. However, the relative hepatic levels of cyp2b10 mRNA measured in our study were very low or below the limit of quantification yielding a comparison analysis unreliable. In addition, our results showed that hepatic cyp2c metabolic activities, using repaglinide and tolbutamide as markers, were significantly decreased in HFD groups. Kim et al. reported that CYP2C catalytic activity determined with diclofenac was decreased in chemically induced diabetes in rats [62]. This finding, in agreement with our study, suggest that CYP2C activities are impaired, thereby lower metabolic clearance can be anticipated for drugs metabolized by CYP2Cs, particularly CYP2C8 or CYP2C9, under conditions associated with pre-diabetes or diabetes.

Our results indicate that cyp2e1 mRNA expression levels and activity remained unchanged and comparable among all groups (HFD and ND). In the same way, expression levels of cyp2e1 mRNA were reported to be unchanged in DIO mice [38,59]. In addition, activity of cyp2e1 was also unaffected in DIO and db/db mice [37,38], but increased activity was shown in ZDF [42]. No alteration in hepatic levels of cyp2e1 was found in streptozocin-induced diabetic mice [41]. These differences in cyp2e1 activity modulation could be function of the animal model of diabetes used and the stage of the disease.

Our data demonstrated a tissue-specific modulation of cyp2b activities by HFD. Indeed, no significant difference was observed for the hydroxylation of bupropion in liver microsomes. However, bupropion hydroxylation was significantly decreased in HFD groups, particularly in the lungs, the heart and kidneys (HDR group only).

To our knowledge, no study has been conducted to assess the impact of HFD induced obesity as a model of early diabetes stage in humans on CYP450s expression or activity in extrahepatic tissues. Although the magnitude of metabolic capacity and significance in total body clearance of extrahepatic CYP450s metabolism are much lower in comparison to hepatic CYP450s, extrahepatic CYP450s metabolism may affect the local exposure to xenobiotics and thus, influence their pharmacological and toxicological effects. For instance, renal cyp450 metabolites of arachidonic acid, 20-HETE and EET, play an important role in the control of blood pressure and the development of acute kidney injury [63]. In fact, arachidonic acid is metabolized by CYP4A and CYP4F families to 20-HETE (vasoconstrictor) and by CYP2C and CYP2J families to EETs (vasodilator). Our results showed a significant decrease in renal activity of cyp4a and cyp2j in the HDR group using dodecanoic acid and ebastine hydroxylation as marker, respectively. This finding indicates that diabetes could influence homeostasis by affecting local biotransformation of endogenous compounds. In high fat diet induced hypertension rats, CYP2C and CYP4A activities were found to be decreased [64]. The discrepancy observed for CYP2C activity can be explained by using different substrate markers (arachidonic acid being not specific for CYP2C but, also a CYP2J substrate).

Little is known about the effects of obesity and diabetes on CYP450 catalytic activities in the lungs, in both humans and animals. Our data showed extensive metabolic activities in lung microsomes for midazolam, bupropion, ebastine and chlorzoxazone corresponding to cyp3a, cyp2b, cyp2j and cyp2e1, respectively. In lung microsomes, HFD was associated with modulation of cyp450 catalytic activity for certain isoforms independently of patterns observed in the liver or in the kidneys. These findings support the concept that CYP450s expressed in the lungs may contribute to drug metabolism for drugs administered intravenously or locally as well as contribute to the first pass metabolism.

In conclusion, the major finding of this study was that HFD affects CYP450 expression and activities in an isoform- and tissue-dependent fashion. Our results clearly indicate that cyp3a and cyp2c metabolic activities were reduced in DIO-T2D mice (Table S5). In humans, these two CYP450 isoenzymes are involved in the metabolism of 80% of medications prescribed in clinical settings. We speculate that modulation of hepatic CYP450s by T2D diabetes may alter drug pharmacokinetics leading to intersubject variability in drug response. In addition, modulation in CYP450s expressed in extra-hepatic organs can cause variations in tissue concentrations of drugs or endogenous compounds leading to impaired pharmacological action of drugs as well as disruption of homeostasis. Therefore, variation in hepatic and extra-hepatic CYP450s makes patients with pre-diabetes and obesity more prone to adverse drug effect, toxicity or inefficacy (e.g., for prodrugs).

Acknowledgments: Sarah Maximos was the recipient of a studentship from the Faculté des études supérieures et post-doctorales de l'Université de Montréal and Sophie Gravel was the recipient of a studentship from the Fonds de la Recherche du Québec en Santé (FRQS). This work was supported by Canadian Institutes of Health Research (CIHR) under the grant #299309. Veronique Michaud is the recipient of a research scholarship from FRQS in partnership with the Institut national d'excellence en santé et en services sociaux (INESSS). We thank Thierry Alquier and the CRCHUM Animal core facility for technical support and the experimental protocol for the DIO mice model. We thank Fleur Gaudette and the CRCHUM pharmacokinetics Core Facility for technical support and analytical method development. We are also grateful to Francois Belanger for his excellent technical assistance providing support in the qPCR analysis.

Author Contributions: Veronique Michaud and Jacques Turgeon conceived and designed the experiments; Sarah Maximos, Michel Chamoun (mRNA experiments) and Sophie Gravel (training for microsome and in vitro incubation protocols) performed the experiments; Sarah Maximos, Veronique Michaud and Jacques Turgeon analyzed and interpreted the data; and Sarah Maximos, Veronique Michaud and Jacques Turgeon wrote the paper.

Abbreviations

DIO	diet-induced obesity
DMSO	dimethyl sulfoxide
G6P	glucose-6-phosphate
G6PD	glucose-6-phosphate dehydrogenase
HDR	high-diet responders
HFD	high-fat diet
IFN-γ	interferon-γ
IL-1β	interleukin-1β
IL-6	interleukin-6
LC-MS/MS	liquid chromatography–tandem mass spectrometry
LDR	low-diet responders
NADP	Nicotinamide-Adenine Dinucleotide Phosphate
P450	cytochrome P450
PMSF	phenylmethanesulfonyl

RT-qPCR	real time quantitative polymerase chain reaction
T2D	type 2 diabetes
VHDR	very high-diet responders

References

1. Whiting, D.R.; Guariguata, L.; Weil, C.; Shaw, J. IDF diabetes atlas: Global estimates of the prevalence of diabetes for 2011 and 2030. *Diabetes Res. Clin. Pract.* **2011**, *94*, 311–321. [CrossRef] [PubMed]
2. Centers for Disease Control and Prevention. *National Diabetes Statistics Report: Estimates of Diabetes and Its Burden in the United States, 2014*; U.S. Department of Health and Human Services: Atlanta, GA, USA, 2014.
3. American Diabetes Association. Standards of medical care in diabetes—2015: summary of revisions. *Diabetes Care* **2015**, *38* (Suppl. 1), S4.
4. Pacanowski, M.A.; Hopley, C.W.; Aquilante, C.L. Interindividual variability in oral antidiabetic drug disposition and response: The role of drug transporter polymorphisms. *Expert Opin. Drug Metab. Toxicol.* **2008**, *4*, 529–544. [CrossRef] [PubMed]
5. Nathan, D.M.; Buse, J.B.; Davidson, M.B.; Ferrannini, E.; Holman, R.R.; Sherwin, R.; Zinman, B. Medical management of hyperglycaemia in type 2 diabetes mellitus: A consensus algorithm for the initiation and adjustment of therapy: A consensus statement from the American Diabetes Association and the European Association for the Study of Diabetes. *Diabetologia* **2009**, *52*, 17–30. [CrossRef] [PubMed]
6. Morrish, G.A.; Pai, M.P.; Green, B. The effects of obesity on drug pharmacokinetics in humans. *Expert Opin. Drug Metab. Toxicol.* **2011**, *7*, 697–706. [CrossRef] [PubMed]
7. Cheymol, G. Effects of obesity on pharmacokinetics implications for drug therapy. *Clin. Pharmacokinet.* **2000**, *39*, 215–231. [CrossRef] [PubMed]
8. Akhlaghi, F.; Dostalek, M.; Falck, P.; Mendonza, A.E.; Amundsen, R.; Gohh, R.Y.; Asberg, A. The concentration of cyclosporine metabolites is significantly lower in kidney transplant recipients with diabetes mellitus. *Ther. Drug Monit.* **2012**, *34*, 38–45. [CrossRef] [PubMed]
9. Marques, M.P.; Coelho, E.B.; Dos Santos, N.A.; Geleilete, T.J.; Lanchote, V.L. Dynamic and kinetic disposition of nisoldipine enantiomers in hypertensive patients presenting with type-2 diabetes mellitus. *Eur. J. Clin. Pharmacol.* **2002**, *58*, 607–614. [CrossRef] [PubMed]
10. Kazui, M.; Nishiya, Y.; Ishizuka, T.; Hagihara, K.; Farid, N.A.; Okazaki, O.; Ikeda, T.; Kurihara, A. Identification of the human cytochrome P450 enzymes involved in the two oxidative steps in the bioactivation of clopidogrel to its pharmacologically active metabolite. *Drug Metab. Dispos.* **2010**, *38*, 92–99. [CrossRef] [PubMed]
11. Lenzini, P.; Wadelius, M.; Kimmel, S.; Anderson, J.L.; Jorgensen, A.L.; Pirmohamed, M.; Caldwell, M.D.; Limdi, N.; Burmester, J.K.; Dowd, M.B.; et al. Integration of genetic, clinical, and INR data to refine warfarin dosing. *Clin. Pharmacol. Ther.* **2010**, *87*, 572–578. [CrossRef] [PubMed]
12. Hall, H.M.; Banerjee, S.; McGuire, D.K. Variability of clopidogrel response in patients with type 2 diabetes mellitus. *Diabetes Vasc. Dis. Res.* **2011**, *8*, 245–253. [CrossRef] [PubMed]
13. Jacobson, P.A.; Oetting, W.S.; Brearley, A.M.; Leduc, R.; Guan, W.; Schladt, D.; Matas, A.J.; Lamba, V.; Julian, B.A.; Mannon, R.B.; et al. Novel polymorphisms associated with tacrolimus trough concentrations: Results from a multicenter kidney transplant consortium. *Transplantation* **2011**, *91*, 300–308. [CrossRef] [PubMed]
14. Dostalek, M.; Sam, W.J.; Paryani, K.R.; Macwan, J.S.; Gohh, R.Y.; Akhlaghi, F. Diabetes mellitus reduces the clearance of atorvastatin lactone: Results of a population pharmacokinetic analysis in renal transplant recipients and in vitro studies using human liver microsomes. *Clin. Pharmacokinet.* **2012**, *51*, 591–606. [CrossRef] [PubMed]
15. Manolopoulos, V.G.; Ragia, G.; Tavridou, A. Pharmacogenomics of oral antidiabetic medications: Current data and pharmacoepigenomic perspective. *Pharmacogenomics* **2011**, *12*, 1161–1191. [CrossRef] [PubMed]
16. Manolopoulos, V.G. Pharmacogenomics and adverse drug reactions in diagnostic and clinical practice. *Clin. Chem. Lab. Med.* **2007**, *45*, 801–814. [CrossRef] [PubMed]
17. Holstein, A.; Beil, W. Oral antidiabetic drug metabolism: Pharmacogenomics and drug interactions. *Expert Opin. Drug Metab. Toxicol.* **2009**, *5*, 225–241. [CrossRef] [PubMed]

18. Bano, G. Glucose homeostasis, obesity and diabetes. *Best Pract. Res. Clin. Obstet. Gynaecol.* **2013**, *27*, 715–726. [CrossRef] [PubMed]
19. Paragh, G.; Seres, I.; Harangi, M.; Fulop, P. Dynamic interplay between metabolic syndrome and immunity. *Adv. Exp. Med. Biol.* **2014**, *824*, 171–190. [PubMed]
20. Dandona, P.; Aljada, A.; Bandyopadhyay, A. Inflammation: The link between insulin resistance, obesity and diabetes. *Trends Immunol.* **2004**, *25*, 4–7. [CrossRef] [PubMed]
21. Morgan, E.T. Impact of infectious and inflammatory disease on cytochrome P450-mediated drug metabolism and pharmacokinetics. *Clin. Pharmacol. Ther.* **2009**, *85*, 434–438. [CrossRef] [PubMed]
22. Rendic, S.; Guengerich, F.P. Update information on drug metabolism systems—2009, part II: Summary of information on the effects of diseases and environmental factors on human cytochrome P450 (CYP) enzymes and transporters. *Curr. Drug Metab.* **2010**, *11*, 4–84. [CrossRef] [PubMed]
23. Du Souich, P.; Fradette, C. The effect and clinical consequences of hypoxia on cytochrome P450, membrane carrier proteins activity and expression. *Expert Opin. Drug Metab. Toxicol.* **2011**, *7*, 1083–1100. [CrossRef] [PubMed]
24. Hameed, I.; Masoodi, S.R.; Mir, S.A.; Nabi, M.; Ghazanfar, K.; Ganai, B.A. Type 2 diabetes mellitus: From a metabolic disorder to an inflammatory condition. *World J. Diabetes* **2015**, *6*, 598–612. [PubMed]
25. Sunman, J.A.; Hawke, R.L.; LeCluyse, E.L.; Kashuba, A.D. Kupffer cell-mediated IL-2 suppression of CYP3A activity in human hepatocytes. *Drug Metab. Dispos.* **2004**, *32*, 359–363. [CrossRef] [PubMed]
26. Donato, M.T.; Guillen, M.I.; Jover, R.; Castell, J.V.; Gomez-Lechon, M.J. Nitric oxide-mediated inhibition of cytochrome P450 by interferon-gamma in human hepatocytes. *J. Pharmacol. Exp. Ther.* **1997**, *281*, 484–490. [PubMed]
27. Jover, R.; Bort, R.; Gomez-Lechon, M.J.; Castell, J.V. Down-regulation of human CYP3A4 by the inflammatory signal interleukin-6: Molecular mechanism and transcription factors involved. *FASEB J. Off. Publ. Fed. Am. Soc. Exp. Biol.* **2002**, *16*, 1799–1801. [CrossRef] [PubMed]
28. Kotlyar, M.; Carson, S.W. Effects of obesity on the cytochrome P450 enzyme system. *Int. J. Clin. Pharmacol. Ther.* **1999**, *37*, 8–19. [PubMed]
29. Cheng, P.Y.; Morgan, E.T. Hepatic cytochrome P450 regulation in disease states. *Curr. Drug Metab.* **2001**, *2*, 165–183. [CrossRef] [PubMed]
30. Wang, M.; Tian, X.; Leung, L.; Wang, J.; Houvig, N.; Xiang, J.; Wan, Z.K.; Saiah, E.; Hahm, S.; Suri, V.; et al. Comparative pharmacokinetics and metabolism studies in lean and diet- induced obese mice: An animal efficacy model for 11beta-hydroxysteroid dehydrogenase type 1 (11beta-HSD1) inhibitors. *Drug Metab. Lett.* **2011**, *5*, 55–63. [CrossRef] [PubMed]
31. O'Shea, D.; Davis, S.N.; Kim, R.B.; Wilkinson, G.R. Effect of fasting and obesity in humans on the 6-hydroxylation of chlorzoxazone: A putative probe of CYP2E1 activity. *Clin. Pharmacol. Ther.* **1994**, *56*, 359–367. [CrossRef] [PubMed]
32. Emery, M.G.; Fisher, J.M.; Chien, J.Y.; Kharasch, E.D.; Dellinger, E.P.; Kowdley, K.V.; Thummel, K.E. CYP2E1 activity before and after weight loss in morbidly obese subjects with nonalcoholic fatty liver disease. *Hepatology* **2003**, *38*, 428–435. [CrossRef] [PubMed]
33. Wang, Z.; Hall, S.D.; Maya, J.F.; Li, L.; Asghar, A.; Gorski, J.C. Diabetes mellitus increases the in vivo activity of cytochrome P450 2E1 in humans. *Br. J. Clin. Pharmacol.* **2003**, *55*, 77–85. [CrossRef] [PubMed]
34. Fisher, C.D.; Lickteig, A.J.; Augustine, L.M.; Ranger-Moore, J.; Jackson, J.P.; Ferguson, S.S.; Cherrington, N.J. Hepatic cytochrome P450 enzyme alterations in humans with progressive stages of nonalcoholic fatty liver disease. *Drug Metab. Dispos.* **2009**, *37*, 2087–2094. [CrossRef] [PubMed]
35. Woolsey, S.J.; Mansell, S.E.; Kim, R.B.; Tirona, R.G.; Beaton, M.D. CYP3A activity and expression in nonalcoholic fatty liver disease. *Drug Metab. Dispos.* **2015**, *43*, 1484–1490. [CrossRef] [PubMed]
36. Kudo, T.; Shimada, T.; Toda, T.; Igeta, S.; Suzuki, W.; Ikarashi, N.; Ochiai, W.; Ito, K.; Aburada, M.; Sugiyama, K. Altered expression of CYP in TSOD mice: A model of type 2 diabetes and obesity. *Xenobiotica* **2009**, *39*, 889–902. [CrossRef] [PubMed]
37. Lam, J.L.; Jiang, Y.; Zhang, T.; Zhang, E.Y.; Smith, B.J. Expression and functional analysis of hepatic cytochromes P450, nuclear receptors, and membrane transporters in 10- and 25-week-old db/db mice. *Drug Metab. Dispos.* **2010**, *38*, 2252–2258. [CrossRef] [PubMed]

38. Ghose, R.; Omoluabi, O.; Gandhi, A.; Shah, P.; Strohacker, K.; Carpenter, K.C.; McFarlin, B.; Guo, T. Role of high-fat diet in regulation of gene expression of drug metabolizing enzymes and transporters. *Life Sci.* **2011**, *89*, 57–64. [CrossRef] [PubMed]
39. Patoine, D.; Petit, M.; Pilote, S.; Picard, F.; Drolet, B.; Simard, C. Modulation of CYP3a expression and activity in mice models of type 1 and type 2 diabetes. *Pharmacol. Res. Perspect.* **2014**, *2*, e00082. [CrossRef] [PubMed]
40. Zhou, X.; Rougee, L.R.; Bedwell, D.W.; Cramer, J.W.; Mohutsky, M.A.; Calvert, N.A.; Moulton, R.D.; Cassidy, K.C.; Yumibe, N.P.; Adams, L.A.; et al. Difference in the pharmacokinetics and hepatic metabolism of antidiabetic drugs in zucker diabetic fatty and sprague-dawley rats. *Drug Metab. Dispos.* **2016**, *44*, 1184–1192. [CrossRef] [PubMed]
41. Sakuma, T.; Honma, R.; Maguchi, S.; Tamaki, H.; Nemoto, N. Different expression of hepatic and renal cytochrome P450s between the streptozotocin-induced diabetic mouse and rat. *Xenobiotica* **2001**, *31*, 223–237. [CrossRef] [PubMed]
42. Khemawoot, P.; Yokogawa, K.; Shimada, T.; Miyamoto, K. Obesity-induced increase of CYP2E1 activity and its effect on disposition kinetics of chlorzoxazone in Zucker rats. *Biochem. Pharmacol.* **2007**, *73*, 155–162. [CrossRef] [PubMed]
43. Oh, S.J.; Choi, J.M.; Yun, K.U.; Oh, J.M.; Kwak, H.C.; Oh, J.G.; Lee, K.S.; Kim, B.H.; Heo, T.H.; Kim, S.K. Hepatic expression of cytochrome P450 in type 2 diabetic Goto-Kakizaki rats. *Chem. Biol. Interact.* **2012**, *195*, 173–179. [CrossRef] [PubMed]
44. Song, B.J.; Matsunaga, T.; Hardwick, J.P.; Park, S.S.; Veech, R.L.; Yang, C.S.; Gelboin, H.V.; Gonzalez, F.J. Stabilization of cytochrome P450j messenger ribonucleic acid in the diabetic rat. *Mol. Endocrinol.* **1987**, *1*, 542–547. [CrossRef] [PubMed]
45. Dong, Z.G.; Hong, J.Y.; Ma, Q.A.; Li, D.C.; Bullock, J.; Gonzalez, F.J.; Park, S.S.; Gelboin, H.V.; Yang, C.S. Mechanism of induction of cytochrome P-450ac (P-450j) in chemically induced and spontaneously diabetic rats. *Arch. Biochem. Biophys.* **1988**, *263*, 29–35. [CrossRef]
46. Yamazoe, Y.; Murayama, N.; Shimada, M.; Yamauchi, K.; Kato, R. Cytochrome P450 in livers of diabetic rats: Regulation by growth hormone and insulin. *Arch. Biochem. Biophys.* **1989**, *268*, 567–575. [CrossRef]
47. Thummel, K.E.; Schenkman, J.B. Effects of testosterone and growth hormone treatment on hepatic microsomal P450 expression in the diabetic rat. *Mol. Pharmacol.* **1990**, *37*, 119–129. [PubMed]
48. Raza, H.; Ahmed, I.; Lakhani, M.S.; Sharma, A.K.; Pallot, D.; Montague, W. Effect of bitter melon (Momordica charantia) fruit juice on the hepatic cytochrome P450-dependent monooxygenases and glutathione S-transferases in streptozotocin-induced diabetic rats. *Biochem. Pharmacol.* **1996**, *52*, 1639–1642. [CrossRef]
49. Li, L.; Zhang, Y. Changes of CYP2E1 activity in diabetic rat model. *Acta Pharm. Sin.* **1998**, *33*, 891–895.
50. Karlgren, M.; Miura, S.; Ingelman-Sundberg, M. Novel extrahepatic cytochrome P450s. *Toxicol. Appl. Pharmacol.* **2005**, *207*, 57–61. [CrossRef] [PubMed]
51. Peyot, M.L.; Pepin, E.; Lamontagne, J.; Latour, M.G.; Zarrouki, B.; Lussier, R.; Pineda, M.; Jetton, T.L.; Madiraju, S.R.; Joly, E.; et al. Beta-cell failure in diet-induced obese mice stratified according to body weight gain: Secretory dysfunction and altered islet lipid metabolism without steatosis or reduced beta-cell mass. *Diabetes* **2010**, *59*, 2178–2187. [CrossRef] [PubMed]
52. Livak, K.J.; Td, S. Analysis of relative gene expression data using real-time quantitative PCR and the 2(-Delta Delta C(T)) Method. *Methods* **2001**, *25*, 402–408. [CrossRef] [PubMed]
53. Schmittgen, T.D.; Livak, K.J. Analyzing real-time PCR data by the comparative C(T) method. *Nat. Protoc.* **2008**, *3*, 1101–1108. [CrossRef] [PubMed]
54. Michaud, V.; Frappier, M.; Dumas, M.C.; Turgeon, J. Metabolic activity and mRNA levels of human cardiac CYP450s involved in drug metabolism. *PLoS ONE* **2010**, *5*, e15666. [CrossRef] [PubMed]
55. Shayeganpour, A.; Korashy, H.; Patel, J.P.; El-Kadi, A.O.; Brocks, D.R. The impact of experimental hyperlipidemia on the distribution and metabolism of amiodarone in rat. *Int. J. Pharm.* **2008**, *361*, 78–86. [CrossRef] [PubMed]
56. Dostalek, M.; Court, M.H.; Yan, B.; Akhlaghi, F. Significantly reduced cytochrome P450 3A4 expression and activity in liver from humans with diabetes mellitus. *Br. J. Pharmacol.* **2011**, *163*, 937–947. [CrossRef] [PubMed]

57. Patoine, D.; Levac, X.; Pilote, S.; Drolet, B.; Simard, C. Decreased CYP3A expression and activity in guinea pig models of diet-induced metabolic syndrome: Is fatty liver infiltration involved? *Drug Metab. Dispos.* **2013**, *41*, 952–957. [CrossRef] [PubMed]
58. Smith, H.S. Opioid Metabolism. *Mayo Clin. Proc.* **2009**, *84*, 613–624. [CrossRef]
59. Yoshinari, K.; Takagi, S.; Yoshimasa, T.; Sugatani, J.; Miwa, M. Hepatic CYP3A expression is attenuated in obese mice fed a high-fat diet. *Pharm. Res.* **2006**, *23*, 1188–1200. [CrossRef] [PubMed]
60. Guo, Y.; Cui, J.Y.; Lu, H.; Klaassen, C.D. Effect of various diets on the expression of phase-I drug-metabolizing enzymes in livers of mice. *Xenobiotica* **2015**, *45*, 586–597. [CrossRef] [PubMed]
61. Gravel, S.; Grangeon, A.; Gaudette, F.; Chiasson, J.-L.; Dallaire, S.; Langelier, H.; Turgeon, J.; Michaud, V. Type 2 Diabetes modulates CYP450 metabolic activities; an important variability factor in drug response. In Proceedings of the ASCPT 2016, San Diego, CA, USA, 8–12 March 2016.
62. Kim, Y.C.; Oh, E.Y.; Kim, S.H.; Lee, M.G. Pharmacokinetics of diclofenac in rat model of diabetes mellitus induced by alloxan or steptozotocin. *Biopharm. Drug Dispos.* **2006**, *27*, 85–92. [CrossRef] [PubMed]
63. Fan, F.; Muroya, Y.; Roman, R.J. Cytochrome P450 eicosanoids in hypertension and renal disease. *Curr. Opin. Nephrol. Hypertens.* **2015**, *24*, 37–46. [CrossRef] [PubMed]
64. Wang, M.H.; Smith, A.; Zhou, Y.; Chang, H.H.; Lin, S.; Zhao, X.; Imig, J.D.; Dorrance, A.M. Downregulation of renal CYP-derived eicosanoid synthesis in rats with diet-induced hypertension. *Hypertension* **2003**, *42*, 594–599. [CrossRef] [PubMed]

6

Pharmacokinetics and Anti-Gastric Ulceration Activity of Oral Administration of Aceclofenac and Esomeprazole in Rats

Tae Hwan Kim [1], Subindra Kazi Thapa [2], Da Young Lee [3], Seung Eun Chung [3], Jun Young Lim [3], Hyeon Myeong Jeong [3], Chang Ho Song [3], Youn-Woong Choi [4], Sang-Min Cho [4], Kyu-Yeol Nam [4], Won-Ho Kang [4], Soyoung Shin [2] and Beom Soo Shin [3,*]

1. College of Pharmacy, Catholic University of Daegu, Gyeongsan, Gyeongbuk 38430, Korea; thkim@cu.ac.kr
2. College of Pharmacy, Wonkwang University, Iksan, Jeonbuk 54538, Korea; thapasubindra@gmail.com (S.K.T.); shins@wku.ac.kr (S.S.)
3. School of Pharmacy, Sungkyunkwan University, Suwon, Gyeonggi 16419, Korea; dayoung717@skku.edu (D.Y.L.); jsehome08@skku.edu (S.E.C.); panacea89@skku.edu (J.Y.L.); wise219143@skku.edu (H.M.J.); sky84312@skku.edu (C.H.S.)
4. Korea United Pharm. Inc., Seoul 06116, Korea; choi0528@kup.co.kr (Y.-W.C.); sweety1723@kup.co.kr (S.-M.C.); kynam@kup.co.kr (K.-Y.N.); kangwonho@kup.co.kr (W.-H.K.)

* Correspondence: bsshin@skku.edu

Abstract: This study examined the effects of esomeprazole on aceclofenac pharmacokinetics and gastrointestinal complications in rats. Aceclofenac alone, or in combination with esomeprazole, was orally administered to male Sprague-Dawley rats. Plasma concentrations of aceclofenac, its major metabolite diclofenac, and esomeprazole were simultaneously determined by a novel liquid chromatography-tandem mass spectrometry method. Gastrointestinal damage was determined by measuring ulcer area and ulcer lesion index of the stomach. Oral administration of aceclofenac induced significant gastric ulceration, which was inhibited by esomeprazole administration. Following concurrent administration of aceclofenac and esomeprazole, overall pharmacokinetic profiles of aceclofenac and metabolic conversion to diclofenac were unaffected by esomeprazole. Aceclofenac metabolism and pharmacokinetics were not subject to significant food effects, whereas bioavailability of esomeprazole decreased in fed compared to fasting conditions. In contrast, the pharmacokinetics of aceclofenac and esomeprazole were significantly altered by different dosing vehicles. These results suggest that co-administration of esomeprazole with aceclofenac may reduce aceclofenac-induced gastrointestinal complications without significant pharmacokinetic interactions. The optimal combination and clinical significance of the benefits of the combination of aceclofenac and esomeprazole need to be further evaluated.

Keywords: aceclofenac; diclofenac; esomeprazole; pharmacokinetics; gastric ulcer

1. Introduction

Aceclofenac is one of the most popular oral nonsteroidal anti-inflammatory drugs (NSAIDs), and has proven effective in the treatment of osteoarthritis [1], rheumatoid arthritis [2], ankylosing spondylitis [3], and pain [4,5]. The absolute oral bioavailability of aceclofenac is 15% in rats [6] due to extensive metabolism. However, metabolism of aceclofenac is species-specific [7]. While aceclofenac is mainly metabolized to 4′-hydroxyaceclofenac in humans, the major metabolite in rats is diclofenac [7]. Aceclofenac and its metabolites exert anti-inflammatory effects by inhibition of prostaglandin E2 (PGE2) production via cyclooxygenases COX-1 and COX-2. Aceclofenac and 4′-hydroxyaceclofenac are selective COX-2 inhibitors with IC50 of 0.77 and 36 μM, respectively. Aceclofenac and 4′-hydroxyaceclofenac have IC50 > 100 μM for COX-1 in human whole blood [8]. In contrast, diclofenac inhibits both COX-1 (IC50 = 0.6 μM) and COX-2 (IC50 = 0.04 μM) [8]. Therefore, although diclofenac is present at lower levels in the plasma following aceclofenac administration in humans, diclofenac may contribute to the pharmacological action of aceclofenac in both humans and rats based on low IC50 values.

In general, selective COX-2 inhibitors exert less adverse effects on the gastrointestinal (GI) tract because COX-1 plays a protective role by stimulating the secretion of mucus and bicarbonate, increasing mucosal blood flow, and promoting epithelial proliferation [9]. Nevertheless, the superior clinical safety of aceclofenac related to GI adverse events is controversial. Aceclofenac was well tolerated, and the incidence of adverse GI events was generally lower than that of other NSAIDs [10]. Several clinical studies have shown that the overall withdrawal rate in aceclofenac recipients was lower than that in patients treated with tenoxicam [11], ketoprofen [2], and diclofenac [12]. Conversely, adverse events associated with aceclofenac use are still observed and include nausea, diarrhea, flatulence, gastritis, constipation, vomiting, and ulcerative stomatitis. No significant differences in GI event rates were reported between aceclofenac and other NSAIDs in individual clinical trials [1–3,11–19]. The number of patients with fecal blood loss did not differ significantly between aceclofenac and similar drugs such as tenoxicam [11,19], diclofenac [12,13], piroxicam [16], or indomethacin [3].

Gastroprotective therapy, such as with proton pump inhibitors (PPIs) in combination with NSAIDs, has been recommended for patients who are at risk for GI complications [20]. Among PPIs, esomeprazole, the S-isomer of omeprazole, has been shown to be useful in the prevention and healing of NSAID-induced gastric injury in clinical studies [21–25]. Nevertheless, co-therapy with NSAIDs and gastroprotective agents often results in poor clinical outcomes due to inadequate dosing and low patient compliance [26,27]. To improve patient compliance and clinical outcomes, a fixed-dose combination of an NSAID (naproxen) and esomeprazole magnesium (VIMOVO®) was approved by the United States FDA in 2010.

Despite relatively low frequency and severity of GI complications with aceclofenac treatment alone, aceclofenac therapy may benefit when combined with esomeprazole. However, potential pharmacokinetic and pharmacodynamic interactions between aceclofenac and esomeprazole are not well characterized. To our knowledge, no reports are available on the effects of esomeprazole on the prevention or healing of aceclofenac-induced GI ulceration in preclinical and clinical studies.

Therefore, the present study evaluated pharmacokinetic interactions between aceclofenac and esomeprazole, as well as effects of esomeprazole on aceclofenac-induced gastric ulceration in rats. Food effects on the pharmacokinetics of aceclofenac and esomeprazole were also studied.

2. Materials and Methods

2.1. Chemicals

Aceclofenac and esomeprazole magnesium dihydrate were supplied by Korea United Pharm. Inc. (Seoul, Korea). Diclofenac, lansoprazole, ammonium formate, sodium bicarbonate, and methylcellulose were purchased from Sigma-Aldrich Co. (St. Louis, MO, USA). HPLC grade acetonitrile, methanol, and distilled water were purchased from J.T. Baker, Inc. (Philipsburg, NJ, USA). Polyethylene glycol (PEG) 200 and citric acid were obtained from Junsei Chemical Co. (Tokyo, Japan), dimethyl sulfoxide (DMSO) was purchased from Kanto Chemical Co. (Tokyo, Japan), and urea was purchased from USB Co. (Cleveland, OH, USA).

2.2. Animals

Male Sprague-Dawley rats (8–10 weeks; body weight 220–282 g) were purchased from Samtako (Osan, Korea) and kept in plastic cages with free access to water and standard rat diet. The rats were maintained at a temperature of 23 ± 2 °C with a 12 h light-dark cycle and relative humidity of 50 ± 10%. They were acclimatized for at least one week prior to experimentation. All animal care and the protocols were conducted according to the Guidelines for the Care and Use of Animals which was approved by the Catholic University of Daegu (IACUC-2016-006; 29 April 2016) and Wonkwang University (WKU17-02; 10 January 2017).

2.3. Pharmacokinetic Studies

Aceclofenac and esomeprazole were prepared in four different vehicles, i.e., DMSO:PEG200:distilled water = 10:70:20 (vehicle A), 0.5% methylcellulose suspension in distilled water (vehicle B), citric urea buffer which consisted of urea (20 g/mL) and trisodium citrate (10 g/mL) for aceclofenac and 0.5% methylcellulose suspension containing 0.25 mM $NaHCO_3$ for esomeprazole (vehicle C), and DMSO:citric urea buffer = 1:14 solution for aceclofenac and DMSO:citric urea buffer = 1:9 solution for esomeprazole (vehicle D).

The rats were fasted for 12 h prior to the drug administration except for the rats for the fed condition in which the rats were allowed free access to standard rat diet to examine food effect. Aceclofenac and esomeprazole solutions or suspensions were administered to rats by oral gavage. For vehicles A and B, aceclofenac and esomeprazole were dissolved or suspended together in the vehicle and simultaneously administered to rats. For vehicle C, aceclofenac in the citric urea buffer, esomeprazole in 0.5% methylcellulose suspension, and 0.25 mM $NaHCO_3$ were sequentially administered with a 5 min interval. For vehicle D, esomeprazole solution was administered first, and aceclofenac solution was administered 10 min after the esomeprazole dose. Approximately 200 μL of venous blood was collected predose and 0.25, 0.5, 1, 2, 3, 4, 6, 8, 12, 18, and 24 h postdose from the jugular vein. Plasma samples were obtained by centrifugation of the blood samples at 4000× *g* for 10 min and stored at −70 °C until analysis. The stomach was collected for measurement of gastric lesions.

2.4. Measurement of Gastric Lesions

To evaluate the effects of esomeprazole on gastric damage associated with aceclofenac administration, rats were separated into six groups, i.e., control group (blank vehicle D, $n = 7$), positive control group (200 mg/kg of aceclofenac, $n = 7$), and four test groups (200 mg/kg of aceclofenac + 5, 10, 20, or 40 mg/kg of esomeprazole, $n = 3$ or 4). The rats were fasted 24 h before aceclofenac and esomeprazole doses. Esomeprazole solution was administered 10 min prior to aceclofenac (200 mg/kg) administration. At 6 h after the aceclofenac dose, rats were sacrificed, the stomach was excised, and gastric damage was examined. Since this study was conducted by two separate experiments and each experiment has the control and positive control, the number of animals included for the control ($n = 7$) and positive control ($n = 7$) was higher than test groups ($n = 3$–4). Except for the esomeprazole doses, all experimental protocols were identical between the two studies.

The gastric damage by aceclofenac was measured by calculation of ulcerative lesion area and ulcer index. After sacrificing the animal, the stomach was dissected along its greater curvature and fixed on a board. The stomach was then macroscopically examined, and the area of the lesion was quantified using an image analysis program, Image J (National Institutes of Health, Bethesda, MD, USA). The extent of ulceration was also assessed by calculation of an ulcer index according to the method of Andrade et al. [28,29]. Ulcers were first classified as ulcer area < 1 mm^2 (Level I), ulcer area = 1–3 mm^2 (Level II), and ulcer area > 3 mm^2 (Level III), and the ulcer indexes were calculated:

$$\begin{aligned}&\textit{Ulcer index}\\&= 1 \times (\textit{number of Level I ulcer}) + 2 \times (\textit{number of Level II ulcer}) + 3 \times (\textit{number of Level III ulcer})\end{aligned}$$

2.5. Liquid Chromatography-Tandem Mass Spectrometry (LC-MS/MS)

Concentrations of aceclofenac, its metabolite, diclofenac, and esomeprazole in the rat plasma were determined by a newly developed LC-MS/MS assay. Calibration samples were prepared by spiking 50 μL of blank rat plasma with 50 μL of the standard aceclofenac, diclofenac, and esomeprazole working standard solutions in methanol followed by addition of 50 μL of the internal standard (IS) solution (lansoprazole, 100 ng/mL in methanol) and 350 μL of methanol as precipitation solvent. The final calibration samples yielded concentrations of 5, 10, 50, 100, 500, 1000, 5000, and 10,000 ng/mL for aceclofenac, 10, 50, 100, 500, 1000, 5000, and 10,000 ng/mL for diclofenac, and 0.25, 0.5, 2.5, 5, 25, 50, 250, and 500 ng/mL for esomeprazole. For plasma sample preparation, 50 µL of the IS and 400 µL of methanol were added to 50 µL of the rat plasma samples. The mixture was then mixed on a vortex mixer for 1 min and centrifuged at 34,220× g for 10 min. After centrifugation, 100 µL of the supernatant was diluted with the same volume of 25 mM ammonium formate, and a volume of 2 µL was injected into the LC-MS/MS.

The LC-MS/MS comprised an Agilent 6430 coupled with an Agilent 1200 HPLC system (Agilent, Santa Clara, CA, USA). Chromatographic separations were achieved on a Kinetex C18 column 50 × 2.10 mm i.d., 2.0 µm (Phenomenex, Torrence, CA, USA) with a Security Guard Cartridge (Phenomenex, Torrence, CA, USA). The mobile phase (MP) consisted of a mixture of 25 mM ammonium formate with 0.2% formic acid (MP-A) and acetonitrile (MP-B). The initial condition of 77% MP-A and 23% MP-B was held for 4 min followed by a linear increase of MP-B to 90% in the next 0.3 min. The flow rate of the mobile phase was set at 0.35 mL/min at the initial condition. The composition of 10:90 of MP-A:MP-B was maintained for 1 min, and the flow rate was 0.6 mL/min. The system was brought back to the initial condition of 77% MP-A by a linear gradient in 0.3 min and a flow rate of 0.35 mL/min and maintained for 3 min before the next injection. The column oven temperature was 40 °C. The mass spectrometer was operated using electron spray ionization (ESI) in positive ion mode with a dwell time of 100 ms. The fragmentor voltage was 85 V for aceclofenac, esomeprazole, and the IS, and 80 V for diclofenac. The collision energy was 40 V for aceclofenac, 34 V for diclofenac, 5 V for esomeprazole, and 5 V for the IS. Gas temperature, gas flow rate, and nebulizer gas pressure were set at 350 °C, 10 L/min, and 20 psi, respectively. The transition of the precursors to the product ion was monitored at m/z 354.0→214.0 for aceclofenac, 296.0→214.0 for diclofenac, 346.3→198.0 for esomeprazole, and 370.1→252.0 for the IS.

The lower limit of quantification (LLOQ) of the assay was 5 ng/mL, 10 ng/mL, and 0.25 ng/mL for aceclofenac, diclofenac, and esomeprazole, respectively, in the rat plasma. The intra- and inter-day accuracy was 103.0–110.8% for aceclofenac, 95.2–108.8% for diclofenac, and 90.4–111.0% for esomeprazole (n = 4, each). The intra- and inter-day precision was below 11.0% for aceclofenac, 12.1% for diclofenac, and 13.2% for esomeprazole (n = 4, each). The recovery calculated by comparing the peak area obtained from the standard solution spiked in the blank plasma followed by a protein precipitation process to that obtained from the matrix-free solvent was 97.2 ± 6.8% for aceclofenac, 89.9 ± 5.0% for diclofenac, 109.3 ± 2.0% for esomeprazole, and 107.5 ± 3.1% for the IS (n = 3).

2.6. Non-Compartmental Analysis

The non-compartmental pharmacokinetic parameters were estimated by Phoenix® WinNonlin® 6.4 (Certara, Princeton, NJ, USA). These parameters included terminal half-life ($t_{1/2}$), peak plasma concentration (C_{max}) and time to reach C_{max} (T_{max}), areas under the plasma concentration vs. time curve from time zero to the last observation time (AUC_{all}) and from time zero to infinity (AUC_{∞}), and systemic clearance (CL/F).

2.7. Statistical Analysis

The obtained data were analyzed with unpaired t-tests for comparisons between two means of unpaired data or one-way analyses of variance followed by Tukey's post hoc test for comparisons among more than two means of unpaired data. Data were expressed as the mean ± standard deviation (SD). The statistical significance level was set at $p < 0.05$ (SPSS Statistics 17.0, SPSS Inc., Chicago, IL, USA).

3. Results

3.1. Effects of Esomeprazole on Aceclofenac Induced Gastric Damage

Figure 1 shows ulcer index and ulcer areas following oral administration of aceclofenac (200 mg/kg) with or without esomeprazole pre-treatments (0, 5, 10, 20, 40 mg/kg). Two separate experiments were conducted, and data from the two studies were pooled together. While minimal gastric ulcers were observed after administration of control vehicle, significantly higher ulcer index and ulcer area were observed following aceclofenac administration at 200 mg/kg. Ulcer index was significantly reduced by administration of esomeprazole (Figure 1A). However, no statistically significant dose-dependent differences across esomeprazole doses of 5–40 mg/kg were observed, and increasing the dose of esomeprazole to 40 mg/kg did not result in an increased reduction of aceclofenac-induced gastric lesions. Both absolute gastric ulcer area (mm^2) and relative ulceration area compared to total stomach area (%) showed a trend similar to the ulcer index. Significantly higher ulcer areas were observed with aceclofenac treatment, with reduction by esomeprazole co-administration at 10 and 20 mg/kg (Figure 1B,C).

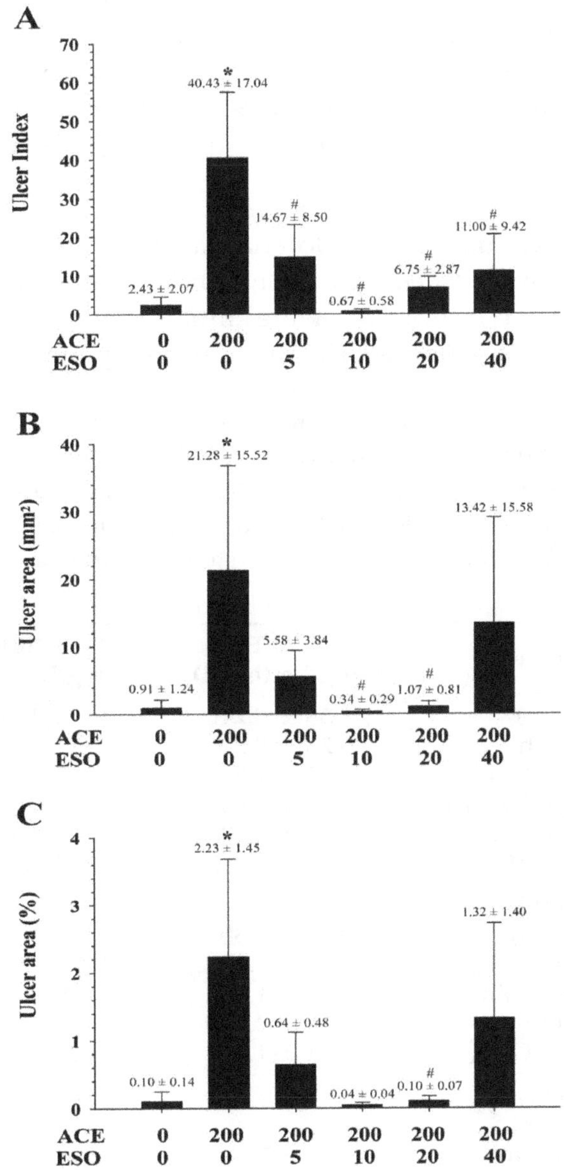

Figure 1. Aceclofenac (ACE) 200 mg/kg-induced gastric ulcers represented by (**A**) ulcer index, (**B**) ulcer area (mm^2), and (**C**) relative ulcer area (%) in the absence or in the presence of pre-treatments with esomeprazole (ESO) 0, 5, 10, 20, 40 mg/kg in rats. Each column represents the mean ± SD. *, $p < 0.05$ vs. control (ACE = 0/ESO = 0 mg/kg); $^{\#}$, $p < 0.05$ vs. ACE = 200/ESO = 0 mg/kg.

3.2. Effects of Esomeprazole on Aceclofenac Pharmacokinetics

Effects of esomeprazole on aceclofenac pharmacokinetics were evaluated after oral administration of aceclofenac (20 mg/kg) in combination with esomeprazole (0, 4, 8 mg/kg) delivered with vehicle C in rats. Average plasma concentration vs. time profiles of aceclofenac, diclofenac, and esomeprazole are shown in Figure 2, and non-compartmental pharmacokinetic parameters are summarized in Table 1. Plasma aceclofenac concentration rapidly increased and reached C_{max} within 0.23 h. Plasma concentration then declined with a mean terminal half-life ($t_{1/2}$) of 0.94–1.39 h. No significant differences in aceclofenac pharmacokinetic parameters were found with esomeprazole co-administration (Table 1).

Diclofenac, a metabolite of aceclofenac, plasma concentrations also rapidly increased following aceclofenac administration to maximum concentrations (C_{max}) of 4.91–10.76 μg/mL with mean T_{max} of 0.23–0.50 h. C_{max} as well as AUC of diclofenac were higher than those of aceclofenac. The $t_{1/2}$ of diclofenac was 3.24–3.84 h. Pharmacokinetic parameters of diclofenac were unaltered by esomeprazole co-administration. The fraction of metabolite formation (AUC_{DIC}/AUC_{ACE}) was also unaltered by esomeprazole administration.

Following oral co-administration of aceclofenac and esomeprazole, esomeprazole plasma concentration rapidly increased and reached C_{max} within 0.15 h, then declined with a $t_{1/2}$ of 3.87–5.67 h (Figure 2C and Table 1). While the $t_{1/2}$ and T_{max} were similar following 4 and 8 mg/kg esomeprazole administration, average C_{max}, AUC_{all}, and AUC_{∞} proportionally increased with the dose increase.

Table 1. Non-compartmental pharmacokinetic parameters of aceclofenac, diclofenac, and esomeprazole obtained after oral administration of aceclofenac (20 mg/kg) and esomeprazole (0, 4 and 8 mg/kg) to rats. Parameters include terminal half-life ($t_{1/2}$), peak plasma concentration (C_{max}), time to reach C_{max} (T_{max}), areas under the plasma concentration vs. time curve from time zero to the last observation time (AUC_{all}) and from time zero to infinity (AUC_{∞}), and systemic clearance (CL/F).

Compound	Parameters	ACE 20/ESO 0 mg/kg (*n* = 4)	ACE 20/ESO 4 mg/kg (*n* = 6)	ACE 20/ESO 8 mg/kg (*n* = 4)
Aceclofenac	$t_{1/2}$ (h)	1.38 ± 0.21	0.94 ± 0.70	1.39 ± 0.72
	T_{max} (h)	0.23 ± 0.20	0.17 ± 0.07	0.19 ± 0.10
	C_{max} (μg/mL)	3.07 ± 1.20	5.12 ± 1.66	5.72 ± 2.55
	AUC_{all} (μg·h/mL)	2.30 ± 0.54	2.54 ± 0.51	2.79 ± 0.61
	AUC_{∞} (μg·h/mL)	2.36 ± 0.52	2.57 ± 0.51	2.83 ± 0.60
	CL/F (mL/min/kg)	146.80 ± 32.40	134.77 ± 32.32	121.94 ± 26.32
Diclofenac	$t_{1/2}$ (h)	3.84 ± 0.32	3.82 ± 1.65	3.24 ± 0.98
	T_{max} (h)	0.50 ± 0.30	0.28 ± 0.11	0.23 ± 0.08
	C_{max} (μg/mL)	4.91 ± 3.19	10.76 ± 2.74	8.89 ± 4.98
	AUC_{all} (μg·h/mL)	7.16 ± 1.98	9.44 ± 1.1	8.56 ± 3.32
	AUC_{∞} (μg·h/mL)	7.76 ± 2.13	10.1 ± 1.35	8.97 ± 3.24
	AUC_{DIC}/AUC_{ACE}	3.94 ± 1.73	4.64 ± 1.32	3.63 ± 0.97
Esomeprazole	$t_{1/2}$ (h)	-	3.87 ± 2.21	5.67 ± 3.68
	T_{max} (h)	-	0.15 ± 0.14	0.13 ± 0.05
	C_{max} (μg/mL)	-	57.14 ± 25.94	142.75 ± 132.71
	AUC_{all} (μg·h/mL)	-	27.68 ± 13.39	64.02 ± 49.78
	AUC_{∞} (μg·h/mL)	-	30.91 ± 12.76	68.71 ± 48.72
	CL/F (mL/min/kg)	-	2442.37 ± 884.54	3087.76 ± 2334.25

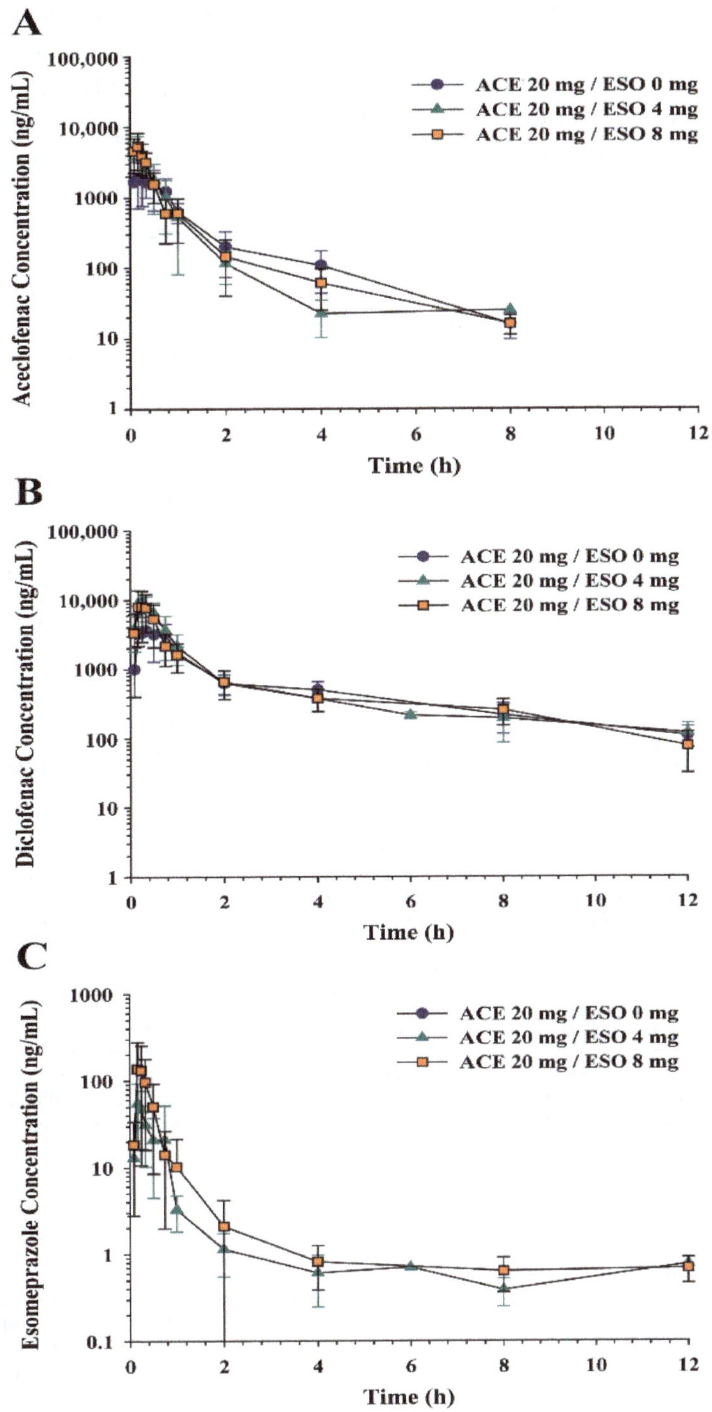

Figure 2. Average plasma concentration-time profiles of (**A**) aceclofenac, (**B**) diclofenac, and (**C**) esomeprazole following oral administration of aceclofenac (20 mg/kg) in combination with esomeprazole (0, 4, 8 mg/kg) in rats. Data represent mean ± SD (n = 4–6).

3.3. Effects of Different Dosing Vehicles on the Pharmacokinetics of Aceclofenac and Esomeprazole

Figure 3 summarizes plasma concentration vs. time profiles of aceclofenac, diclofenac, and esomeprazole following administration of aceclofenac and esomeprazole using different dosing vehicles. The non-compartmental pharmacokinetic parameters are summarized in Table 2. Since different doses were used with vehicles A, B, C (aceclofenac 20 mg/kg and esomeprazole 4 mg/kg), and vehicle D (aceclofenac 200 mg/kg and esomeprazole 20 mg/kg), the systemic exposure parameters C_{max} and AUC were normalized by dose and compared. Statistical comparisons were made only for dose-independent parameters, such as $t_{1/2}$, T_{max}, C_{max}/D, AUC/D, and CL/F.

For aceclofenac, significant differences were found for $t_{1/2}$, C_{max}/D, and AUC_{all}/D depending on the vehicle. Drug $t_{1/2}$ was longer when vehicle B (0.5% methylcellulose suspension in distilled water) was used than when vehicle C was used. Aceclofenac C_{max}/D as well as AUC_{all}/D with vehicle B was also lower than those in other vehicles. The C_{max}/D of aceclofenac was the highest in vehicle C compared to all other vehicles. However, the AUC_{∞}/D of aceclofenac was comparable across all tested vehicles.

Table 2. Non-compartmental pharmacokinetic parameters of aceclofenac and diclofenac obtained after oral administration of vehicle A, B, C, and D containing aceclofenac (20 mg/kg for A, B, and C and 200 mg/kg for D) and esomeprazole (4 mg/kg for A, B, and C and 20 mg/kg for D) to rats.

Compound	Parameters	Vehicle A (n = 5)	Vehicle B (n = 4)	Vehicle C (n = 6)	Vehicle D (n = 6)
Aceclofenac	$t_{1/2}$ (h) [a]	2.13 ± 0.30	6.47 ± 5.59	0.94 ± 0.70	1.89 ± 1.65
	T_{max} (h)	0.57 ± 0.80	0.60 ± 0.93	0.17 ± 0.07	0.27 ± 0.21
	C_{max} (μg/mL)	2.53 ± 0.57	0.69 ± 0.33	5.12 ± 1.66	21.69 ± 6.48
	C_{max} (μg/mL)/D (mg/kg) [b]	0.13 ± 0.03	0.03 ± 0.02	0.26 ± 0.08	0.11 ± 0.03
	AUC_{all} (μg·h/mL)	3.35 ± 1.72	0.88 ± 0.82	2.54 ± 0.51	34.75 ± 9.82
	AUC_{all} (μg·h/mL)/D (mg/kg) [c]	0.37 ± 0.07	0.07 ± 0.06	0.47 ± 0.05	0.63 ± 0.23
	AUC_{∞} (μg·h/mL)	3.53 ± 1.89	1.42 ± 1.14	2.57 ± 0.51	38.16 ± 9.00
	AUC_{∞} (μg·h/mL)/D (mg/kg)	0.18 ± 0.09	0.07 ± 0.06	0.13 ± 0.03	0.19 ± 0.05
	CL/F (mL/min/kg)	116.07 ± 51.38	446.08 ± 358.98	134.77 ± 32.32	91.01 ± 23.36
Diclofenac	$t_{1/2}$ (h) [d]	1.97 ± 0.35	3.04 ± 1.42	3.82 ± 1.65	5.57 ± 3.21
	T_{max} (h)	0.60 ± 0.78	0.69 ± 0.88	0.28 ± 0.11	1.33 ± 1.67
	C_{max} (μg/mL)	5.98 ± 3.06	0.63 ± 0.28	10.76 ± 2.74	43.69 ± 14.61
	AUC_{all} (μg·h/mL)	7.41 ± 1.35	1.46 ± 1.30	9.44 ± 1.10	125.81 ± 46.49
	AUC_{∞} (μg·h/mL)	7.51 ± 1.38	1.58 ± 1.44	10.1 ± 1.35	129.86 ± 44.66
	AUC_{DIC}/AUC_{ACE} [a]	3.04 ± 1.06	2.03 ± 0.24	4.64 ± 1.32	4.33 ± 0.85
Esomeprazole	$t_{1/2}$ (h)	1.69 ± 0.75	5.14 ± 5.30	3.87 ± 2.21	3.72 ± 0.38
	T_{max} (h)	1.80 ± 3.47	0.21 ± 0.08	0.15 ± 0.14	0.21 ± 0.08
	C_{max} (ng/mL)	15.43 ± 3.36	13.54 ± 4.08	57.14 ± 25.94	319 ± 136.81
	C_{max} (ng/mL)/D (mg/kg) [e]	3.86 ± 0.84	3.39 ± 1.02	14.28 ± 6.49	15.95 ± 6.84
	AUC_{all} (ng·h/mL)	33.83 ± 10.1	27.28 ± 6.43	27.68 ± 13.39	143.85 ± 48.71
	AUC_{all} (ng·h/mL)/D (mg/kg)	8.46 ± 2.53	6.82 ± 1.61	6.92 ± 3.35	7.19 ± 2.44
	AUC_{∞} (ng·h/mL)	42.09 ± 19.27	37.03 ± 11.85	30.91 ± 12.76	151.35 ± 51.65
	AUC_{∞} (ng·h/mL)/D (mg/kg)	10.52 ± 4.82	9.26 ± 2.96	7.73 ± 3.19	7.57 ± 2.58
	CL/F (mL/min/kg)	1786.9 ± 670.64	1910.9 ± 518.68	2442.37 ± 884.54	2356.49 ± 602.56

[a] ANOVA ($p < 0.05$, post hoc: Tukey, B vs. C); [b] ANOVA ($p < 0.05$, post hoc: Tukey, C vs. A, B, D); [c] ANOVA ($p < 0.05$, post hoc: Tukey, B vs. A, C, D); [d] ANOVA ($p < 0.05$, post hoc: Tukey, A vs. D; [e] ANOVA ($p < 0.05$, post hoc: Tukey, A, B vs. C, D); * Statistical significance was only presented for dose-independent parameters.

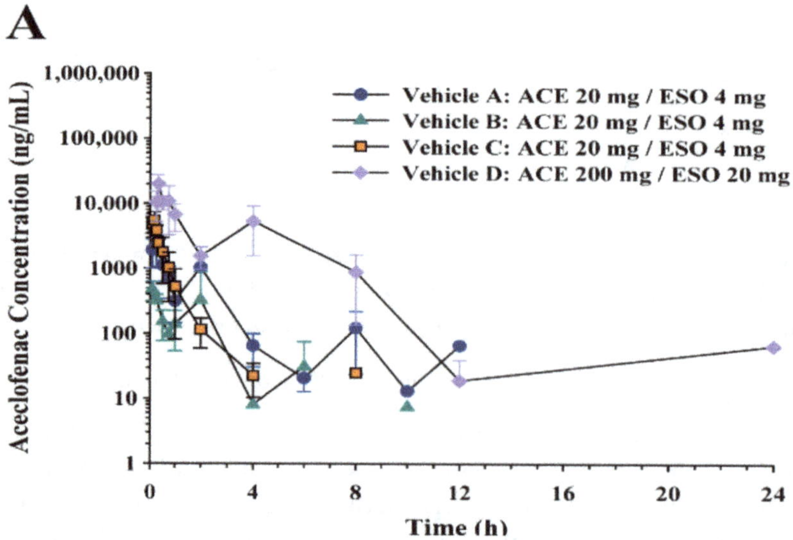

Figure 3. *Cont.*

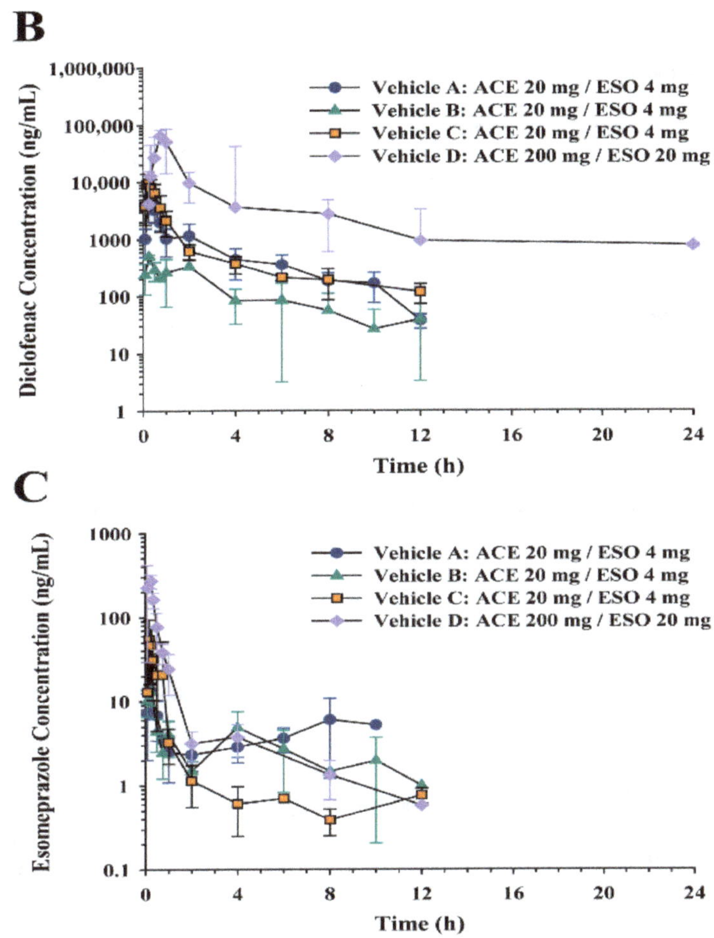

Figure 3. Average plasma concentration-time profiles of (**A**) aceclofenac, (**B**) diclofenac, and (**C**) esomeprazole following oral administration of vehicle A, B, C, and D containing aceclofenac (20 mg/kg for A, B, and C and 200 mg/kg for D) and esomeprazole (4 mg/kg for A, B, and C and 20 mg/kg for D) in rats.

Most pharmacokinetic parameters of diclofenac except $t_{1/2}$ were similar regardless of the dosing vehicle. The fraction metabolized, i.e., AUC_{DIC}/AUC_{ACE}, after aceclofenac administration was higher in vehicle C compared to that in vehicle B.

Most pharmacokinetic parameters of esomeprazole were not changed by different dosing vehicles, except C_{max}/D. The C_{max}/D values were similar between vehicles C and D, which were over 3.7-fold higher than those in vehicles A and B (Table 2).

3.4. Food Effects on the Pharmacokinetics of Aceclofenac and Esomeprazole

To evaluate food effects on aceclofenac and esomeprazole pharmacokinetics, aceclofenac (20 mg/kg) and esomeprazole (4 mg/kg) prepared in vehicle A were orally administered in fasting and fed conditions. Plasma concentration vs. time profiles of aceclofenac, diclofenac, and esomeprazole are shown in Figure 4. Non-compartmental pharmacokinetic parameters of aceclofenac, diclofenac, and esomeprazole in fasting and fed conditions are summarized in Table 3. Although overall plasma concentration vs. time profiles of aceclofenac and diclofenac were similar between fasting and fed conditions (Figure 4A,B), a longer $t_{1/2}$ was observed in fasting conditions for aceclofenac. In contrast, there was no significant difference between the $t_{1/2}$ in the fasting and fed conditions for diclofenac (Table 3). Conversely, overall esomeprazole plasma concentrations were lower in the fed condition than in the fasting condition (Figure 4C). The $t_{1/2}$ was longer and C_{max} and AUC_{all} were significantly lower for esomeprazole in the fed condition (Table 3).

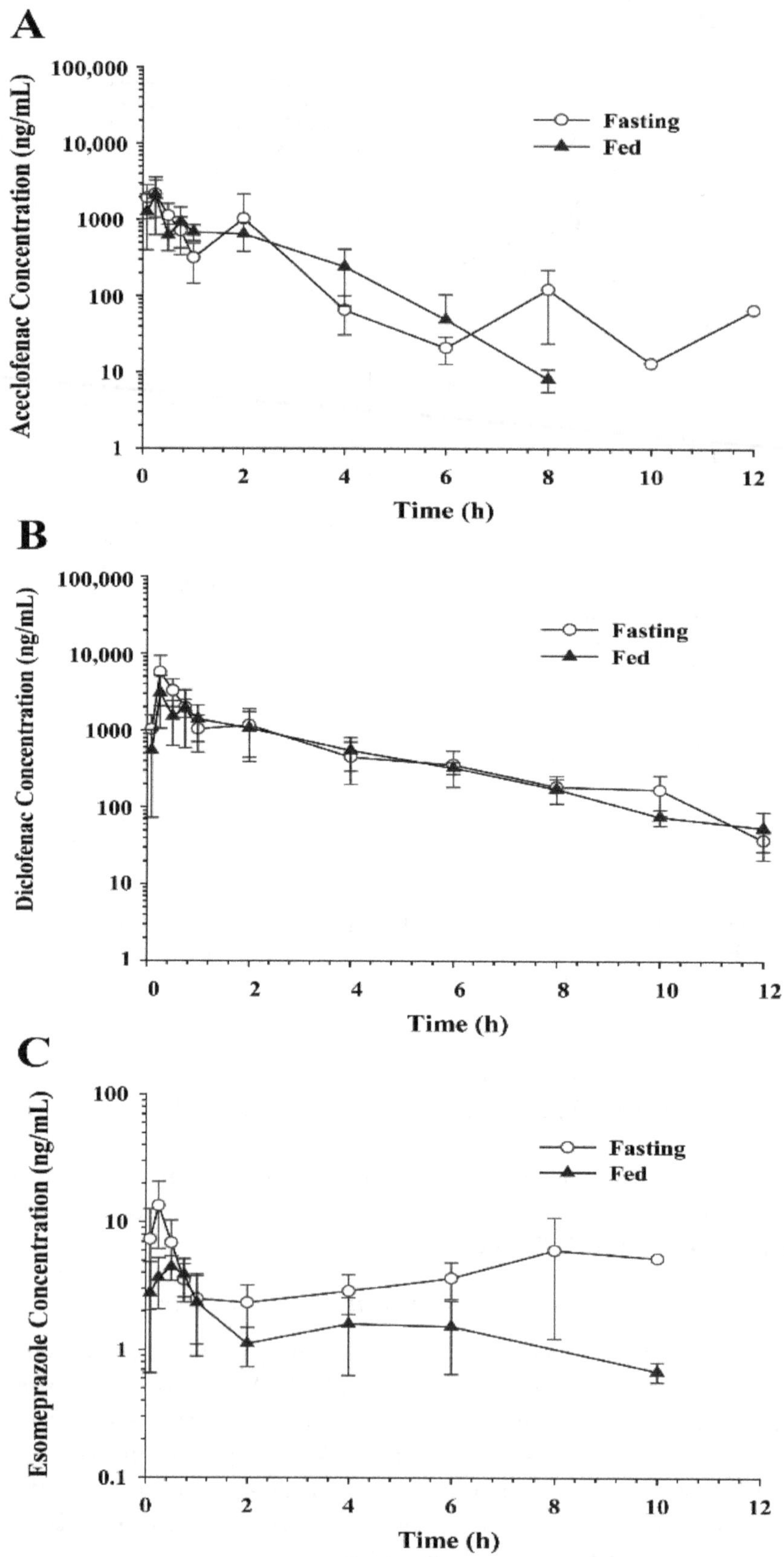

Figure 4. Average plasma concentration-time profiles of (**A**) aceclofenac, (**B**) diclofenac, and (**C**) esomeprazole following oral administration of aceclofenac (20 mg/kg) in combination with esomeprazole (4 mg/kg) in rats with fasting vs. fed conditions. Data represent mean ± SD (n = 4–5).

Table 3. Non-compartmental pharmacokinetic parameters of aceclofenac, diclofenac, and esomeprazole obtained after oral administration of aceclofenac (20 mg/kg) and esomeprazole (4 mg/kg) to rats under fasted and fed state.

Compound	Parameters	Fasted (n = 5)	Fed (n = 4)
Aceclofenac	$t_{1/2}$ (h) *	2.13 ± 0.30	0.81 ± 0.21
	T_{max} (h)	0.57 ± 0.80	0.65 ± 0.91
	C_{max} (μg/mL)	2.53 ± 0.57	2.27 ± 1.38
	AUC_{all} (μg·h/mL)	3.35 ± 1.72	2.95 ± 0.41
	AUC_{∞} (μg·h/mL)	3.53 ± 1.89	2.97 ± 0.41
	CL/F (mL/min/kg)	116.07 ± 51.38	114.1 ± 17.25
Diclofenac	$t_{1/2}$ (h)	1.97 ± 0.35	2.22 ± 0.59
	T_{max} (h)	0.60 ± 0.78	0.69 ± 0.88
	C_{max} (μg/mL)	5.98 ± 3.06	3.12 ± 1.91
	AUC_{all} (μg·h/mL)	7.41 ± 1.35	6.36 ± 1.27
	AUC_{∞} (μg·h/mL)	7.51 ± 1.38	6.56 ± 1.31
	AUC_{DIC}/AUC_{ACE}	3.04 ± 1.06	2.57 ± 0.27
Esomeprazole	$t_{1/2}$ (h) *	1.69 ± 0.75	3.18 ± 1.02
	T_{max} (h)	1.80 ± 3.47	0.40 ± 0.29
	C_{max} (ng/mL) *	15.43 ± 3.36	4.84 ± 0.94
	AUC_{all} (ng·h/mL) *	33.83 ± 10.10	13.96 ± 4.82
	AUC_{∞} (ng·h/mL)	42.09 ± 19.27	17.26 ± 4.42
	CL/F (mL/min/kg)	1786.9 ± 670.64	4061.35 ± 1041.26

* t-test ($p < 0.05$, Fasted vs. Fed).

4. Discussion

This study demonstrated no significant pharmacokinetic interactions between aceclofenac and esomeprazole in rats. Metabolic formation of diclofenac from aceclofenac was fast and extensive, which was consistent with previous reports [6,7]. Aceclofenac metabolism to diclofenac was also largely unaffected by concurrent administration of esomeprazole. Although diclofenac may be present at lower levels in humans than in rats, it significantly inhibits enzymatic activity of COX enzymes and contributes to the pharmacological action of aceclofenac in both humans and rats. Moreover, consistent with results in humans [22,23,25], our results indicate that esomeprazole may suppress gastric mucosal damage induced by aceclofenac in rats.

Substantial lesions were observed in the gastric mucosa following single dose oral administration of aceclofenac at 200 mg/kg in rats compared to that following vehicle administration (Figure 1). Co-administration of esomeprazole significantly suppressed gastric mucosal damage. Similarly, esomeprazole has demonstrated efficacy in the prevention and treatment of NSAIDs-induced gastric ulcers in humans [22,23,25] and experimental animals [30]. However, esomeprazole prevention of gastric ulcers was not dose-dependent in our study (Figure 1). While gastric ulceration induced by aceclofenac was almost entirely prevented by co-administration with esomeprazole at 10 and 20 mg/kg, no additional benefit was seen at the higher esomeprazole dose (40 mg/kg).

The gastro-protective effects of esomeprazole in combination with NSAIDs are potentially attributed to multiple mechanisms. Both acid-dependent and acid-independent mechanisms were proposed. Esomeprazole significantly inhibited gastric acid secretion in parallel with a significant reduction in mucosal damage in rats treated with indomethacin for 2 weeks [30]. In addition, esomeprazole restored proliferating cell nuclear antigen (PCNA) and Ki-67 expression and decreased malondialdehyde (MDA) levels and caspase-3 expression [30]. Reduction of oxidative tissue damage may also contribute to the gastroprotective actions of esomeprazole [31,32]. Digestive effects of esomeprazole may also confer gastroprotection [31]. Although the present study mainly focused on apparent gastric injury, we also analyzed the biomarkers that may contribute to gastric injury in mucosal samples. However, measured levels of MDA and protein expression of NF-κB, PCNA, and caspase-3 were variable and not dependent on aceclofenac administration. Minor changes in these biomarkers were observed with esomeprazole co-administration. It is possible that mucosal samples may be damaged during macroscopic examination in the present experimental setting. In addition, experimental conditions (i.e., a single dose administration of aceclofenac and esomeprazole) are different from studies that examined the effects of repeated exposures of indomethacin for two weeks followed by one week of esomeprazole co-administration [30]. The mechanism of gastroprotective effects of esomeprazole in combination with aceclofenac should be evaluated in further studies.

When pharmacokinetics of aceclofenac and esomeprazole were compared in fed vs. fasted conditions, the $t_{1/2}$ of aceclofenac was longer in fasting conditions. Multiple peaks were observed in the plasma concentration vs. time profiles and were more prominent in the fasting conditions (Figure 4A). These results agree with those of previous studies in which multiple peaks were present [6]. The multiple-peak phenomenon may result from the presence of either enterohepatic recirculation or a complicated absorption process [33,34], which may be favorable in fasting conditions [6]. The pharmacokinetics of the metabolite diclofenac were not altered by the presence of food. However, a significant reduction in systemic exposure to esomeprazole was observed in the fed versus fasting condition (Table 3). This is consistent with previous reports that the mean exposure after administration of a single dose of esomeprazole was decreased by 43–53% after food intake compared to fasting conditions resulting in the recommendation for esomeprazole to be taken at least one hour before meals [35].

During the present study, we also found that both aceclofenac and esomeprazole pharmacokinetics were significantly dependent on dosing vehicles. Among four different dosing vehicles, vehicle C (citric urea buffer solution) allowed for the most rapid absorption of aceclofenac, as evidenced by the highest C_{max}/D with a short T_{max} (Table 2). A previous study reported that a mixture of urea and sodium citrate similar to vehicle C markedly increased aceclofenac water solubility [6]. Increased water solubility may have contributed to the increased rate of aceclofenac absorption. On the contrary, vehicle B (0.5% methylcellulose suspension in distilled water) induced lower C_{max}/D and AUC_{all}/D with a longer $t_{1/2}$ compared to the solution vehicle, which may be due to slower absorption of the suspension. However, the overall extent of absorption and AUC_{∞} of aceclofenac were comparable across suspension and solution vehicles. For esomeprazole, a significantly higher C_{max} was observed when esomeprazole was dosed in vehicles C and D than in vehicles A and B (Table 2). Esomeprazole stability is pH-dependent, and it degrades rapidly in an acidic environment [35]. Vehicles C and D contained neutral buffers, which may have prevented acid-catalyzed degradation of esomeprazole in the stomach leading to a higher C_{max}. When omeprazole was given in combination with sodium bicarbonate, bioavailability was reported to increase by 2-fold [36].

5. Conclusions

Potential interactions between aceclofenac and esomeprazole were evaluated with regard to pharmacokinetics and GI adverse effects. While metabolism and pharmacokinetic profiles of aceclofenac were mostly unaltered, gastric ulceration associated with aceclofenac was significantly inhibited by concurrent administration of esomeprazole. The clinical benefits, as well as the optimal dose of the combination of aceclofenac and esomeprazole, should be evaluated in further studies. Since both aceclofenac and esomeprazole absorption was affected by dosing vehicles, design of optimal formulations may provide further advantages with regard to pharmacokinetics and efficacy.

Author Contributions: Conceptualization, T.H.K., S.S., and B.S.S.; Methodology, T.H.K., S.K.T., Y.-W.C., S.-M.C., K.-Y.N., W.-H.K., S.S., and B.S.S.; Investigation, T.H.K., S.K.T., D.Y.L., S.E.C., J.Y.L., H.M.J., C.H.S., and B.S.S.; Formal analysis, T.H.K., S.K.T., S.S., and B.S.S.; Resources, S.S. and B.S.S.; Writing-Original Draft Preparation, T.H.K., S.S., and B.S.S.; Writing-Review and Editing, T.H.K., S.S., and B.S.S. Supervision, B.S.S.; Funding Acquisition, S.S., Y.-W.C., W.-H.K., and B.S.S.

References

1. Ward, D.E.; Veys, E.M.; Bowdler, J.M.; Roma, J. Comparison of aceclofenac with diclofenac in the treatment of osteoarthritis. *Clin. Rheumatol.* **1995**, *14*, 656–662. [CrossRef] [PubMed]

2. Martin-Mola, E.; Gijon-Banos, J.; Ansoleaga, J.J. Aceclofenac in comparison to ketoprofen in the treatment of rheumatoid arthritis. *Rheumatol. Int.* **1995**, *15*, 111–116. [CrossRef] [PubMed]
3. Batlle-Gualda, E.; Figueroa, M.; Ivorra, J.; Raber, A. The efficacy and tolerability of aceclofenac in the treatment of patients with ankylosing spondylitis: A multicenter controlled clinical trial. Aceclofenac indomethacin study group. *J. Rheumatol.* **1996**, *23*, 1200–1206. [PubMed]
4. Schattenkirchner, M.; Milachowski, K.A. A double-blind, multicentre, randomised clinical trial comparing the efficacy and tolerability of aceclofenac with diclofenac resinate in patients with acute low back pain. *Clin. Rheumatol.* **2003**, *22*, 127–135. [CrossRef] [PubMed]
5. Movilia, P.G. Evaluation of the analgesic activity and tolerability of aceclofenac in the treatment of post-episiotomy pain. *Drugs Exp. Clin. Res.* **1989**, *15*, 47–51. [PubMed]
6. Noh, K.; Shin, B.S.; Kwon, K.I.; Yun, H.Y.; Kim, E.; Jeong, T.C.; Kang, W. Absolute bioavailability and metabolism of aceclofenac in rats. *Arch. Pharm. Res.* **2015**, *38*, 68–72. [CrossRef] [PubMed]
7. Bort, R.; Ponsoda, X.; Carrasco, E.; Gomez-Lechon, M.J.; Castell, J.V. Comparative metabolism of the nonsteroidal antiinflammatory drug, aceclofenac, in the rat, monkey, and human. *Drug Metab. Dispos.* **1996**, *24*, 969–975. [PubMed]
8. Henrotin, Y.; de Leval, X.; Mathy-Hartet, M.; Mouithys-Mickalad, A.; Deby-Dupont, G.; Dogne, J.M.; Delarge, J.; Reginster, J.Y. In vitro effects of aceclofenac and its metabolites on the production by chondrocytes of inflammatory mediators. *Inflamm. Res.* **2001**, *50*, 391–399. [CrossRef] [PubMed]
9. Scheiman, J.M. Nsaids, gastrointestinal injury, and cytoprotection. *Gastroenterol. Clin. North Am.* **1996**, *25*, 279–298. [CrossRef]
10. Dooley, M.; Spencer, C.M.; Dunn, C.J. Aceclofenac: A reappraisal of its use in the management of pain and rheumatic disease. *Drugs* **2001**, *61*, 1351–1378. [CrossRef] [PubMed]
11. Perez-Ruiz, F.; Alonso-Ruiz, A.; Ansoleaga, J.J. Comparative study of the efficacy and safety of aceclofenac and tenoxicam in rheumatoid arthritis. *Clin. Rheumatol.* **1996**, *15*, 473–477. [CrossRef] [PubMed]
12. Diaz, C.; Rodriguez de la Serna, A.; Geli, C.; Gras, X. Efficacy and tolerability of aceclofenac versus diclofenac in the treatment of knee osteoarthritis: A multicentre study. *Eur. J. Rheumatol. Inflamm.* **1996**, *16*, 17–22.
13. Pasero, G.; Marcolongo, R.; Serni, U.; Parnham, M.J.; Ferrer, F. A multi-centre, double-blind comparative study of the efficacy and safety of aceclofenac and diclofenac in the treatment of rheumatoid arthritis. *Curr. Med. Res. Opin.* **1995**, *13*, 305–315. [CrossRef] [PubMed]
14. Torri, G.; Vignati, C.; Agrifoglio, E.; Benvenuti, M.; Ceciliani, L.; Raschella, B.F.; Letizia, G.; Martorana, U.; Tessari, L.; Thovez, G.; et al. Aceclofenac versus piroxicam in the management of osteoarthritis of the knee: A double-blind controlled study. *Curr. Ther. Res.* **1994**, *55*, 576–583. [CrossRef]
15. Pasero, G.; Ruju, G.; Marcolongo, R.; Senesi, M.; Seni, U.; Mannoni, A.; Accardo, S.; Seriolo, B.; Colombo, B.; Ligniere, G.C.; et al. Aceclofenac versus naproxen in the treatment of ankylosing spondylitis: A double-blind, controlled study. *Curr. Ther. Res.* **1994**, *55*, 833–842. [CrossRef]
16. Perez Busquier, M.; Calero, E.; Rodriguez, M.; Castellon Arce, P.; Bermudez, A.; Linares, L.F.; Mesa, J.; Ffernandez Crisostomos, C.; Garcia, C.; Garcia Lopez, A.; et al. Comparison of aceclofenac with piroxicam in the treatment of osteoarthritis. *Clin. Rheumatol.* **1997**, *16*, 154–159. [CrossRef] [PubMed]
17. Kornasoff, D.; Frerick, H.; Bowdler, J.; Montull, E. Aceclofenac is a well-tolerated alternative to naproxen in the treatment of osteoarthritis. *Clin. Rheumatol.* **1997**, *16*, 32–38. [CrossRef] [PubMed]
18. Kornasoff, D.; Maisenbacher, J.; Bowdler, J.; Raber, A. The efficacy and tolerability of aceclofenac compared to indomethacin in patients with rheumatoid arthritis. *Rheumatol. Int.* **1996**, *15*, 225–230. [CrossRef] [PubMed]
19. Villa Alcazar, L.F.; de Buergo, M.; Rico Lenza, H.; Montull Fruitos, E. Aceclofenac is as safe and effective as tenoxicam in the treatment of ankylosing spondylitis: A 3 month multicenter comparative trial. Spanish study group on aceclofenac in ankylosing spondylitis. *J. Rheumatol.* **1996**, *23*, 1194–1199. [PubMed]
20. Lanza, F.L.; Chan, F.K.; Quigley, E.M. Practice Parameters Committee of the American College of, G. Guidelines for prevention of nsaid-related ulcer complications. *Am. J. Gastroenterol.* **2009**, *104*, 728–738. [CrossRef] [PubMed]
21. Agrawal, N.M.; Campbell, D.R.; Safdi, M.A.; Lukasik, N.L.; Huang, B.; Haber, M.M. Superiority of lansoprazole vs ranitidine in healing nonsteroidal anti-inflammatory drug-associated gastric ulcers: Results of a double-blind, randomized, multicenter study. Nsaid-associated gastric ulcer study group. *Arch. Intern. Med.* **2000**, *160*, 1455–1461. [CrossRef] [PubMed]

22. Goldstein, J.L.; Johanson, J.F.; Suchower, L.J.; Brown, K.A. Healing of gastric ulcers with esomeprazole versus ranitidine in patients who continued to receive nsaid therapy: A randomized trial. *Am. J. Gastroenterol.* **2005**, *100*, 2650–2657. [CrossRef] [PubMed]
23. Hawkey, C.; Talley, N.J.; Yeomans, N.D.; Jones, R.; Sung, J.J.; Langstrom, G.; Naesdal, J.; Scheiman, J.M.; Group, N.S.S. Improvements with esomeprazole in patients with upper gastrointestinal symptoms taking non-steroidal antiinflammatory drugs, including selective cox-2 inhibitors. *Am. J. Gastroenterol.* **2005**, *100*, 1028–1036. [CrossRef] [PubMed]
24. Morgner, A.; Miehlke, S.; Labenz, J. Esomeprazole: Prevention and treatment of nsaid-induced symptoms and ulcers. *Expert Opin. Pharmacother.* **2007**, *8*, 975–988. [CrossRef] [PubMed]
25. Scheiman, J.M.; Yeomans, N.D.; Talley, N.J.; Vakil, N.; Chan, F.K.; Tulassay, Z.; Rainoldi, J.L.; Szczepanski, L.; Ung, K.A.; Kleczkowski, D.; et al. Prevention of ulcers by esomeprazole in at-risk patients using non-selective nsaids and cox-2 inhibitors. *Am. J. Gastroenterol.* **2006**, *101*, 701–710. [CrossRef] [PubMed]
26. Lanas, A.; Polo-Tomas, M.; Roncales, P.; Gonzalez, M.A.; Zapardiel, J. Prescription of and adherence to non-steroidal anti-inflammatory drugs and gastroprotective agents in at-risk gastrointestinal patients. *Am. J. Gastroenterol.* **2012**, *107*, 707–714. [CrossRef] [PubMed]
27. Dries, A.M.; Richardson, P.; Cavazos, J.; Abraham, N.S. Therapeutic intent of proton pump inhibitor prescription among elderly nonsteroidal anti-inflammatory drug users. *Aliment. Pharmacol. Ther.* **2009**, *30*, 652–661. [CrossRef] [PubMed]
28. Andrade, S.F.; Antoniolli, D.; Comunello, E.; Cardoso, L.G.V.; Carvalho, J.C.T.; Bastos, J.K. Antiulcerogenic activity of crude extract, fractions and populnoic acid isolated from austroplenckia populnea (celastraceae). *Z. Naturforsch. C* **2006**, *61*, 329–333. [CrossRef] [PubMed]
29. Adinortey, M.B.; Ansah, C.; Galyuon, I.; Nyarko, A. In vivo models used for evaluation of potential antigastroduodenal ulcer agents. *Ulcers* **2013**, *2013*, 12. [CrossRef]
30. Fornai, M.; Colucci, R.; Antonioli, L.; Awwad, O.; Ugolini, C.; Tuccori, M.; Fulceri, F.; Natale, G.; Basolo, F.; Blandizzi, C. Effects of esomeprazole on healing of nonsteroidal anti-inflammatory drug (nsaid)-induced gastric ulcers in the presence of a continued nsaid treatment: Characterization of molecular mechanisms. *Pharmacol. Res.* **2011**, *63*, 59–67. [CrossRef] [PubMed]
31. Suzuki, H.; Hibi, T. Novel effects other than antisecretory action and off-label use of proton pump inhibitors. *Expert Opin. Pharmacother.* **2005**, *6*, 59–67. [CrossRef] [PubMed]
32. Pastoris, O.; Verri, M.; Boschi, F.; Kastsiuchenka, O.; Balestra, B.; Pace, F.; Tonini, M.; Natale, G. Effects of esomeprazole on glutathione levels and mitochondrial oxidative phosphorylation in the gastric mucosa of rats treated with indomethacin. *Naunyn Schmiedebergs Arch. Pharmacol.* **2008**, *378*, 421–429. [CrossRef] [PubMed]
33. Metsugi, Y.; Miyaji, Y.; Ogawara, K.; Higaki, K.; Kimura, T. Appearance of double peaks in plasma concentration-time profile after oral administration depends on gastric emptying profile and weight function. *Pharm. Res.* **2008**, *25*, 886–895. [CrossRef] [PubMed]
34. Kim, T.H.; Shin, S.; Landersdorfer, C.B.; Chi, Y.H.; Paik, S.H.; Myung, J.; Yadav, R.; Horkovics-Kovats, S.; Bulitta, J.B.; Shin, B.S. Population pharmacokinetic modeling of the enterohepatic recirculation of fimasartan in rats, dogs, and humans. *AAPS J.* **2015**, *17*, 1210–1223. [CrossRef] [PubMed]
35. U.S. FDA, NDA 21-153/S-022: Nexium (esomeprazole magnesium) delayed-release capsules. 2001. Available online: http://www.accessdata.fda.gov/drugsatfda_docs/label/2006/021153s022lbl.pdf (accessed on 31 July 2018).
36. Pilbrant, A.; Cederberg, C. Development of an oral formulation of omeprazole. *Scand. J. Gastroenterol. Suppl.* **1985**, *108*, 113–120. [CrossRef] [PubMed]

7

Identification of Catalposide Metabolites in Human Liver and Intestinal Preparations and Characterization of the Relevant Sulfotransferase, UDP-Glucuronosyltransferase and Carboxylesterase Enzymes

Deok-Kyu Hwang [1,†], Ju-Hyun Kim [2,†], Yongho Shin [1], Won-Gu Choi [1], Sunjoo Kim [1], Yong-Yeon Cho [1], Joo Young Lee [1], Han Chang Kang [1] and Hye Suk Lee [1,*]

1 BK21 PLUS Team for Creative Leader Program for Pharmacomics-based Future Pharmacy, College of Pharmacy, The Catholic University of Korea, Bucheon 14662, Korea
2 College of Pharmacy, Yeungnam University, Gyeongsan 38541, Korea
* Correspondence: sianalee@catholic.ac.kr
† These authors contributed equally to this work.

Abstract: Catalposide, an active component of *Veronica* species such as *Catalpa ovata* and *Pseudolysimachion lingifolium*, exhibits anti-inflammatory, antinociceptic, anti-oxidant, hepatoprotective, and cytostatic activities. We characterized the in vitro metabolic pathways of catalposide to predict its pharmacokinetics. Catalposide was metabolized to catalposide sulfate (M1), 4-hydroxybenzoic acid (M2), 4-hydroxybenzoic acid glucuronide (M3), and catalposide glucuronide (M4) by human hepatocytes, liver S9 fractions, and intestinal microsomes. M1 formation from catalposide was catalyzed by sulfotransferases (SULTs) 1C4, SULT1A1*1, SULT1A1*2, and SULT1E1. Catalposide glucuronidation to M4 was catalyzed by gastrointestine-specific UDP-glucuronosyltransferases (UGTs) 1A8 and UGT1A10; M4 was not detected after incubation of catalposide with human liver preparations. Hydrolysis of catalposide to M2 was catalyzed by carboxylesterases (CESs) 1 and 2, and M2 was further metabolized to M3 by UGT1A6 and UGT1A9 enzymes. Catalposide was also metabolized in extrahepatic tissues; genetic polymorphisms of the carboxylesterase (CES), UDP-glucuronosyltransferase (UGT), and sulfotransferase (SULT) enzymes responsible for catalposide metabolism may cause inter-individual variability in terms of catalposide pharmacokinetics.

Keywords: catalposide; in vitro human metabolism; UDP-glucuronosyltransferase; sulfotransferase; carboxylesterase

---

1. Introduction

Catalposide is an active iridoid glycoside of *Veronica* species including *Catalpa ovata* and *Pseudolysimachion lingifolium* [1–3]. Catalposide exhibits various biological effects including anti-inflammatory [4–9], anti-oxidant [10], antinociceptic [8], cytostatic [11], hypolipidemic via peroxisome proliferator-activated receptor-α activation [12], and hepatoprotective activities [13].

Catalposide had a short half-life (19.3 ± 9.5 min), and exhibited high systemic clearance (96.7 ± 44.1 mL/min/kg), and low urinary excretion (9.9 ± 4.1% of the dose) after intravenous administration of 10 mg/kg to male Sprague-Dawley rats [14]. This indicated that catalposide might be extensively metabolized in rats. However, catalposide remained stable after 1 h incubation with rat liver microsomes in the presence of NADPH [14]. Thus, catalposide may be catabolized via non-cytochrome P450 (CYP)-mediated mechanism. Catalposide was the substrate of OAT3, OATP1B1, and OATP1B3 transporters and weakly inhibited their transport activities with IC_{50} values of 83, 200, and 235 μM, respectively, suggesting that OAT3, OATP1B1, and OATP1B3 may regulate the pharmacokinetics and drug interactions of catalposide [15].

Pharmacokinetics and metabolism of potential active constituents in herbal drugs is helpful for the determination of dosage regimens and interpretation of pharmacological effects under clinical conditions [16]. It is important to establish the comparative metabolism and drug-metabolizing enzymes of active constituents for a full characterization of its pharmacokinetics, pharmacodynamics, and toxicity. The characterization of drug-metabolizing enzymes such as CYPs, carboxylesterases (CESs), UDP-glucuronosyltransferases (UGTs), and sulfotransferases (SULTs) responsible for the metabolism of a drug may reveal inter-individual variability in drug metabolism and the potential drug interactions [17–19]. However, catalposide metabolism has not been studied in humans and animals. We identified catalposide metabolites and drug-metabolizing enzymes involved to predict its pharmacokinetics and possible drug interactions.

We identified catalposide metabolites formed from in vitro incubations of catalposide with human hepatocytes, intestinal microsomes, and liver S9 fractions using liquid chromatography-high resolution mass spectrometry (LC-HRMS) and characterized the CES, UGT, and SULT enzymes involved in catalposide metabolism using human cDNA-expressed CES, UGT, and SULT supersomes, respectively.

2. Materials and Methods

2.1. Materials and Reagents

Catalposide (purity, 98%) was obtained from Aobious Inc. (Gloucester, MA, USA). Alamethicin, 3-phosphoadenosine-5-phosphosulfate (PAPS), and uridine 5′-diphosphoglucuronic acid (UDPGA) were from Sigma-Aldrich Co. (St. Louis, MO, USA). 4-hydroxybenzoic acid and 4-hydroxybenzoic acid glucuronide were purchased from Toronto Research Chemicals (North York, ON, Canada). Pooled human intestinal microsomes; pooled human liver S9 fractions; human cDNA-expressed UGTs 1A1/3/4/6/7/8/9/10 and 2B4/7/15/17 supersomes; human cDNA-expressed CESs 1b, 1c, and 2 supersomes; cryopreserved human hepatocytes; and hepatocyte purification kits were obtained from Corning Life Sciences (Woburn, MA, USA). Human cDNA-expressed SULT 1A1*1, 1A1*2, 1A2, 1A3, 1B1, 1C2, 1C4, 1E1, and 2A1 supersomes were purchased from Cypex Ltd. (Dundee, UK). Methanol (HPLC grade) was from Burdick & Jackson Inc. (SK Chemicals, Ulsan, Korea), and all other chemicals were of the highest quality available. Calibration mixtures for Exactive MS [ProteoMass LTQ/FT-hybrid ESI positive mode Cal Mix (MSCAL5) and negative mode Cal Mix (MSCAL6)] were obtained from Supelco (Bellefonte, PA, USA).

2.2. In Vitro Metabolism of Catalposide in Cryopreserved Human Hepatocytes

Cryopreserved human hepatocytes were recovered with the aid of a hepatocyte purification kit, and viable cells were resuspended in William's E buffer at a final concentration of 1.28×10^6 cells/mL [20]. Human hepatocyte suspensions (62.5 μL, 8.00×10^4 cells) and 62.5 μL of 400 μM catalposide in William's E buffer were added to the wells of a 96-well plate and the mixture was incubated for 120 min at 37 °C in a CO_2 incubator. Methanol (250 μL) was added to each well and the mixture was centrifuged at 3000× *g* for 10 min. Aliquots of the supernatants (250 μL) were evaporated to dryness using a vacuum evaporator (Genevac Ltd., Ipswich, UK). Each residue was dissolved in 100 μL of 5% methanol and an aliquot (5 μL) was injected into the LC-HRMS system.

2.3. In Vitro Metabolism of Catalposide in Human Liver S9 Fractions and Intestinal Microsomes

Each reaction mixture contained 50 mM potassium phosphate buffer (pH 7.4), 10 mM magnesium chloride, human liver S9 fractions or human intestinal microsomes (100 μg protein), 2 mM UDPGA or

200 μM PAPS, 200 μM catalposide or a possible metabolite, and 1000 μM 4-hydroxybenzoic acid in a volume of 200 μL. Samples lacking UDPGA and PAPS served as controls. The mixtures were incubated at 37 °C for 60 min and the reactions were then quenched by adding 500 μL of methanol. The tubes were centrifuged and the supernatants evaporated to dryness using a vacuum concentrator. The residues were dissolved in 100 μL of 5% methanol and 5 μL aliquots were injected into the LC-HRMS system.

2.4. Characterization of Human SULTs Involved in Catalposide Sulfation

To screen for SULT enzymes involved in catalposide sulfation, each 100 μL of reaction mixture contained 20 μM PAPS; 10 mM dithiothreitol; 5 mM magnesium chloride; 50 mM phosphate buffer (pH 7.4); 150 μM catalposide; and the human liver S9 fraction (40 μg protein) or human cDNA-expressed SULT 1A1*1, 1A1*2, 1A2, 1A3, 2A1, 1B1, 1C2, 1C4, or 1E1 supersomes [1A1*1 (0.25), 1A1*2 (0.5), 1A2 (0.25), 1A3 (0.2), 2A1 (1.25), 1B1 (0.5), 1C2 (2.5), 1C4 (0.1), 1E1 (0.2 μg protein)]. Incubation proceeded at 37 °C for 5 min. The reactions were stopped by adding 100 μL of methanol containing 30 ng/mL 4-methylumbelliferone (an internal standard). After vortex-mixing and centrifugation, 50 μL of each supernatant was diluted with 50 μL deionized water. The mixture was transferred to an injection vial, and an aliquot (5 μL) was injected into the LC-HRMS system.

To explore the kinetics of the metabolism of catalposide to catalposide sulfate, various concentrations of catalposide (10 to 2000 μM) were incubated in duplicate with pooled human liver S9 fractions (40 μg protein) or human cDNA-expressed SULT1A1*1 (0.5 μg protein), SULT1A1*2 (0.5 μg protein), SULT1C4 (0.1 μg protein), or SULT1E1 (0.2 μg protein) in the presence of 20 μM PAPS, 10 mM dithiothreitol, and 5 mM magnesium chloride at 37 °C for 5 min to obtain K_m and V_{max} values.

2.5. Characterization of Human UGTs Involved in Catalposide and 4-Hydroxybenzoic Acid Glucuronidation

To identify the UGT enzymes responsible for formation of catalposide glucuronide (M4) from catalposide and 4-hydroxybenzoic acid glucuronide (M3) from 4-hydroxybenzoic acid (M2), 100 μL reaction mixtures containing human intestinal microsomes (40 μg protein), or human cDNA-expressed UGTs 1A1, 1A3, 1A4, 1A6, 1A7, 1A8, 1A9, 1A10, 2B4, 2B7, 2B15, or 2B17 (10 μg protein); 2 mM UDPGA; 0.025 mg/mL alamethicin; and 400 μM catalposide or 500 μM 4-hydroxybenzoic acid in 50 mM Tris buffer (pH 7.4) were incubated at 37 °C for 60 min. The reactions were stopped by addition of 100 μL methanol containing 30 ng/mL 4-methylumbelliferone (an internal standard). After vortex-mixing and centrifugation, 50 μL of each supernatant was diluted with an equal volume of water and a 5 μL aliquot was injected into the LC-HRMS system.

To explore the kinetics of the metabolism of catalposide to catalposide glucuronide, various concentrations of catalposide (10, 25, 100, 400, 800, 1200, 1600, and 2000 μM) were incubated in duplicate with 2 mM UDPGA, 0.025 mg/mL alamethicin, pooled human intestinal microsomes (40 μg protein), or human cDNA-expressed UGT1A8 or UGT1A10 supersomes (20 μg protein), to obtain K_m and V_{max} values.

2.6. Characterization of Carboxylesterases Involved in the Formation of 4-Hydroxybenzoic Acid from Catalposide

To identify the CES enzymes involved in hydrolysis of catalposide to 4-hydroxybenzoic acid, 100 μL reaction mixtures containing human liver S9 fractions; human intestinal microsomes; or human CES1b, CES1c, or CES2 enzymes (50 μg protein), and catalposide (200 or 400 μM) in 50 mM phosphate buffer (pH 7.4) were incubated at 37 °C for 30 min. Reactions were stopped by addition of 100 μL 4-methylumbelliferone (internal standard, 10 ng/mL) in methanol. After vortex-mixing and centrifugation, 50 μL of each supernatant was diluted with 50 μL of deionized water. Each mixture was transferred to an injection vial, and a 5 μL aliquot was injected into the LC-HRMS system.

2.7. LC-HRMS Analysis of Catalposide and Metabolites

To separate and identify catalposide and its metabolites, we used a Q-Exactive Orbitrap mass spectrometer coupled to an Accela UPLC system (Thermo Scientific, Waltham, MA, USA). Catalposide and its metabolites were optimally separated on a Halo C18 column via gradient elution using 5% (*v/v*) methanol in 1 mM ammonium formate (pH 3.1) (mobile phase A) and methanol (mobile phase B) at a flow rate of 0.5 mL/min: 5% mobile phase B for 2 min, 5–20% mobile phase B over 11.5 min, 20–90% mobile phase B over 0.5 min, 90% mobile phase B for 3 min, 90–5% mobile phase B over 0.5 min, and 5% mobile phase B for 2.5 min. The column and the autosampler were maintained at 40 and 6 °C, respectively. Accurate mass measurements of catalposide and its metabolites were derived via electrospray ionization in the negative mode using the following electrospray source settings: ion transfer capillary temperature, 330 °C; needle spray voltage, −3000 V; capillary voltage, −47.5 V; nitrogen sheath gas, 50 arbitrary units; auxiliary gas, 15 arbitrary units. The resolution and automatic gain control were scaled to 70,000 and 1,000,000, respectively. MS data were obtained using external calibration over the scan range *m/z* 100–700 and processed using Xcalibur software version 2.2 (Thermo Scientific). The Q-Exactive Orbitrap MS was calibrated using MSCAL5 and MSCAL6 for the positive and negative ion modes, respectively. Nitrogen gas was employed for higher-energy collision dissociation (HCD) at an energy of 25 eV to obtain product ion spectra of catalposide and its metabolites. Structures were determined using Mass Frontier software (version 6.0; HighChem Ltd., Bratislava, Slovakia). We used the extracted ion monitoring mode for quantification: *m/z* 481.1349 for catalposide, *m/z* 657.1674 for catalposide glucuronide, *m/z* 561.0921 for catalposide sulfate, *m/z* 137.0239 for 4-hydroxybenzoic acid, *m/z* 313.0569 for 4-hydroxybenzoic acid glucuronide, and *m/z* 175.0410 for 4-methylumbelliferone (the internal standard). The peak areas of all components were integrated using Xcalibur software. The calibration curve was linear over the catalposide concentration range 0.5–200 pmol. The concentrations of catalposide glucuronide and catalposide sulfate were calculated using the calibration curve for catalposide because we had no authentic standards.

2.8. Data Analysis

All results are the average of two determinations obtained using pooled human intestinal microsomes, pooled human liver S9 fractions, UGTs, and SULTs. The apparent kinetic parameters (K_m, V_{max}, n, and K_i) for formation of catalposide glucuronide or catalposide sulfate by human intestinal microsomes, liver S9 fractions, UGTs, or SULTs were determined by fitting the Hill equation model [$V = V_{max}S^n/(K_m{}^n + S^n)$], the substrate inhibition model [$V = V_{max}/(1 + K_m/S + S/K_i)$], or the single enzyme model [$V = V_{max}S/(K_m + S)$] to the unweighted formation rates of catalposide glucuronide and catalposide sulfate, respectively, over a range of catalposide concentrations using Enzyme Kinetics software (version 1.1 SPSS Science Inc., Chicago, IL, USA). In the above equations, V is the velocity of the reaction at substrate concentration [S], V_{max} is the maximum velocity, n is the Hill constant, K_m is the substrate concentration at which the reaction velocity is 50% of V_{max}, and K_i is the dissociation constant of the substrate binding to the inhibitory region within the enzyme active site.

3. Results

3.1. In Vitro Metabolic Profiles of Catalposide Incubated with Human Hepatocytes and Intestinal Microsomes

LC-HRMS analysis of extracts after incubation of catalposide with human hepatocytes revealed three metabolites (M1–M3) and residual catalposide (Figure 1A). LC-HRMS analysis of reaction mixtures after incubation of catalposide with human intestinal microsomes in the presence of UDPGA yielded M2, M3, and a new metabolite M4 (Figure 1B).

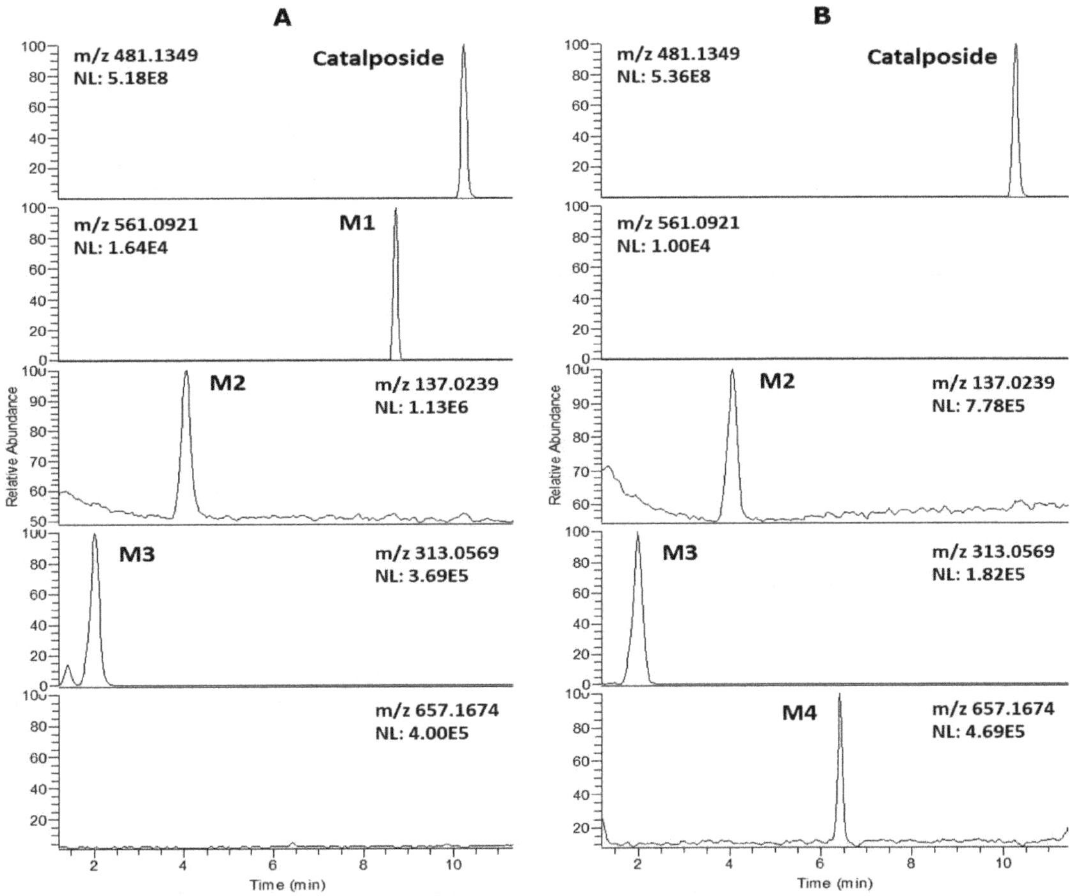

Figure 1. Extracted ion chromatograms of catalposide and its possible metabolites after incubation of 200 μM catalposide with (**A**) human hepatocytes for 2 h at 37 °C in a CO_2 incubator and (**B**) human intestinal microsomes in the presence of UDPGA at 37 °C for 1 h (mass accuracy: 5 ppm). The extracted ion chromatograms were reconstructed based on the $[M–H]^-$ ions: *m/z* 481.1349 for catalposide, *m/z* 561.0921 for M1 (catalposide sulfate), *m/z* 137.0239 for M2 (4-hydroxybenzoic acid), *m/z* 313.0569 for M3 (4-hydroxybenzoic acid glucuronide), and *m/z* 657.1674 for M4 (catalposide glucuronide).

The formulae, deprotonated molecular ions ($[M–H]^-$), mass errors, and retention times of catalposide and its four metabolites, M1–M4, are shown in Table 1. The four metabolite peaks were identified using the accurate mass values and the characteristic product ions of the product scan spectra (Table 1, Figure 2). The mass errors between the theoretical and observed *m/z* values for each metabolite were less than 5 ppm, indicating good correlations between the calculated theoretical masses and the experimentally observed masses obtained after full-scan MS analysis.

Table 1. Molecular formulae, deprotonated molecular ions ($[M–H]^-$), mass errors, retention times (t_R), and product ions of catalposide and its metabolites were identified after incubation of catalposide with human hepatocytes and intestinal microsomes.

Metabolite	Formula	Exact Mass $[M–H]^-$ (*m/z*)	Error (ppm)	t_R (min)	Product Ions (*m/z*)
Catalposide	$C_{22}H_{26}O_{12}$	481.1349	−0.6	10.26	319.0822, 205.0497, 137.0239
M1	$C_{22}H_{26}SO_{15}$	561.0921	0.2	8.74	481.1349, 319.0822, 205.0499, 137.0239
M2	$C_7H_6O_3$	137.0239	−3.6	4.07	93.0339
M3	$C_{13}H_{14}O_9$	313.0569	1.3	2.02	193.0345, 175.0240, 137.0239, 113.0239, 85.0283
M4	$C_{28}H_{34}O_{18}$	657.1674	0.3	6.41	481.1353, 319.0823, 205.0499, 175.0240, 137.0239, 113. 0238, 85.0283

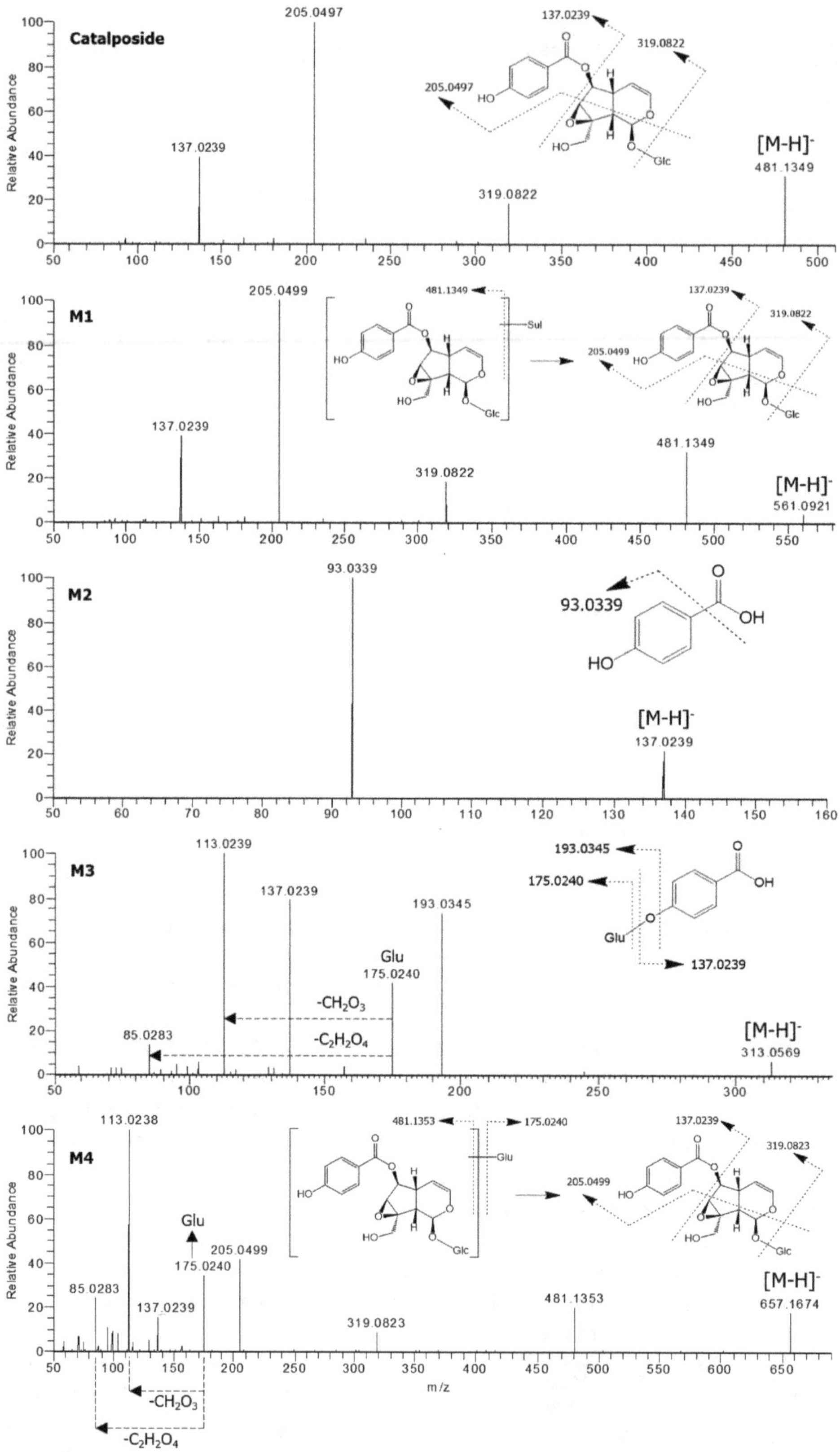

Figure 2. Product scan spectra of catalposide and its four metabolites, M1–M4 obtained via liquid chromatography-high resolution mass spectrometry (LC-HRMS) analysis of reaction mixtures obtained after incubation of catalposide with human intestinal microsomes in the presence of uridine 5′-diphosphoglucuronic acid (UDPGA) or human hepatocytes. Glc: glucose; Glu: glucuronosyl.

The product scan spectra of catalposide exhibiting the [M−H]$^-$ ion at *m/z* 481.1349 generated characteristic product ions at *m/z* 319.0822 (reflecting loss of glucose from the [M−H]$^-$ ion), *m/z* 205.0497 (loss of $C_5H_6O_3$ caused by the breakdown of the iridoid moiety of *m/z* 319.0822), and *m/z* 137.0239 (the 4-hydroxybenzoyl moiety) (Figure 2).

M1 exhibited an [M−H]$^-$ ion at *m/z* 561.0921, that is, 80 amu higher than the [M−H]$^-$ ion of catalposide, indicating that M1 was catalposide sulfate. The product scan spectra of M1 generated the characteristic product ions at *m/z* 481.1349 (loss of SO_3 from the [M−H]$^-$ ion), *m/z* 319.0822 (loss of glucose from *m/z* 481.1349), *m/z* 205.0499, and *m/z* 137.0239 (Figure 2). M1 was also formed from catalposide after incubation with human liver S9 fractions in the presence of PAPS. Thus, M1 was identified as catalposide sulfate.

M2 exhibited an [M−H]$^-$ ion at *m/z* 137.0239 and generated a characteristic product ion at *m/z* 93.0339 (reflecting loss of a carboxyl group from the [M−H]$^-$ ion)(Figure 2). M2 was identified as 4-hydroxybenzoic acid by comparison with the mass, retention time, and product ion of the authentic standard.

M3 exhibited an [M−H]$^-$ ion at *m/z* 313.0569, that is, 176 amu higher than the [M−H]$^-$ ion of M2 (4-hydroxybenzoic acid), reflecting glucuronidation of M2. In the product scan spectrum of M3, characteristic product ions were observed at *m/z* 137.0239 (reflecting loss of the glucuronosyl moiety from the [M−H]$^-$ ion), *m/z* 175.0240 (the glucuronosyl moiety), and *m/z* 113.0239 (loss of CO_2 and H_2O from *m/z* 175.0240) (Figure 2). Incubation of 4-hydroxybenzoic acid (M2) with human liver S9 fractions or intestinal microsomes in the presence of UDPGA yielded M3, which was identified as 4-hydroxybenzoic acid glucuronide by comparison with the mass, retention time, and product ions of the authentic standard.

M4 exhibited an [M−H]$^-$ ion at *m/z* 657.1674, that is, 176 amu higher than the [M−H]$^-$ ion of catalposide, reflecting catalposide glucuronidation. M4 yielded characteristic product ions at *m/z* 481.1353 (reflecting loss of the glucuronosyl moiety from the [M−H]$^-$ ion), *m/z* 319.0823 (loss of glucose from *m/z* 481.1353), *m/z* 205.0499, *m/z* 175.0240, *m/z* 113.0238, and *m/z* 85.0283 (Figure 2). Thus, M4 was identified as catalposide glucuronide.

The possible in vitro metabolic pathways of catalposide in humans are shown in Figure 3. Catalposide is metabolized to catalposide sulfate (M1), catalposide glucuronide (M4), and 4-hydroxybenzoic acid (M2); the latter is then further metabolized to 4-hydroxybenzoic acid glucuronide (M3).

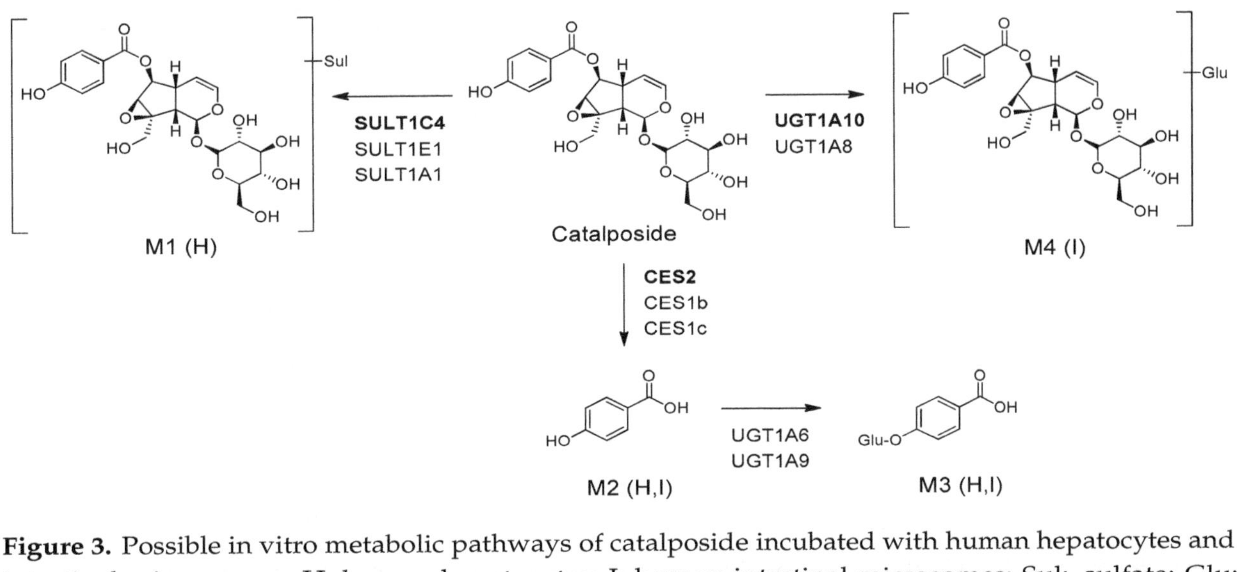

Figure 3. Possible in vitro metabolic pathways of catalposide incubated with human hepatocytes and intestinal microsomes. H: human hepatocytes; I: human intestinal microsomes; Sul: sulfate; Glu: glucuronic acid; CES: carboxylesterase; UGT: UDP-glucuronosyltransferase; SULT: sulfotransferase.

3.2. Characterization of Human SULT, UGT, and CES Enzymes Involved in Catalposide Metabolism

A screen using human cDNA-expressed SULTs 1A1*1, 1A1*2, 1A2, 1A3, 1B1, 1C2, 1C4, 1E1, and 2A1 to assess the formation of catalposide sulfate (M1) from catalposide identified possible roles for SULTs 1A1*1, 1A1*2, 1C4, and 1E1 (Figure 4).

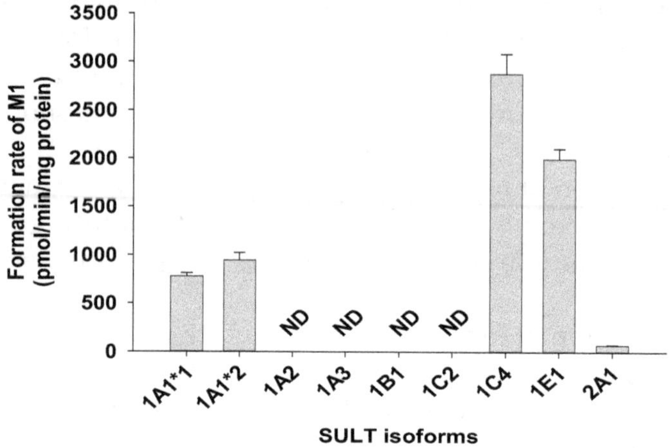

Figure 4. Rate of formation of catalposide sulfate (M1) from 150 μM catalposide by human cDNA-expressed SULT enzymes. All data are means ± SD (n = 3). ND: <32 pmol/min/mg protein.

The formation of catalposide sulfate from catalposide catalyzed by SULTs 1A1*1, 1A1*2, and 1E1 exhibited substrate inhibition kinetics, but the activities of SULT1C4 and pooled human liver S9 fractions fitted the Hill equation (Figure 5). The enzyme kinetic parameters for the formation of catalposide sulfate from catalposide are listed in Table 2. SULT1C4 exhibited a higher affinity for catalposide and more rapid sulfation than did SULT1A1*1, SULT1A1*2, and SULT1E1.

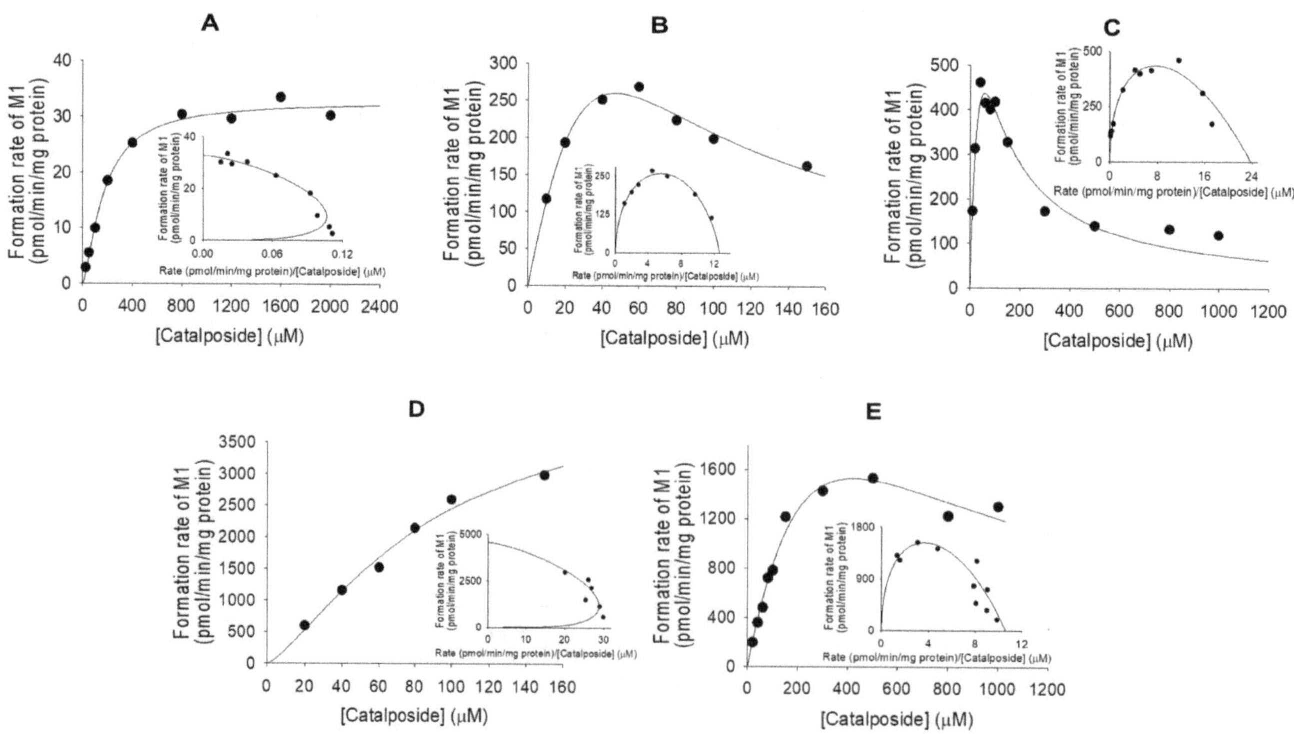

Figure 5. Michaelis–Menten plots of the sulfation of catalposide to catalposide sulfate (M1) by pooled human liver S9 fractions (**A**) and human cDNA-expressed SULT1A1*1 (**B**), SULT1A1*2 (**C**), SULT1C4 (**D**), and SULT1E1 (**E**). Insets: Eadie–Hofstee plots. Each data point represents the average of two determinations.

Table 2. Kinetic parameters for the formation of catalposide sulfate (M1) and catalposide glucuronide (M4) from catalposide in pooled human liver S9 fractions, intestinal microsomes, and human cDNA-expressed sulfotransferase (SULT) or UDP-glucuronosyltransferase (UGT) enzymes.

Enzyme	K_m (μM)	V_{max}	K_i (μM)	n	Cl_{int}
Sulfation of catalposide to M1					
SULT1A1*1	162.0	2046.8	13.7	-	12.6
SULT1A1*2	50.5	1203.2	65.5	-	23.8
SULT1C4	89.8	4576.2	-	1.4	51.0
SULT1E1	456.6	4840.0	391.4	-	10.6
Human liver S9 fractions	169.7	32.8	-	1.4	0.19
Glucuronidation of catalposide to M4					
UGT1A8	1230.1	48.7	-	0.9221	0.0396
UGT1A10	641.7	218.1	-	2.3	0.3399
Human intestinal microsomes	1341.3	106.2	-	-	0.0792

V_{max}: pmol/min/mg protein; Cl_{int}: μL/min/mg protein; n: Hill coefficient.

A screen using human cDNA-expressed UGTs 1A1, 1A3, 1A4, 1A6, 1A7, 1A8, 1A9, 1A10, 2B4, 2B7, 2B15, and 2B17 supersomes for the metabolism of 4-hydroxybenzoic acid (M2) to 4-hydroxybenzoic acid glucuronide (M3) identified possible roles of UGT1A6 and UGT1A9 (Figure 6A). The results show that 4-hydroxybenzoic acid glucuronide (M3) was produced on incubation of catalposide with human hepatocytes, liver S9 fractions, and intestinal microsomes.

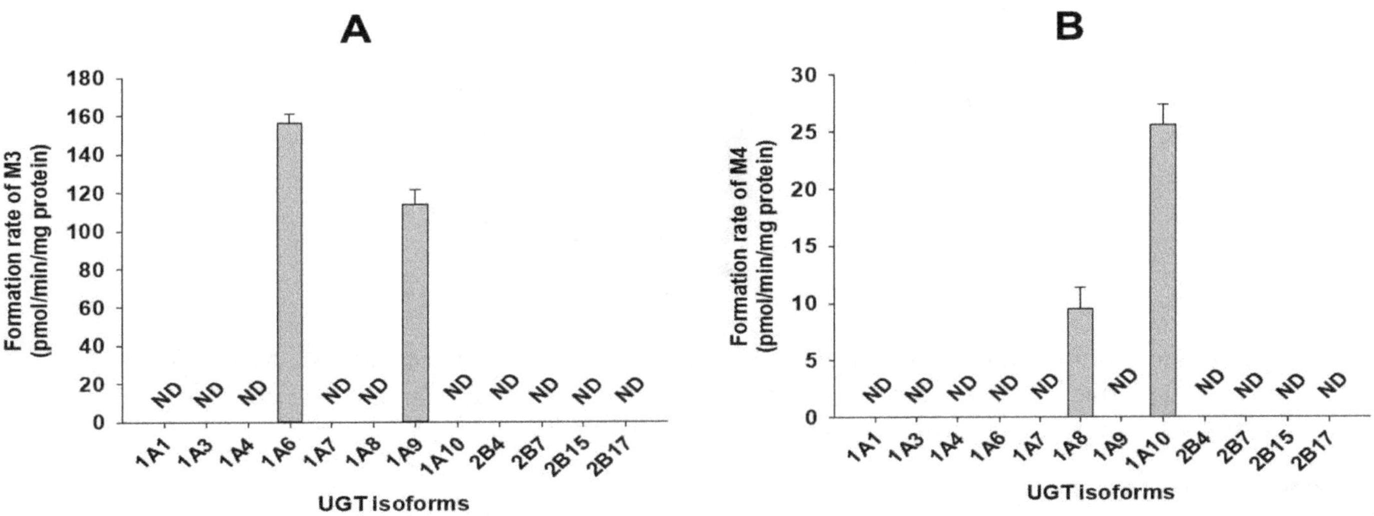

Figure 6. Rates of formation of (**A**) 4-hydroxybenzoic acid glucuronide (M3) from 500 μM 4-hydroxybenzoic acid (M2) and (**B**) catalposide glucuronide (M4) from 400 μM catalposide by human cDNA-expressed UGT enzymes. All data are means ± SD (n = 3). ND: <27 pmol/min/mg protein for M3, <0.83 pmol/min/mg protein for M4.

A screen using twelve human cDNA-expressed UGT supersomes, to assess the metabolism of catalposide to catalposide glucuronide (M4), identified possible roles of gastrointestinal tract-specific UGT1A8 and UGT1A10 (Figure 6B). The results show that catalposide glucuronide (M4) was produced after incubation of catalposide with pooled human intestinal microsomes, but not human liver S9 fractions.

Formation of catalposide glucuronide (M4) from catalposide by pooled human intestinal microsomes followed single enzyme kinetics; formation via UGT1A8 and UGT1A10 exhibited Hill equation kinetics (Figure 7, Table 2).

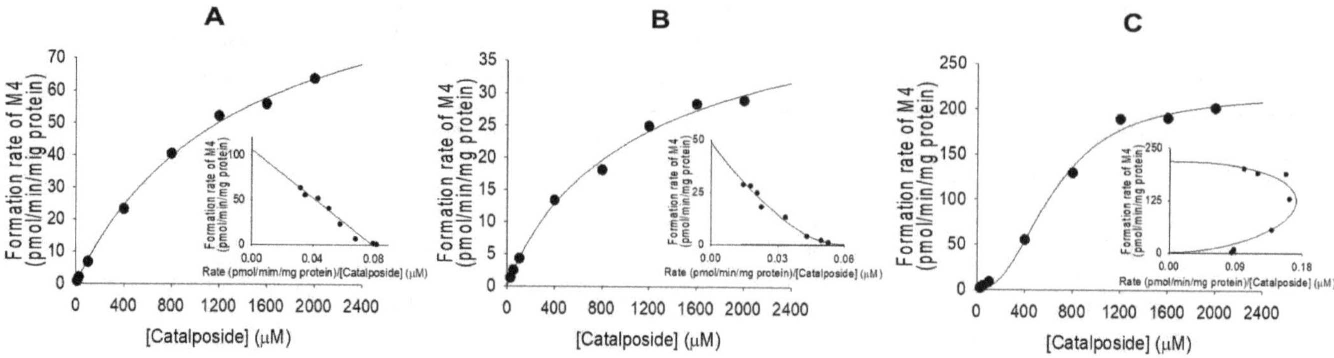

Figure 7. Michaelis–Menten plots for glucuronidation of catalposide to catalposide glucuronide (M4) by pooled human intestinal microsomes (**A**) and human cDNA-expressed UGT1A8 (**B**) and UGT1A10 (**C**). Insets: Eadie–Hofstee plots. Each data point represents the average of two determinations.

4-Hydroxybenzoic acid (M2) was formed from catalposide by pooled human liver S9 fractions; intestinal microsomes; and the CES1b, CES1c, and CES2 enzymes (Figure 8). The rate of formation of 4-hydroxybenzoic acid (M2) after incubation of catalposide with pooled human intestinal microsomes was higher than that after incubation with pooled human liver S9 fractions (Figure 8).

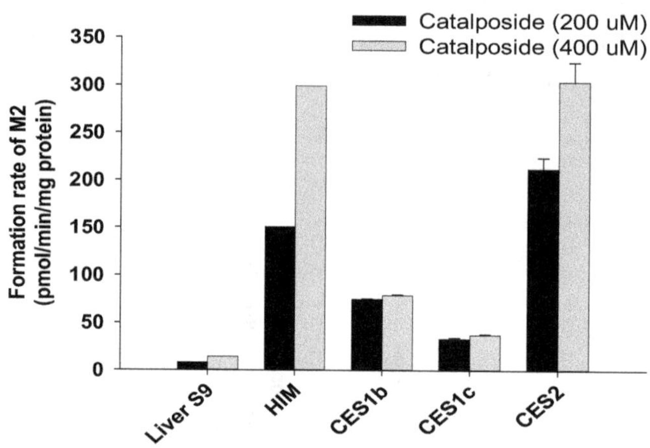

Figure 8. Rates of formation of 4-hydroxybenzoic acid (M2) from 200 μM and 400 μM catalposide in human liver S9 fractions (Liver S9); human intestinal microsomes (HIM); and human cDNA-expressed CES1b, CES1c, and CES2 enzymes. All data are means ± SD (n = 3).

4. Discussion

Catalposide was metabolized to catalposide sulfate (M1), catalposide glucuronide (M4), 4-hydroxybenzoic acid (M2), and M2 glucuronide (M3) by human hepatocytes or intestinal microsomes (Figure 3). On the basis of the kinetics of catalposide sulfate (M1) formation from catalposide catalyzed by human cDNA-expressed SULTs 1A1*1, 1A1*2, 1C4, and 1E1 (Figure 4, Table 2), we suggest that SULT1A1, SULT1C4, and SULT1E1 may play major roles in this metabolism. SULT1C4 exhibited higher activity (Cl_{int}, 51.0 μL/min/mg protein) in terms of catalposide sulfation than did SULT1A1*1, SULT1A1*2, or SULT1E1 (Cl_{int}, 10.6~23.8 μL/min/mg protein) (Table 2). SULT1C4 is highly expressed in the fetal lung and kidney, and at lower levels in the fetal heart, adult kidney, ovary, brain, and spinal cord [21–23]. SULT1A1 is the major hepatic SULT (53% of total hepatic SULTs), but is also present in substantial quantities in the small intestine (19% of total SULTs) [23,24]. SULT1E1 is expressed at relatively low levels in the liver (6% of total SULTs) and small intestine (8% of total SULTs), but is the most abundant enzyme in the lung (40% of total SULTs) [23,24]. Catalposide was metabolized to M1 by cytosolic SULTs of both hepatic and extrahepatic tissues. There may be inter-individual variability in catalposide sulfation, given that SULT1A1, SULT1C4, and SULT1E1 polymorphisms are known in humans [25]. SULT1A1, SULT1C4, and SULT1E1 are induced or inhibited by various drugs and chemicals [26,27]; therefore, co-administration of drugs that inhibit or induce expression of these enzymes may affect catalposide sulfation and thus catalposide pharmacokinetics.

Metabolism of catalposide to catalposide glucuronide (M4) was mediated by human cDNA-expressed UGT1A8 and UGT1A10 enzymes, which are confined to the gastrointestinal tract [28–32] (Figure 7), indicating that catalposide glucuronidation was gastrointestinal tract-specific; glucuronidation was not detected after incubation of catalposide with human hepatocytes and liver S9 fractions. UGT1A10-catalyzed catalposide glucuronidation was more extensive (Cl_{int}, 0.3399 μL/min/mg protein) than UGT1A8-catalyzed glucuronidation (Cl_{int}, 0.0396 μL/min/mg protein) (Table 2). UGT1A10 is more abundant than UGT1A8 in the small intestine (17.3% vs. 0.8% of total UGT protein) and colon (27.4% vs. 1.5% of total UGT protein) [32]. Thus, UGT1A10 may play the major role in glucuronidation of catalposide and UGT1A8 only a minor role. The human UGT1A8 and UGT1A10 enzymes are inhibited by various drugs [30,32–35]. Therefore, co-administration of drugs that inhibit or induce UGT1A8 and UGT1A10 may affect catalposide glucuronidation.

CES2, the predominant CES of the intestine, was more active in terms of hydrolysis of catalposide to 4-hydroxybenzoic acid (M2) than were the hepato-predominant CES1b and CES1c enzymes [32,36]. Thus, the rate of formation of 4-hydroxybenzoic acid (M2) was higher when catalposide was incubated with pooled human intestinal microsomes than with pooled human liver S9 fractions.

UGT1A6 and UGT1A9 play major roles in the formation of 4-hydroxybenzoic acid glucuronide (M3) from 4-hydroxybenzoic acid (Figure 6A). Abbas et al. [37] found that UGT1A9 played the major role in metabolism of 4-hydroxybenzoic acid to 4-hydroxybenzoic acid glucuronide. UGT1A6 and UGT1A9 are major enzymes of both the liver and intestine; therefore, 4-hydroxybenzoic acid glucuronide (M3) was identified after incubation of catalposide with either human hepatocytes or intestinal microsomes.

5. Conclusions

Catalposide was metabolized to catalposide sulfate (M1), 4-hydroxybenzoic acid (M2), M2 glucuronide (M3), and catalposide glucuronide (M4) via sulfation, glucuronidation, and hydrolysis, on incubation with human hepatocytes, liver S9 fractions, or intestinal microsomes. SULT1A1, SULT1C4, and SULT1E1 formed catalposide sulfate (M1) from catalposide. Gastrointestine-specific UGT1A8 and UGT1A10 played major roles in formation of catalposide glucuronide (M4). CES2 and CES1 catalyzed hydrolysis of catalposide to 4-hydroxybenzoic acid (M2), which was further metabolized to M2 glucuronide (M3) by UGT1A6 and UGT1A9. These results suggest that SULT1A1, SULT1C4, SULT1E1, UGT1A8, UGT1A10, CES2, and CES1 enzymes may play important roles in the pharmacokinetics and drug–drug interaction of catalposide in humans. The pharmacokinetics of catalposide may be dramatically affected by the co-administration of inhibitors or inducers of UGTs, CESs, or SULTs.

Author Contributions: Conceptualization, D.-K.H. and H.S.L.; methodology, D.-K.H., W.-G.C., Y.S., and S.K.; software, D.-K.H. and J.-H.K.; investigation, D.-K.H., W.-G.C., Y.S., and S.K.; data curation, D.-K.H., Y.S., J.-H.K., and H.S.L.; writing—original draft preparation, D.-K.H., J.-H.K., and Y.S.; writing—review and editing, Y.-Y.C., J.Y.L., H.C.K., and H.S.L.; supervision, H.S.L.; project administration, H.S.L.; funding acquisition, H.C.K. and H.S.L.

References

1. Harput, U.S.; Saracoglu, I.; Inoue, M.; Ogihara, Y. Phenylethanoid and Iridoid Glycosides from Veronica persica. *Chem. Pharm. Bull.* **2002**, *50*, 869–871. [CrossRef] [PubMed]
2. Harput, U.S.; Saracoglu, I.; Nagatsu, A.; Ogihara, Y. Iridoid Glucosides from Veronica hederifolia. *Chem. Pharm. Bull.* **2002**, *50*, 1106–1108. [CrossRef] [PubMed]
3. Harput, U.; Varel, M.; Nagatsu, A.; Saracoglu, I. Acylated iridoid glucosides from Veronica anagallis-aquatica. *Phytochemistry* **2004**, *65*, 2135–2139. [CrossRef] [PubMed]
4. Oh, H.; Pae, H.O.; Oh, G.S.; Lee, S.Y.; Chai, K.Y.; Song, C.E.; Kwon, T.O.; Chung, H.T.; Lee, H.S. Inhibition of Inducible Nitric Oxide Synthesis by Catalposide from Catalpa ovata. *Planta Med.* **2002**, *68*, 685–689. [CrossRef] [PubMed]

5. An, S.; Pae, H.; Oh, G.; Choi, B.; Jeong, S.; Jang, S.; Oh, H.; Kwon, T.; Song, C.E.; Chung, H. Inhibition of TNF-α, IL-1β, and IL-6 productions and NF-κB activation in lipopolysaccharide-activated RAW 264.7 macrophages by catalposide, an iridoid glycoside isolated from Catalpa ovata G. Don (Bignoniaceae). *Int. Immunopharmacol.* **2002**, *2*, 1173–1181. [CrossRef]
6. Moon, M.K.; Choi, B.M.; Oh, G.S.; Pae, H.O.; Kim, J.D.; Oh, H.; Oh, C.S.; Kim, D.H.; Rho, Y.D.; Shin, M.K.; et al. Catalposide protects Neuro 2A cells from hydrogen peroxide-induced cytotoxicity via the expression of heme oxygenase-1. *Toxicol. Lett.* **2003**, *145*, 46–54. [CrossRef]
7. Kim, S.W.; Choi, S.C.; Choi, E.Y.; Kim, K.S.; Oh, J.M.; Lee, H.J.; Oh, H.M.; Kim, S.; Oh, B.S.; Kimm, K.C.; et al. Catalposide, a Compound Isolated from Catalpa Ovata, Attenuates Induction of Intestinal Epithelial Proinflammatory Gene Expression and Reduces the Severity of Trinitrobenzene Sulfonic Acid-Induced Colitis in Mice. *Inflamm. Bowel Dis.* **2004**, *10*, 564–572. [CrossRef]
8. Kupeli, E.; Harput, U.S.; Varel, M.; Yesilada, E.; Saracoglu, I. Bioassay-guided isolation of iridoid glucosides with antinociceptive and anti-inflammatory activities from *Veronica anagallis-aquatica* L. *J. Ethnopharmacol.* **2005**, *102*, 170–176. [CrossRef]
9. Lu, Q.; Sun, Y.; Shu, Y.; Tan, S.; Yin, L.; Guo, Y.; Tang, L. HSCCC Separation of the Two Iridoid Glycosides and Three Phenolic Compounds from Veronica ciliata and Their in Vitro Antioxidant and Anti-Hepatocarcinoma Activities. *Molecules* **2016**, *21*, 1234. [CrossRef]
10. Kwak, J.H.; Kim, H.J.; Lee, K.H.; Kang, S.C.; Zee, O.P. Antioxidative iridoid glycosides and phenolic compounds from Veronica peregrina. *Arch. Pharmacal Res.* **2009**, *32*, 207–213. [CrossRef]
11. Saracoglu, I.; Harput, U.S. In vitro cytotoxic activity and structure activity relationships of iridoid glucosides derived from Veronica species. *Phytother. Res.* **2012**, *26*, 148–152. [CrossRef] [PubMed]
12. Lee, J.H.; Jun, H.J.; Hoang, M.H.; Jia, Y.; Han, X.H.; Lee, D.H.; Lee, H.J.; Hwang, B.Y.; Lee, S.J. Catalposide is a natural agonistic ligand of peroxisome proliferator-activated receptor-α. *Biochem. Biophys. Res. Commun.* **2012**, *422*, 568–572. [CrossRef] [PubMed]
13. Tan, S.; Lu, Q.; Shu, Y.; Sun, Y.; Chen, F.; Tang, L. Iridoid Glycosides Fraction Isolated from Veronica ciliata Fisch. Protects against Acetaminophen-Induced Liver Injury in Mice. *Evid. Based Complement. Alternat. Med.* **2017**, *2017*. [CrossRef] [PubMed]
14. Ji, H.Y.; Lee, H.W.; Kim, H.H.; Lee, H.I.; Chung, H.T.; Lee, H.S. Determination of Catalposide in Rat Plasma by Liquid Chromatography-Mass Spectrometry. *Anal. Lett.* **2003**, *36*, 2999–3009. [CrossRef]
15. Jeong, H.U.; Kwon, M.; Lee, Y.; Yoo, J.S.; Shin, D.H.; Song, I.S.; Lee, H.S. Organic anion transporter 3- and organic anion transporting polypeptides 1B1- and 1B3-mediated transport of catalposide. *Drug Des. Dev. Ther.* **2015**, *9*, 643–653.
16. Choi, W.G.; Kim, J.H.; Kim, D.K.; Lee, Y.; Yoo, J.S.; Shin, D.H.; Lee, H.S. Simultaneous Determination of Chlorogenic Acid Isomers and Metabolites in Rat Plasma Using LC-MS/MS and Its Application to A Pharmacokinetic Study Following Oral Administration of Stauntonia Hexaphylla Leaf Extract (YRA-1909) to Rats. *Pharmaceutics* **2018**, *10*, 143. [CrossRef] [PubMed]
17. Cerny, M.A. Prevalence of Non-Cytochrome P450-Mediated Metabolism in Food and Drug Administration-Approved Oral and Intravenous Drugs: 2006–2015. *Drug Metab. Dispos.* **2016**, *44*, 1246–1252. [CrossRef] [PubMed]
18. Foti, R.S.; Dalvie, D.K. Cytochrome P450 and non-Cytochrome P450 Oxidative Metabolism: Contributions to the Pharmacokinetics, Safety and Efficacy of Xenobiotics. *Drug Metab. Dispos.* **2016**, *44*, 1229–1245. [CrossRef] [PubMed]
19. Kim, J.H.; Hwang, D.K.; Moon, J.Y.; Lee, Y.; Yoo, J.S.; Shin, D.H.; Lee, H.S. Multiple UDP-Glucuronosyltransferase and Sulfotransferase Enzymes are Responsible for the Metabolism of Verproside in Human Liver Preparations. *Molecules* **2017**, *22*, 670. [CrossRef] [PubMed]
20. Jeong, H.U.; Kim, J.H.; Kong, T.Y.; Choi, W.G.; Lee, H.S. Comparative metabolism of honokiol in mouse, rat, dog, monkey, and human hepatocytes. *Arch. Pharmacal Res.* **2016**, *39*, 516–530. [CrossRef] [PubMed]
21. Suiko, M.; Kurogi, K.; Hashiguchi, T.; Sakakibara, Y.; Liu, M.C. Updated perspectives on the cytosolic sulfotransferases (SULTs) and SULT-mediated sulfation. *Biosci. Biotech. Biochem.* **2017**, *81*, 63–72. [CrossRef] [PubMed]

22. Guidry, A.L.; Tibbs, Z.E.; Runge-Morris, M.; Falany, C.N. Expression, Purification, and Characterization of Human Cytosolic Sulfotransferase (Sult) 1c4. *Horm. Mol. Boil. Clin. Investig.* **2017**, *29*, 27–36. [CrossRef] [PubMed]
23. Coughtrie, M.W. Function and organization of the human cytosolic sulfotransferase (SULT) family. *Chem. Interact.* **2016**, *259*, 2–7. [CrossRef] [PubMed]
24. Riches, Z.; Stanley, E.L.; Bloomer, J.C.; Coughtrie, M.W.H. Quantitative Evaluation of the Expression and Activity of Five Major Sulfotransferases (SULTs) in Human Tissues: The SULT "Pie". *Drug Metab. Dispos.* **2009**, *37*, 2255–2261. [CrossRef] [PubMed]
25. Marto, N.; Morello, J.; Monteiro, E.C.; Pereira, S.A.; Morello, J.B. Implications of Sulfotransferase Activity in Interindividual Variability in Drug Response: Clinical Perspective on Current Knowledge. *Drug Metab. Rev.* **2017**, *49*, 357–371. [CrossRef] [PubMed]
26. James, M.O.; Ambadapadi, S. Interactions of cytosolic sulfotransferases with xenobiotics. *Drug Metab. Rev.* **2013**, *45*, 401–414. [CrossRef] [PubMed]
27. Zhou, T.; Chen, Y.; Huang, C.; Chen, G. Caffeine Induction of Sulfotransferases in Rat Liver and Intestine. *J. Appl. Toxicol.* **2012**, *32*, 804–809. [CrossRef] [PubMed]
28. Lv, X.; Zhang, J.B.; Hou, J.; Dou, T.Y.; Ge, G.B.; Hu, W.Z.; Yang, L. Chemical probes fpr human UDP-glucuronosyltransferases: A comprehensive review. *Biotechnol. J.* **2019**, *14*. [CrossRef] [PubMed]
29. Wang, H.; Cao, G.; Wang, G.; Hao, H. Regulation of Mammalian UDP-Glucuronosyltransferases. *Curr. Drug Metab.* **2018**, *19*, 490–501. [CrossRef]
30. Meech, R.; Hu, D.G.; McKinnon, R.A.; Mubarokah, S.N.; Haines, A.Z.; Nair, P.C.; Rowland, A.; MacKenzie, P.I. The UDP-Glycosyltransferase (UGT) Superfamily: New Members, New Functions, and Novel Paradigms. *Physiol. Rev.* **2019**, *99*, 1153–1222. [CrossRef]
31. Fallon, J.K.; Neubert, H.; Goosen, T.C.; Smith, P.C. Targeted Precise Quantification of 12 Human Recombinant Uridine-Diphosphate Glucuronosyl Transferase 1A and 2B Isoforms Using Nano-Ultra-High-Performance Liquid Chromatography/Tandem Mass Spectrometry with Selected Reaction Monitoring. *Drug Metab. Dispos.* **2013**, *41*, 2076–2080. [CrossRef] [PubMed]
32. Argikar, U.A.; Potter, P.M.; Hutzler, J.M.; Marathe, P.H. Challenges and opportunities with Non-CYP enzymes aldehyde oxidase, carboxylesterase, and UDP-Glucuronosyltransferase: Focus on reaction phenotyping and prediction of human clearance. *AAPS J.* **2016**, *18*, 1391–1405. [CrossRef] [PubMed]
33. Kiang, T.K.; Ensom, M.H.; Chang, T.K. UDP-glucuronosyltransferases and clinical drug-drug interactions. *Pharmacol. Ther.* **2005**, *106*, 97–132. [CrossRef]
34. Miners, J.O.; Mackenzie, P.I.; Knights, K.M. The prediction of drug-glucuronidation parameters in humans: UDP-glucuronosyltransferase enzyme-selective substrate and inhibitor probes for reaction phenotyping and in vitro-in vivo extrapolation of drug clearance and drug-drug interaction potential. *Drug Metab. Rev.* **2010**, *42*, 196–208. [CrossRef]
35. Parkinson, A.; Kazmi, F.; Buckley, D.B.; Yerino, P.; Ogilvie, B.W.; Paris, B.L. System-Dependent Outcomes during the Evaluation of Drug Candidates as Inhibitors of Cytochrome P450 (CYP) and Uridine Diphosphate Glucuronosyltransferase (UGT) Enzymes: Human Hepatocytes versus Liver Microsomes versus Recombinant Enzymes. *Drug Metab. Pharmacok.* **2010**, *25*, 16–27. [CrossRef]
36. Chen, F.; Zhang, B.; Parker, R.B.; Laizure, S.C. Clinical implications of genetic variation in carboxylesterase drug metabolism. *Expert Opin. Drug Metab. Toxicol.* **2018**, *14*, 131–142. [CrossRef]
37. Abbas, S.; Greige-Gerges, H.; Karam, N.; Piet, M.H.; Netter, P.; Magdalou, J. Metabolism of Parabens (4-Hydroxybenzoic Acid Esters) by Hepatic Esterases and UDP-Glucuronosyltransferases in Man. *Drug Metab. Pharmacok.* **2010**, *25*, 568–577. [CrossRef]

8

Pharmacokinetic and Toxicodynamic Characterization of a Novel Doxorubicin Derivative

Samaa Alrushaid [1], Casey L. Sayre [1,2], Jaime A. Yáñez [3], M. Laird Forrest [4], Sanjeewa N. Senadheera [4], Frank J. Burczynski [1], Raimar Löbenberg [5] and Neal M. Davies [5,*]

1. College of Pharmacy, Rady Faculty of Health Sciences, University of Manitoba, Winnipeg, MB R3E 0T5, Canada; umalrush@myumanitoba.ca (S.A.); csayre@roseman.edu (C.L.S.); Frank.Burczynski@umanitoba.ca (F.J.B.)
2. College of Pharmacy, Roseman University of Health Sciences, South Jordan, UT 84096, USA
3. YARI International Group, New Brunswick, NJ 08901 and INDETEC Corp., Lima, Peru; jaimeyanez@gmail.com
4. Department of Pharmaceutical Chemistry, School of Pharmacy, University of Kansas, Lawrence, KS 66047, USA; mforrest@ku.edu (M.L.F.); nilendrasns@yahoo.com (S.N.S.)
5. Faculty of Pharmacy and Pharmaceutical Sciences, University of Alberta, Edmonton, AB T6G 2R3, Canada; raimar@ualberta.ca

* Correspondence: ndavies@ualberta.ca

Abstract: Doxorubicin (Dox) is an effective anti-cancer medication with poor oral bioavailability and systemic toxicities. DoxQ was developed by conjugating Dox to the lymphatically absorbed antioxidant quercetin to improve Dox's bioavailability and tolerability. The purpose of this study was to characterize the pharmacokinetics and safety of Dox after intravenous (IV) and oral (PO) administration of DoxQ or Dox (10 mg/kg) and investigate the intestinal lymphatic delivery of Dox after PO DoxQ administration in male Sprague–Dawley rats. Drug concentrations in serum, urine, and lymph were quantified by HPLC with fluorescence detection. DoxQ intact IV showed a 5-fold increase in the area under the curve (AUC)—18.6 $\pm$ 1.98 compared to 3.97 $\pm$ 0.71 µg * h/mL after Dox—and a significant reduction in the volume of distribution (V_{ss}): 0.138 $\pm$ 0.015 versus 6.35 $\pm$ 1.06 L/kg. The fraction excreted unchanged in urine (f_e) of IV DoxQ and Dox was ~5% and ~11%, respectively. Cumulative amounts of Dox in the mesenteric lymph fluid after oral DoxQ were twice as high as Dox in a mesenteric lymph duct cannulation rat model. Oral DoxQ increased AUC of Dox by ~1.5-fold compared to after oral Dox. Concentrations of β-N-Acetylglucosaminidase (NAG) but not cardiac troponin (cTnI) were lower after IV DoxQ than Dox. DoxQ altered the pharmacokinetic disposition of Dox, improved its renal safety and oral bioavailability, and is in part transported through intestinal lymphatics.

Keywords: doxorubicin; quercetin; pharmacokinetics; bioavailability; lymphatics transport; toxicity

1. Introduction

Doxorubicin (Dox) is an effective anti-cancer medication that has been clinically used to treat a variety of cancers including breast, ovarian, and lymphoma [1–5]. Despite the clinical effectiveness of Dox, its use is limited by off-target adverse effects, particularly dose-related cardiotoxicity and renal toxicity, which involve free radical formation and tissue damage. Dox formulations that are pegylated and in liposomes are utilized in medications, including Doxil™ and Caelyx™ [6]. Pegylated (polyethylene glycol coated) liposome-encapsulated forms of Dox result in an increased concentration of Dox in the skin and a side effect called palmar plantar erythrodysesthesia or hand–foot syndrome [7]. Non-pegylated liposomal Dox called Myocet™ does not have a polyethylene glycol coating, and therefore does not result in the same rate of hand–foot syndrome. This liposomal encapsulation of Dox limits but does not eliminate the cardiotoxic effects of the drug. This damage is caused by the generation of reactive oxidative species (ROS) such as superoxide and hydrogen peroxide upon the reduction of Dox to form electron-deficient semiquinone [8]. Various additional drug delivery approaches have been undertaken to overcome the toxicity limitations of Dox, such as utilization of micelles [9], synthetic polymer conjugates [10], and antibody targeted carriers [11], with varied degrees of success. We have previously demonstrated that hyaluronan, a biopolymeric nanocarrier, improves survival and reduces the toxicity of Dox in xenografts of human breast cancer through the localization of Dox into the lymphatics [8].

Dox is a substrate of both the P–glycoprotein (P–gp) efflux pump [12] and cytochrome P450 metabolic enzymes [13], both of which contribute to its overall disposition, poor oral absorption, and low oral bioavailability. For this reason, Dox is only currently available as a parenteral treatment administered intravenously. We have previously reported the synthesis of a Dox-quercetin derivative designed to overcome P–gp efflux and CYP inhibition [14] as quercetin is a natural flavonoid that exhibits inhibitory effects on CYP3A4 and P–gp [15] and an antioxidant that scavenges free radicals. Our in vitro investigation of DoxQ [14] revealed that both Dox and quercetin are released from the conjugate over time. Furthermore, DoxQ inhibited CYP3A4, a major metabolic enzyme involved in the first pass effect, and demonstrated higher cellular uptake by P–gp-positive (MDCK–MDR) cells compared to free Dox. The inhibitory effects of DoxQ on CYP3A4 and P–gp may improve the oral absorption and bioavailability of Dox in vivo. Additionally, DoxQ retained anti-cancer activity in a triple negative murine breast cancer cell line and was less toxic to both rat and human cardiomyocytes. The cardioprotective mechanism of DoxQ involved scavenging ROS, suppression of oxidative stress, and cardiac hypertrophy markers, and also inhibitory effects on CYP1B1, all of which contribute to Dox's induced cardiotoxicity. Taken together, the in vitro results of DoxQ showed promise at mitigating the cardiotoxicity of Dox and may also mitigate its poor oral bioavailability in vivo by inhibiting CYP3A4 and P–gp [14]. The antioxidant effects of DoxQ may also mitigate the renal toxicity induced by Dox and improve its overall tolerability in vivo.

In addition to quercetin's antioxidant activity and inhibitory effects on CYP3A4 and P–gp, it is naturally absorbed into intestinal lymphatics after gastric or intraduodenal administration [16–18]; this property may be utilized as a novel strategy to deliver Dox into lymphatics. Following oral administration, molecules and drugs are either absorbed from the intestinal mucosa into the blood stream via the hepatic portal vein or into lymphatics via the intestinal lymphatic pathway. Most small molecules and drugs administered orally enter systemic circulation via blood capillaries and become subject to hepatic metabolism before entering the vasculature. In contrast, highly lipophilic molecules and macromolecules such as proteins associate with chylomicrons in the intestinal mucosa and enter systemic circulation via the intestinal lymphatics pathway [19]. These lipophilic molecules and macromolecules are absorbed via lymphatic capillaries, which collect into the mesenteric lymph duct, followed by the thoracic lymph duct, and then drain into systemic circulation at the junction of the left subclavian and left jugular veins [19,20]. Therefore, molecules that are absorbed via the intestinal lymphatic pathway enter systemic circulation without passing through the liver. This alternative absorptive pathway may be of particular importance in drug delivery and may serve as a novel drug delivery approach to minimize the first-pass effect while increasing lymphatic exposure and ultimately improving overall systemic drug exposure [21]. Lipophilic drugs with LogP > 5 and solubility of >50 mg per g in long-chain triglyceride will likely have preferential absorption towards lymphatics owing to their ability to incorporate with intestinal lipoproteins [19]. If the drug of interest does not meet these criteria, it is also possible to alter the physicochemical properties of a small drug molecule by chemically modifying its lipophilicity, utilizing a lipid-based drug delivery system or designing a lipophilic prodrug where the parent drug is chemically conjugated to a lipophilic moiety via a linker that can be easily cleaved in vivo [19–22]. In this study, we utilized a novel Dox–quercetin conjugate where quercetin is designed to act as a lymphatically targeted carrier and may facilitate the intestinal transport of Dox into systemic circulation after oral administration and may also affect its disposition as well as overall systemic exposure after intravenous administration.

In the light of the studies discussed above and our promising DoxQ observations in vitro, this study was conducted to investigate the feasibility of utilizing the antioxidant quercetin as a lymphatically targeted carrier for Dox with the potential to improve its disposition, oral bioavailability, and tolerability in vivo. We hypothesize that the presence of quercetin in DoxQ, intact or when released from the conjugate, will act as a carrier to transport Dox into lymphatics, at least partially, thus bypassing systemic circulation and increasing the overall bioavailability of Dox. The release of quercetin from DoxQ will likely have a beneficial effect and limit the cardiotoxic and renal side effects of doxorubicin. In addition, the synthesis and change in physicochemical properties of DoxQ may alter its pharmacokinetics and metabolism; the release of quercetin from DoxQ or DoxQ intact may also have effects on CYP3A4 and P–gp, which could further augment the disposition and bioavailability of Dox in vivo. Here, the acute in vivo disposition, safety, and lymphatic uptake of DoxQ are characterized for the first time. The pharmacokinetics, toxicodynamics, and intestinal lymphatic absorption of DoxQ in comparison to free Dox are examined in a rat model. Our results demonstrate that DoxQ improves the disposition of Dox and its oral bioavailability and safety, and is partially transported via lymphatics.

2. Materials and Methods

2.1. Chemicals and Reagents

Doxorubicin, duanorubicin, cycloheximide, PEG-400, and DMSO were purchased from Sigma (St. Louis, MO, USA). Analytical grade formic acid and HPLC grade acetonitrile were purchased from Fisher Scientific (Ottawa, ON, Canada). Ultrapure water from a Milli-Q® system (Millipore, Billerica, MA, USA) was used for the mobile phase. HPLC columns, vials, inserts, and 0.2 um nylon filter membranes were purchased from Phenomenex® (Torrance, CA, USA). Silastic® laboratory tubing was purchased from the Dow Corning Corporation (Midland, MI, USA). Intramedic® polyethylene tubing was purchased from Becton Dickinson Primary Care Diagnostics, Becton Dickinson and Company (Sparks, MD, USA). Monoject® 23 gauge (0.6 × 25 mm) polypropylene hub hypodermic needles were purchased from Sherwood Medical (St. Louis, MO, USA). Synthetic absorbable surgical sutures were purchased from Wilburn Medical US (Kernesville, NC, USA). Sterile heparin/50% dextrose catheter lock solution and blunt needles were obtained from SAI Infusion Technologies, Strategic Applications (Lake Villa, IL, USA).

2.2. Synthesis of the DoxQ Conjugate

DoxQ was synthesized by conjugating Dox to quercetin via a glycine linker, as previously described [14].

2.3. Physicochemical Properties

LogP and LogS values of DoxQ were predicted using an online computer software (VCCLAB, Virtual Computational Chemistry Laboratory) [23,24]. pKa, logP, logD at pH 7.4, intrinsic solubility, and solubility at pH 7.4 were calculated using MarvinSketch v. 17.2.20.0 (ChemAxon Ltd., Cambridge, MA, USA), pKa and logP were calculated using GastroPlus v. 9.0.0007 (Simulations Plus, Inc., Lancaster, CA, USA). Portions of these results were generated by GastroPlus™ software (Version 8.0) provided by Simulations Plus, Inc. (Lancaster, CA, USA). The melting point of DoxQ was experimentally determined by MEL-TEMPII melting point apparatus from Laboratory Devices (Holliston, MA, USA).

2.4. Analytical System and Conditions

The analytical method described in [25] was adapted with some modifications. The HPLC system used was a Shimadzu LC-2010A (Kyoto, Japan) with Fluorescence RF-535 detector at 470/560 nm (excitation/emission) wavelengths. Separation was achieved using C18 Phenomenex

Kintex® (Torrance, CA, USA) column (250 μm, 250 × 4.6 mm) for serum and lymph samples or (2.6 μm, 100 × 4.60 mm) joined to (250 μm, 250 × 4.6 mm) for urine samples. The mobile phase was prepared by mixing acetonitrile with 0.1% formic acid in water (35:65, *v*/*v*), which was filtered through 0.2 μm nylon filter and degassed under reduced pressure prior to use. The separation was carried out isocratically at ambient temperature (22 ± 1 °C) with a flow rate of 0.6 mL/min. Shimadzu EZStart (Version 7.4) software was used for data collection and integration. On the day of the analysis, samples were prepared and injected into the HPLC system.

2.4.1. Preparation of Standard Solutions

Stock solutions of Dox (1 mg/mL) and the internal standard (IS) duanorubicin (1 mg/mL) were prepared in methanol, protected from light and stored at −20 °C between uses for no longer than one week. Using the stock solutions of Dox, calibration standards in serum, urine, and lymph were freshly prepared by sequential dilution with blank rat serum, urine, and lymph. A series of concentrations were obtained, particularly 0.1, 0.5, 1.0, 10.0 and 100 μg/mL.

Stock solutions of intact DoxQ (10 mg/mL) were freshly prepared in DMSO and protected from light. Calibration standards of DoxQ in serum and urine were prepared by serial dilution with blank rat serum or urine to yield concentrations of 1, 10, 20, and 100 μg/mL. The final concentration of DMSO in serum and urine spiked standards did not exceed 1%.

2.4.2. Calibration Curves

Calibration curves of Dox and DoxQ were obtained by plotting the peak area ratio of Dox or DoxQ to the internal standard (duanorubicin) versus calibration standards concentration of Dox or DoxQ through the unweighted least squares linear regression.

2.5. *Animals and Surgical Procedures*

Male Sprague–Dawley rats (250–300 g) were obtained from Charles River Labs (Montreal, QC, Canada) and given food (Purina Rat Chow 5001) and water ad libitum in the animal facility for at least three days before use. Rats were housed in temperature-controlled rooms with a 12 h light/dark cycle. The animal ethics protocol was revised and approved by the Bannatyne Campus Animal Care Committee at the University of Manitoba, (protocol #16-004, approved 29 March 2016).

2.6. *Pharmacokinetic Study*

Eight surgically modified, with exposed jugular vein catheterization (polyurethane–silastic blended catheter), adult male Sprague–Dawley rats (average weight: 250 g) were purchased from Charles River Laboratories (Saint-Constant, QC, Canada). The cannula was flushed daily with a sterile heparin/50% dextrose catheter lock solution to maintain the patency of the cannula, as advised in the technical sheet supplied with the animals from Charles River. Each animal was placed in a separate metabolic cage overnight and fasted for 12 h before dosing. On the day of experiment, the animals were dosed either intravenously or orally with Dox (10 mg/kg) or equimolar DoxQ (n = 4 for each treatment group). Both Dox and DoxQ were freshly reconstituted in 3% DMSO and 97% PEG-400 prior to dosing. Animals received water ad libitum pre- and post-dosing, and food (Purina Rat Chow 5001) was provided 2 h post-dosing. Doses were selected based on previous use in similar pharmacokinetic studies [13,15] and sensitivity of analytical instrumentation. Serial blood samples (0.30 mL) were collected at 0, 1 min, 15 min, and 30 min, then 1, 2, 4, 6, 12, 24, 48 and 72 h after IV administration. The same blood collection time points were applied following oral administration except for 1 min. At 72 h after administration, the animals were euthanized and exsanguinated. Immediately after all the blood collection time points (except the terminal point); the cannula was flushed with the same volume of 0.9% saline to replenish the collected blood volume. The dead volume of the cannula was filled with a small volume (~0.15 mL) of heparinized lock solution after each blood draw to maintain the patency of the cannula. The samples were collected into regular polypropylene microcentrifuge tubes, centrifuged at 15,000 rpm for 5 min (Beckman Microfuge centrifuge, Beckman Coulter Inc., Fullerton, CA, USA), and the serum collected and stored at −20 °C until further sample preparation for HPLC analysis. Urine samples were also collected at 0, 2, 6, 12, 24, 48 and 72 h following Dox or DoxQ administration. The exact urine volume of each sample was recorded then stored at −20 °C until further sample preparation for HPLC analysis.

2.7. *Intestinal Lymphatic Drug Delivery*

The intestinal transport of DoxQ via lymphatics was examined in vivo by two methods. In the first method, mesenteric lymph cannulated rat model was used to directly measure the concentrations of Dox in the lymph after administration of DoxQ or Dox. In the second method cycloheximide, a chylomicron blocking drug, was administered intraperitoneally prior to oral administration of DoxQ or Dox then concentrations of Dox were measured in serum to indirectly assess lymphatic transport.

2.7.1. Mesenteric Lymph Cannulation Surgery

Six male Sprague–Dawley rats (~300 g) were obtained from Charles River Labs (Montreal, QC, Canada) and given food (Purina Rat Chow 5001) and water ad libitum in the animal facility for at least three days before use. On the day of surgical operation, rats were anesthetized by isoflurane and the abdominal hair was shaved. Rats were maintained under inhaled anesthesia on a warm surgical table. A ~2.5 cm abdominal midline skin incision was made and extended through the musculature using blunt dissection beginning the incision at a point just above the xyphoid cartilage and proceeding distally. The intestine and liver were retracted using surgical retractors to locate the superior mesenteric lymph duct, which is filled with opaque white chyle. The lymph duct was isolated from the surrounding connective tissue and a small incision was made with a bent 23 G needle in the ventral wall of the lymph. A catheter was inserted through the incision and secured by placing a small cellulose patch with a drop of Vetbond™ over the point of insertion into the lymph duct. When a gradual and continuous flow of lymph was observed, an initial lymph sample was collected into a normal microtube. A single dose (10 mg/kg) of DoxQ (n = 3) or Dox (n = 3) was administered by oral gavage while the rat was under anesthesia. Thereafter, lymph samples were collected over one hour after dosing. The animals were euthanized after the last lymph sample collection.

2.7.2. Lymph Blockage by Cycloheximide

Cycloheximide (3 mg/kg) was administered intraperitoneally (IP) to jugular vein cannulated male Sprague–Dawley rats (~250 g) (n = 4) 1.5 h prior to oral administration of DoxQ to block the formation of chylomicrons in lymph [26–35]. DoxQ was then administered orally (10 mg/kg). Blood samples were collected at 0 h, 15 min, 30 min, 1 h, 2 h, 6 h, 12 h, 24 h and 48 h. The animals were euthanized after the last blood sample collection.

2.8. *Treatment of Biological Samples for Analysis*

2.8.1. Serum and Lymph Sample Preparation

To a 100 µL serum or lymph sample (except 0 h), 10 µM of the internal standard (duanorubicin) was added then vortexed for 30 s (Vortex Genie–2, VWR Scientific, West Chester, PA, USA). One milliliter of cold HPLC grade acetonitrile (pre-stored at −20 °C) was added to the precipitate proteins, vortexed for 2 min (Vortex Genie–2, VWR Scientific, West Chester, PA, USA), and centrifuged at 15,000 rpm for 5 min; the supernatant was transferred to new, labeled 2 mL centrifuge tubes. The samples were evaporated to dryness using a Savant SPD1010 SpeedVac Concentrator (Thermo Fisher Scientific, Inc., Asheville, NC, USA). The residue was reconstituted with 100 µL of mobile phase, vortexed for 1 min, and centrifuged at 15,000 rpm for 5 min; the supernatant was transferred to HPLC vials and 100 µL were injected into the HPLC system.

2.8.2. Urine Sample Preparation

Two hundred microliters of urine and 10 μM of the internal standard were combined and vortexed for 30 s. The proteins present in the urine samples were precipitated using 1.6 mL cold HPLC-grade acetonitrile (pre-stored at −20 °C), vortexed for 2 min, and centrifuged at 15,000 rpm for 15 min. The supernatant was transferred to new, labeled 2-mL centrifuge tubes. The samples were evaporated to dryness using SpeedVac. The residue was reconstituted with 200 μL of mobile phase, vortexed for 1 min, and centrifuged at 15,000 rpm for 15 min. The supernatant was transferred to HPLC vials and vortexed, and 100 μL was injected into the HPLC system.

2.9. Pharmacokinetic Analysis

Pharmacokinetic analysis was performed using data from individual rats, and the mean and standard error of the mean (SEM) were calculated for each group. The elimination rate constant (k_{el}) was estimated by linear regression of the serum concentrations in the log-linear terminal phase. Non-compartmental modeling of the serum concentration versus time data points was performed using Phoenix® WinNonlin® software (Version 6.3) (Pharsight Corporation, Mountain View, CA, USA) to calculate the pharmacokinetic parameters in the terminal phase, namely mean residence time (MRT), total clearance (CL_{tot}), and volume of distribution (V_{ss}). The initial maximum serum concentration (C_0) was calculated by back extrapolation using WinNonlin software. Based on the cumulative urinary excretion data, the fraction excreted in urine (f_e by dividing the total cumulative amount excreted in urine (ΣXu) by the dose), renal clearance (CL_{renal} by multiplying f_e by CL_{tot}), and hepatic clearance ($CL_{hepatic}$ by subtracting CL_{renal} from CL_{tot}, assuming that hepatic clearance is equivalent to non-renal clearance) were calculated. The fraction of a dose converted to a specific metabolite (F_m) was calculated using the following equation: $F_m = AUC_{(m,D)}/AUC_{(m)}$, where $AUC_{(m,D)}$ is the AUC of the metabolite after IV or PO administration of its precursor (Dox after DoxQ) and $AUC_{(m)}$ is the AUC of the metabolite after IV administration of an equimolar dose of the preformed metabolite (Dox after Dox) [36,37].

2.10. Assessment of Cardiac Toxicity of DoxQ and Dox

The cardiac toxicity was assessed after a single IV dose of Dox or DoxQ utilizing a rat cardiac Troponin-I (cTnI) ultra-sensitive ELISA kit from Life Diagnostics, Inc. (West Chester, PA, USA). Blood samples from pharmacokinetic studies were collected at 0, 12, 24, and 48 h from the jugular vein after a single 10 mg/kg IV dose of Dox (n = 4) or an equimolar dose of DoxQ (n = 4). Samples were centrifuged to obtain the serum and stored at −20 °C in a freezer until analysis. On the day of the analysis, cTnI concentrations were measured in serum samples following the manufacturer's instructions. The area under the effect curve (AUEC) was calculated for cTnI concentrations at 12–48 h post-dosing using the trapezoidal rule [38,39] by WinNonlin® software.

2.11. Assessment of Renal Toxicity of Dox and DoxQ

2.11.1. Urinary Output

The urinary output of rats over 24 h was monitored before and after administration of a single IV dose of Dox (10 mg/kg) or equimolar DoxQ to assess potential renal toxicity. Acute renal toxicity induced by Dox and other drugs may result in a reduction in the total urinary output [40–42]. The total urine volume excreted over 24 h post-dosing was compared to the total urine volume excreted over 24 h pre-dosing.

2.11.2. β-*N*-Acetylglucosaminidase (NAG)

The potential renal toxicity of Dox and DoxQ was determined by measuring β-*N*-acetylglucosaminidase (NAG), a marker of ongoing renal damage, in rat urine [8,43]. Urine samples from pharmacokinetics experiments were collected from metabolic cages at 0 h, 12 h, 24 h, and 48 h and stored at −20 °C until analysis. Concentrations of NAG urine samples were measured using an assay kit from ALPCO Diagnostics (Salem, NH, USA, cat. No. 73-1290050) on a Medica EasyRA automated clinical chemistry analyzer (Medica Corporation, Bedford, MA, USA) [44,45].

2.12. Statistical Analysis

Compiled data were presented as mean and standard error of the mean (mean ± SEM). Where possible, the data were analyzed for statistical significance using SigmaPlot software (v. 13.0, Systat Software, Inc., San Jose, CA, USA). Student's *t*-test was employed for unpaired samples to compare means between two groups, while one-way ANOVA was employed to compare the means of three or more groups, with subsequent *t*-tests between groups if necessary; a value of $p < 0.05$ was considered statistically significant.

3. Results

3.1. Physicochemical Properties

As DoxQ is a chemical derivative of Dox, the change in the chemical structure of Dox will likely alter the physiochemical properties of the parent drug, which may affect its disposition into biological fluids and pharmacokinetic profile. Therefore, exploring the physicochemical properties of DoxQ in comparison to Dox provides insight into the differences in their dispositions and pharmacokinetics. Computer software, namely VCCLAB [23,24], MarvinSketch, and GastroPlus, were used to predict the physicochemical properties of DoxQ and Dox (Table 1). The estimated partition coefficient (LogP) value of DoxQ (2.6–3.8) was 3–5-fold higher than Dox (logP 0.49–1.3), suggesting the higher lipophilicity of DoxQ. The distribution coefficient at pH 7.4 ($LogD_{7.4}$), which takes into account the ionizable groups at specific pH, of DoxQ was 25-fold higher than Dox (0.097) and may be a better predictor of lipophilicity. The predicted LogP and $LogD_{7.4}$ values of DoxQ are in agreement with the low predicted solubility (0.006 mg/mL) of DoxQ compared to Dox (0.243 mg/mL) at physiological pH and higher logS values of DoxQ. The predicted pKa values of DoxQ were also different than those of Dox. Furthermore, the experimentally determined melting point of DoxQ was 175 °C compared to 242 °C. The difference in the predicted pKa values of DoxQ versus Dox as well as other physicochemical properties described above indicate that DoxQ is distinct from Dox and exhibits unique physicochemical properties.

Table 1. Physicochemical properties of Dox, quercetin, and DoxQ.

Compound	Doxorubicin (Free Base)	Quercetin	DoxQ
Structure	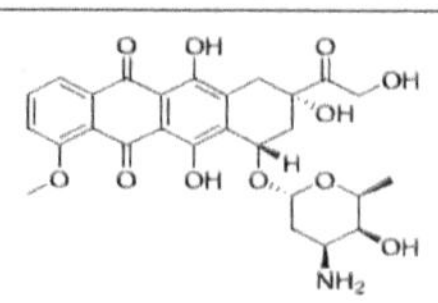	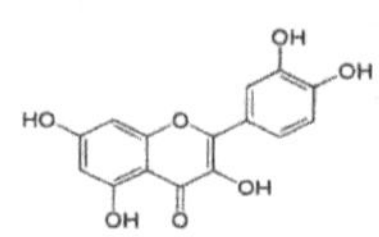	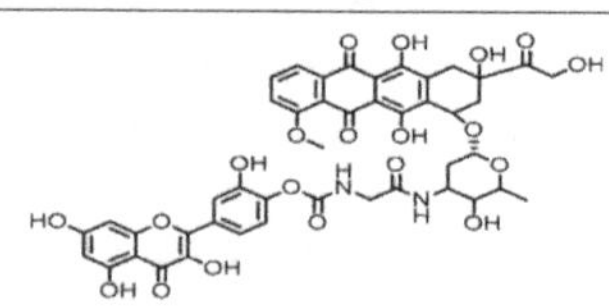
Molecular Weight (g/mol)	543.53	302.238	928.82
Formula	$C_{27}H_{29}NO_{11}$	$C_{15}H_{10}O_7$	$C_{45}H_{40}N_2O_{20}$
pKa (MarvinSketch)	8.00, 9.17, 9.93, 12.67, 13.49, 14.10	6.38, 7.85, 8.63, 10.29, 12.82	6.37, 7.72, 7.94, 8.97, 9.51, 10.21, 12.53, 13.10, 13.57, 14.06, 14.77
pKa (GastroPlus)	6.77, 8.43, 9.5	7.24, 8.15, 9.12, 10.25, 11.35	7.21, 8.08, 8.78, 9.38, 9.91, 10.64, 11.26
pKa (GastroPlus, after fitting solubility)	6.974, 10.08	6.582, 8.15, 10.25, 11.35	7.978, 8.08, 8.78, 9.38, 10.64, 11.26
logP (MarvinSketch)	1.30	1.75	2.60
logP (neutral, GastroPlus)	0.49	1.96	2.61
logP (VCCLAB)	1.3	1.44 ± 0.55	3.8 ± 1.5
$logD_{7.4}$ (MarvinSketch)	0.097	1.00	2.407
Intrinsic solubility (MarvinSketch)	−4.05 logS	−2.49 logS	−6.47 logS
Solubility at pH 7.4 (MarvinSketch)	−3.27 logS	−1.42 logS	−5.34 logS
Solubility at pH 7.4 (MarvinSketch)	0.243 mg/mL	15.15 mg/mL	0.006 mg/mL
logS (VCCLAB)	2.7	2.78	3.43
Melting point (experimental)	242 °C	316.5 °C *	175 °C

* PubChem [46].

3.2. HPLC Analysis of Dox

Optimal separation of Dox, DoxQ, and duanorubicin (IS) in serum, urine, and lymph was achieved with a mobile phase composed of acetonitrile with 0.1% formic acid in water 35:65, v/v and a flow rate of 0.6 mL/min on a C18 Phenomenex Kintex® (Torrance, CA, USA) column. Chromatograms were free of any interfering peaks co-eluted with peaks of interest (Figure 1). Calibration curves of Dox in serum and lymph were linear over the range of 0.05–100 μg/mL in serum and lymph and 0.1–100 μg/mL for urine, with excellent linearity ($r^2 > 0.99$) in all three matrices. Calibration curves of DoxQ in serum and urine were linear over the range of 1–100 μg/mL ($r^2 > 0.99$). The observed maximum serum concentration (C_{max}) of both Dox and DoxQ at 1 min post-dosing was within the linear range. The limit of quantification (LOQ) was 0.05 μg/mL and 1 μg/mL for Dox and DoxQ intact, respectively.

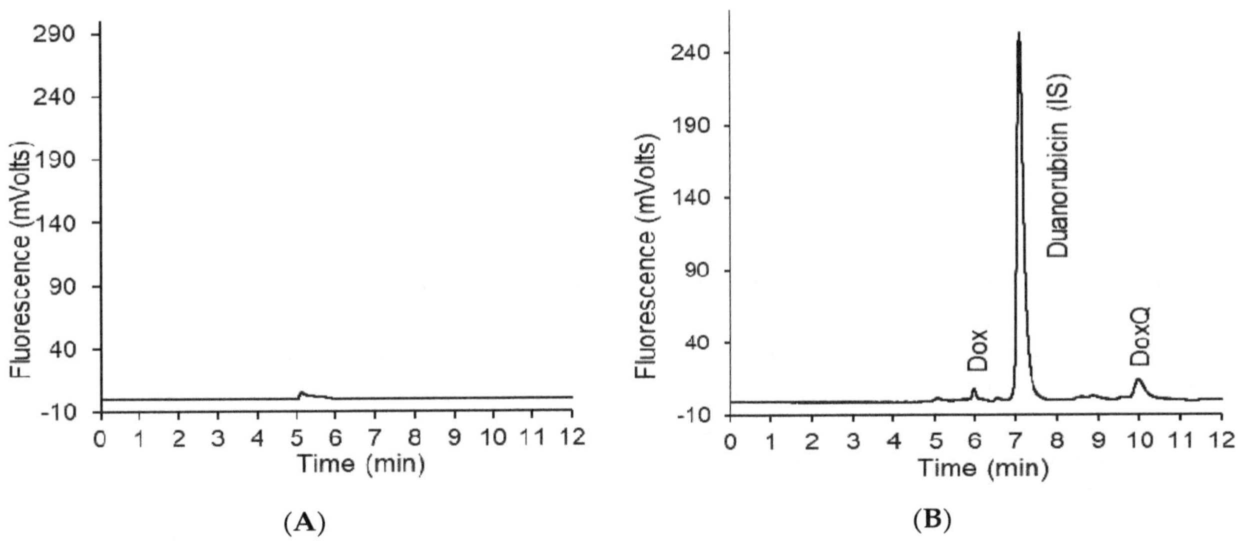

Figure 1. (**A**) Representative chromatogram of blank serum; (**B**) representative chromatogram of Dox, DoxQ, and the internal standard duanorubicin after 30 min of DoxQ IV dosing.

3.3. Pharmacokinetics of Dox and DoxQ

3.3.1. IV Administration

The disposition profiles of Dox and DoxQ intact in serum and urine following a single IV dose of Dox and an equimolar dose of DoxQ were examined (Figures 2 and 3). The serum concentration–time profile of IV DoxQ showed a rapid decline over the first 30 min and was quantifiable up to 1 h post-dosing. The concentrations of Dox after Dox were quantifiable up to 6 h post-dosing (Figure 2), with a maximum serum concentration (C_0) of Dox after Dox of ~25 μg/mL. The disposition profile of Dox after Dox, as well as its pharmacokinetic parameters, are consistent with the literature [13,15,25]. Following IV administration of DoxQ, both DoxQ intact and Dox were detected with maximum serum concentration (C_0) of intact DoxQ of ~108 μg/mL and ~1 μg/mL for free Dox (Table 2). Concentrations of intact DoxQ demonstrated a rapid decline over one hour, while concentrations of Dox after DoxQ dosing showed a slower decline and were quantifiable up to 2 h post-dosing. Notably, the maximum serum concentration (C_0) of intact DoxQ after equimolar IV DoxQ was 4–5-fold higher than C_{max} of Dox after IV Dox. The area under the concentration–time curve (AUC) of intact DoxQ (18.6 ± 1.98 μg * h/mL) was also 5-fold higher than that of Dox (3.97 ± 0.71 μg * h/mL), demonstrating higher systemic exposure to DoxQ. The volume of distribution V_{ss} of Dox was ~80-fold higher than that of DoxQ, suggesting significantly greater tissue distribution of Dox. The fraction of DoxQ metabolized into Dox was ~12%.

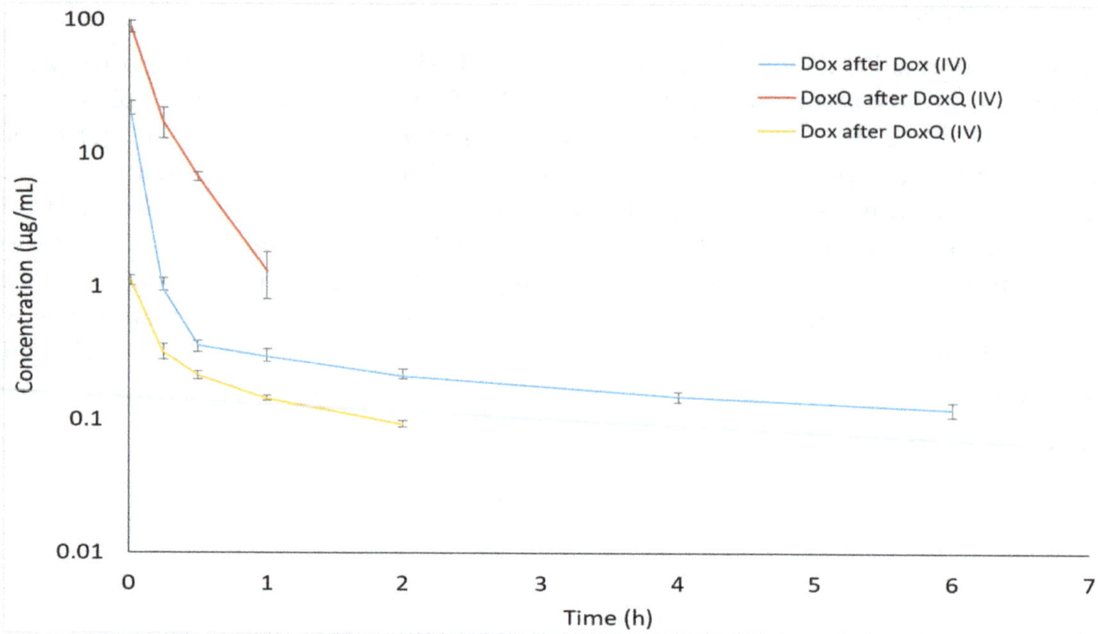

Figure 2. Concentrations of Dox and DoxQ intact after IV administration of Dox (10 mg/kg, $n = 4$ mean ± SEM) or DoxQ (equimolar dose, $n = 3$ mean ± SEM) in rat serum.

Table 2. Pharmacokinetics of Dox and DoxQ intact in rat serum after IV administration of Dox (10 mg/kg) and an equimolar dose of DoxQ (mean ± SEM, $n = 4$ unless otherwise stated).

Pharmacokinetic Parameter	Dox Administered	DoxQ Administered	
	Dox	DoxQ [1]	Dox
C_0 (µg/mL)	24.7 ± 14.2	108 ± 26.4 *	1.23 ± 0.11 +
k_{el} (h^{-1})	0.16 ± 0.02	4.59 ± 0.78 *	0.75 ± 0.076 +
$t_{1/2}$ (h)	4.69 ± 0.8 @	0.16 ± 0.3 *	0.87 ± 0.07
C_{last} (µg/mL)	0.12 ± 0.03	1.11 ± 0.17 *	0.09 ± 0.01 +
T_{last} (h) [2]	6	1	2
AUC_{last} (µg * h/mL)	3.97 ± 0.7 @	18.6 ± 1.98 *	0.46 ± 0.04 +
AUC_{inf} (µg * h/mL)	4.79 ± 1.83	NC	0.62 ± 0.03
V_{ss} (L/kg)	6.35 ± 2.11	0.08 ± 0.015	NA
CL_{renal} (L/h/kg) [1]	0.28 ± 0.84	0.02 ± 0.005	NA
$CL_{hepatic}$ (L/h/kg) [1]	2.35 ± 0.36	0.51 ± 0.06*	NA
CL_{total} (L/h/kg) [1]	2.63 ± 0.39	0.53 ± 0.01 *	NA
f_e (%)	10.73 ± 3.14	4.32 ± 1.005	NA
f_m (%)	NA	NA	11.66 ±0.86

[1] $n = 3$; [2] Median; NC = not calculable because $r^2 < 0.8$ or AUC% extrapolated > 27%; NA = not applicable; * $p < 0.05$ Dox after Dox versus DoxQ after DoxQ, + $p < 0.05$ DoxQ after DoxQ versus Dox after DoxQ, @ $p < 0.05$ Dox after Dox versus Dox after DoxQ.

In the urine, both DoxQ intact and Dox were detected after DoxQ IV dosing. Likewise, Dox was excreted unchanged after Dox IV dosing (Figure 3). The total cumulative urinary excretion plots demonstrate that DoxQ is predominantly excreted as intact DoxQ and, to a much lower extent, as free Dox after DoxQ dosing. The total cumulative amount of free Dox excreted unchanged was much higher after Dox dosing than after DoxQ. The fraction of the dose excreted unchanged in the urine (f_e) of DoxQ and Dox were 4.32 ± 1.005 and 10.73 ± 3.14, respectively, indicating that both drugs are mainly eliminated by non-renal routes.

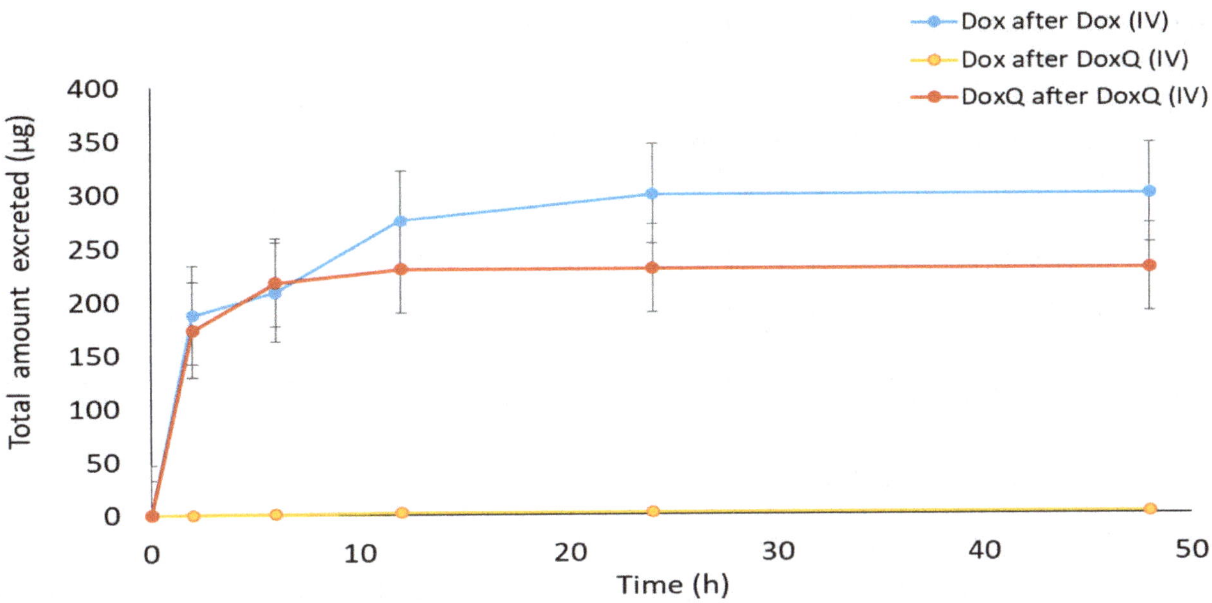

Figure 3. Cumulative amounts of Dox and DoxQ intact excreted unchanged in the urine after IV administration of Dox (10 mg/kg; n = 3 mean ± SEM) and equimolar DoxQ (n = 4 mean ± SEM) during the 48 h post-dosing.

3.3.2. Oral Administration

Following oral administration of DoxQ only the metabolite Dox was detected in serum as opposed to both DoxQ intact and Dox after IV administration (Figure 4). Following oral administration of Dox, Dox was also detected in serum. The serum concentration time plots demonstrate that concentrations of Dox after DoxQ were higher than after Dox at all time points, with resultant higher calculated AUC_{last} values of Dox after DoxQ than Dox after Dox when each was orally administered (Table 3). Bioavailability of Dox after Dox was ~8.5%, while the fraction of DoxQ metabolized into Dox was ~10.3%.

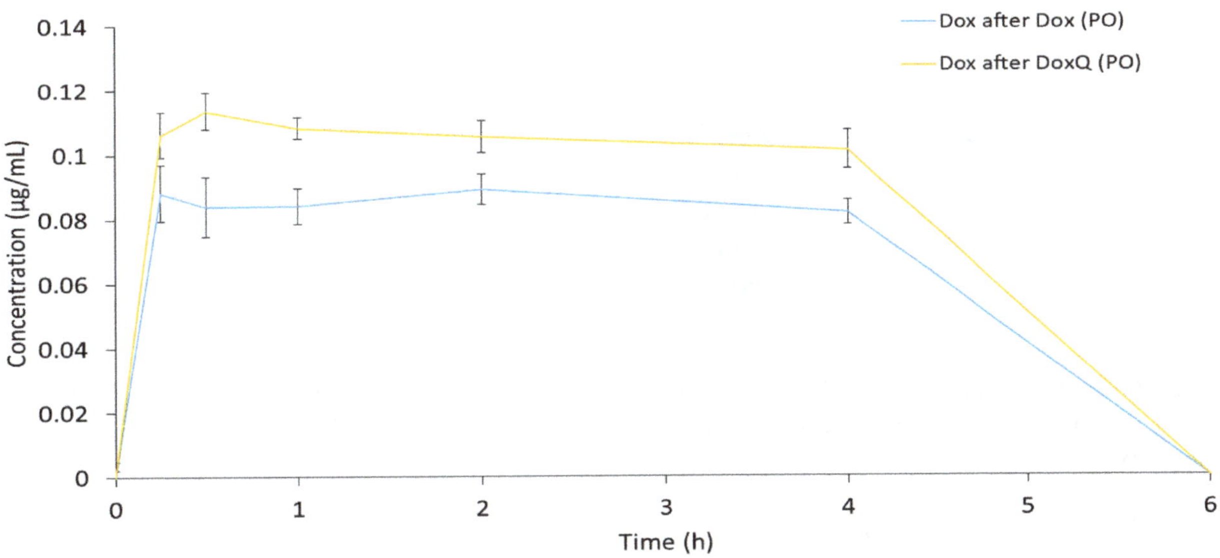

Figure 4. Concentrations of Dox after PO administration of Dox (10 mg/kg) and equimolar DoxQ in rat serum over 6 h. (n = 3 mean ± SEM for Dox, n = 4 mean ± SEM for DoxQ).

Table 3. Pharmacokinetics of Dox after oral administration of 10 mg/kg Dox and equimolar DoxQ in rat serum (mean ± SEM, n = 4 unless otherwise stated).

Pharmacokinetic Parameter	Dox Administered	DoxQ Administered	Cycloheximide + DoxQ Administered
	Dox [1]	Dox	Dox
C_{max} (μg/mL)	0.09 ± 0.01	0.11 ± 0.01 $^{+}$	0.07 ± 0.001
C_{last} (μg/mL)	0.08 ± 0.01	0.10 ± 0.01	0.07 ± 0.02
T_{last} (h) [2]	4	4	4
AUC_{last} (μg * h/mL)	0.33 ± 0.04	0.41 ± 0.03 $^{+}$	0.27 ± 0.005
F_m (%)	NA	10.32 ± 0.42 $^{+}$	6.81 ± 0.14
F (%)	8.57 ± 0.71	NA	NA

[1] n = 3; [2] Median; NA = Not applicable; $^{+}$ $p < 0.05$ Dox after DoxQ versus Dox after Cycloheximide + DoxQ.

3.4. Intestinal Lymphatic Drug Delivery

3.4.1. Mesenteric Lymph Duct Cannulation

The mesenteric lymph duct cannulation rat model is commonly used as to directly examine the transport of drugs after oral administration because it enables the collection of lymphatic fluids as it flows from the intestine [20,35]. The intestinal lymphatic transport of Dox after oral administration DoxQ and Dox was investigated in a mesenteric lymph duct cannulated model to assess whether the presence of quercetin facilitates lymphatic transport of Dox. Following oral DoxQ or Dox dosing, lymph samples were collected up to one hour post-dosing and concentrations of Dox were measured by HPLC. The cumulative amount of Dox in mesenteric lymph fluid after oral DoxQ were two-fold higher than after Dox (Figure 5), suggesting that quercetin in DoxQ, intact or when released, increased the intestinal delivery of Dox into lymphatics.

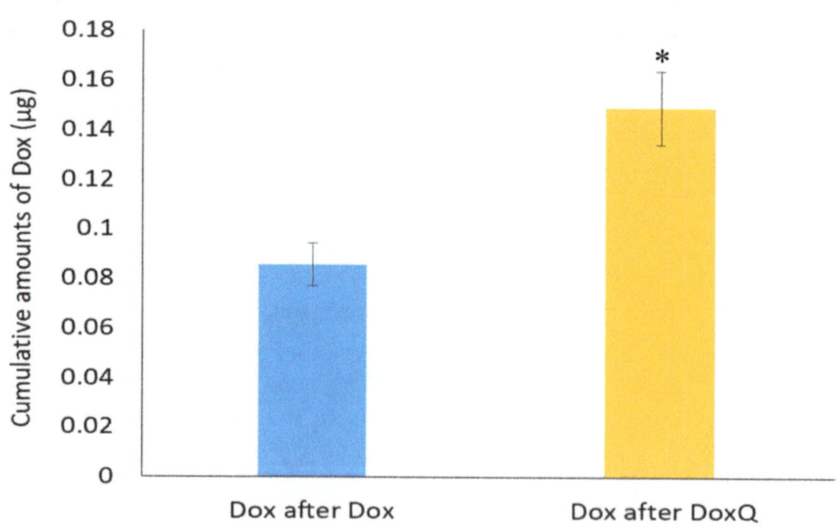

Figure 5. Cumulative amounts of Dox in mesenteric lymph fluid over one hour after oral administration of Dox (10 mg/kg) and equimolar DoxQ (n = 3, mean ± SEM). * $p < 0.05$ Dox after DoxQ versus Dox after Dox.

3.4.2. Lymph Blockage by Cycloheximide

Intestinal lymphatic delivery of Dox was also examined indirectly in the cycloheximide treated rat model. Lymph blockage was achieved by pre-administration of cycloheximide 1.5 h prior to oral administration of DoxQ. A 3 mg/kg intraperitoneal dose of cycloheximide was chosen based on previous studies published in the literature [26–35]. Likewise, a 1.5-h time delay prior to oral DoxQ dosing was chosen to achieve maximum lymph blockage [29].

Figure 6 demonstrates that pre-administration of cycloheximide prior to oral DoxQ reduced the systemic exposure of Dox compared to DoxQ administered alone. Given that quercetin is naturally transported via intestinal lymphatics and could act as a carrier for Dox's (Dox in DoxQ) lymphatic transport, blockage of the intestinal lymphatic pathway may reduce systemic exposure. The results suggest that quercetin in DoxQ, intact or when released from the conjugate, facilitates intestinal lymphatic transport of Dox, and that blocking the lymphatic pathway resulted in lower levels of circulating Dox.

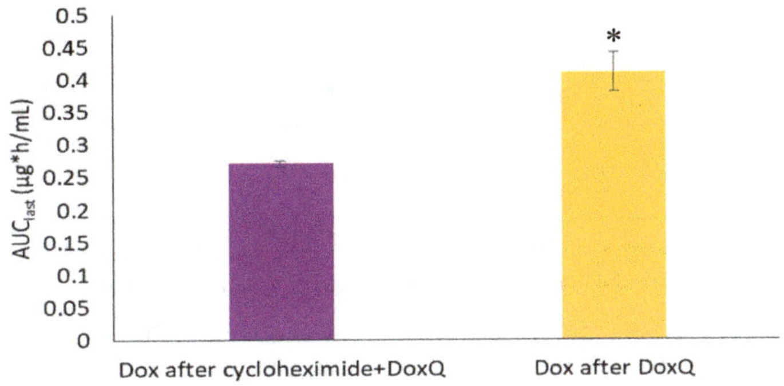

Figure 6. Systemic exposure (AUC$_{last}$) of Dox after PO administration of DoxQ alone or after cycloheximide IP followed by DoxQ PO in rat serum (n = 4 mean ± SEM). * $p < 0.05$ Dox after DoxQ versus Dox after cycloheximide + DoxQ.

3.5. Cardiotoxicity of Dox and Dox

The clinical use of Dox is limited by its dose-related cardiotoxicity, which can result in cardiac muscle injury. The extent of myocardial injury can be assessed by measuring the levels of cardiac troponins in blood. Cardiac troponins are highly sensitive and specific biomarkers of cardiac muscle damage, induced by chemotherapeutics as well as other pathological conditions [47]. cTnI is commonly used as an early marker of cardiotoxicity induced by Dox [8,48] as it is released within 2–3 h of myocardial injury and peaks at 24 h [49,50]. Based on the reported peak troponin concentrations following myocardium injury, levels of cTnI were measured in serum samples from pharmacokinetic study at 12, 24, and 48 h after a single acute IV dose (10 mg/kg) of Dox or equimolar DoxQ utilizing an ELISA kit. Figure 7 illustrates that the concentrations of cTnI at 12, 24, and 48 h post-IV-dosing of DoxQ were lower than after Dox dosing, though this did not reach statistical significance and thus the cardiac toxicity induced by DoxQ and Dox was not different using this biomarker. Although the calculated area under the effect curve (AUEC) of cTnI concentrations at 12–48 h post-DoxQ-dosing (Figure 8) was lower than the AUEC after Dox, it did not result in cardioprotective effects of DoxQ as there were no statistical differences between the treatment groups.

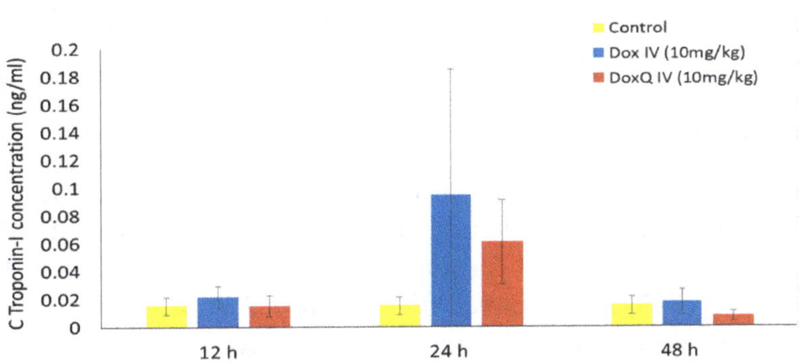

Figure 7. cTnI concentrations after IV (10 mg/kg) administration of Dox and equimolar DoxQ (n = 4 mean ± SEM). Data were not statistically significant.

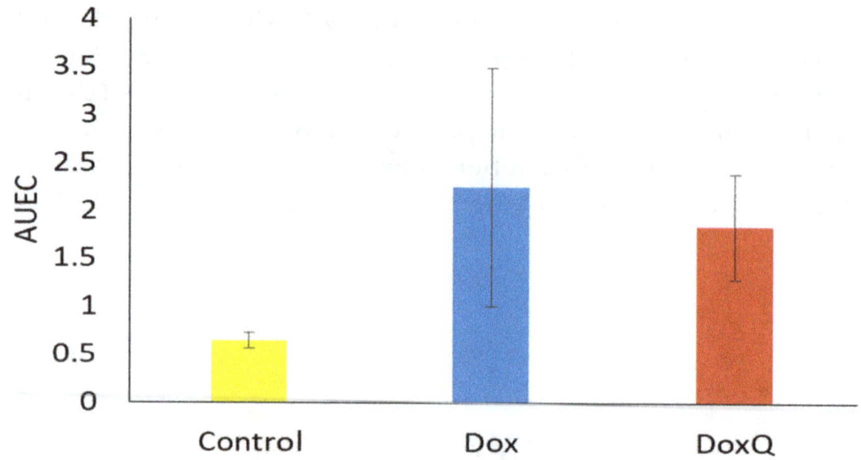

Figure 8. AUEC of cTnI concentrations 12-48 h after IV (10 mg/kg) administration of Dox and equimolar DoxQ ($n = 4$ mean ± SEM). Data were not statistically significant.

3.6. Renal Toxicity of Dox and DoxQ

3.6.1. Urinary Output over 24 h

Dox can also induce renal toxicity, which could be manifested as reduced urinary output. Thus, the effect of DoxQ on the total urinary output of rats over 24 h was examined in comparison to rats treated with Dox after a single acute IV dose. Figure 9 shows that there was no significant difference in the total urine volume over 24 h in rats treated with Dox or an equimolar dose of DoxQ.

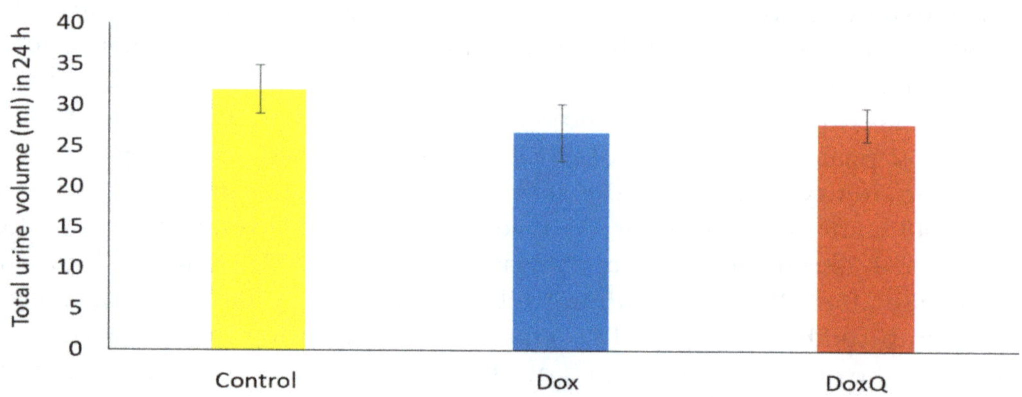

Figure 9. Average total urine volume 24 h post IV Dox (10 mg/Kg) and equimolar DoxQ compared to control untreated. Dox ($n = 3$ Mean ± SEM), DoxQ ($n = 4$ Mean ± SEM), control ($n = 7$ Mean ± SEM). Data were not statistically significant.

3.6.2. β-N-Acetylglucosaminidase (NAG)

The potential renal toxicity of Dox and DoxQ was determined by measuring β-*N*-acetylglucosaminidase (NAG), a lysosomal enzyme found in large concentrations in kidney tubules and a sensitive and early marker of renal damage [8,51,52]. Urine samples from pharmacokinetic studies after a single IV dose of DoxQ or Dox collected at 0, 2, 6, 12, 24 and 48 h were analyzed on a Medica easy RA analyzer for NAG concentrations. Cumulative amounts of NAG in 24 h after DoxQ dosing were lower than after Dox (Figure 10), suggesting lower renal toxicity induced after DoxQ administration compared to Dox.

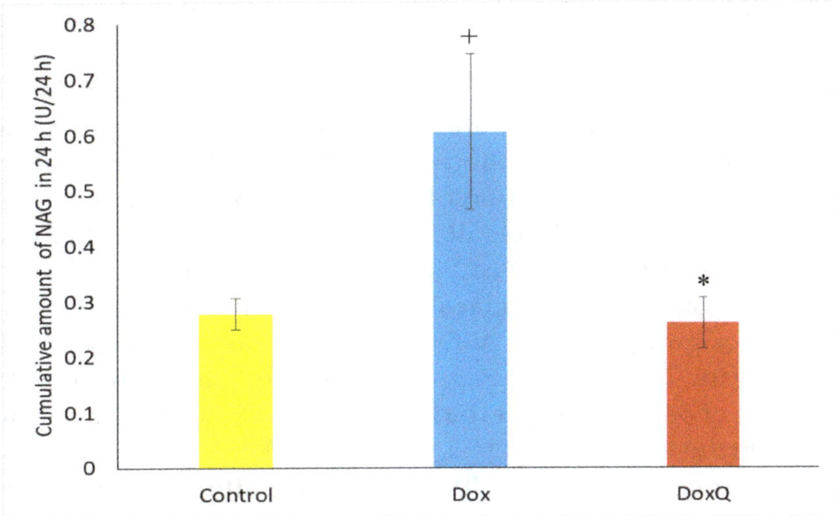

Figure 10. Total amount of NAG excreted in urine after IV administration of Dox (10 mg/kg) mean ± SEM) and equimolar DoxQ compared to control untreated ($n = 4$, mean ± SEM). + $p < 0.05$ Dox versus control ,* $p < 0.05$ DoxQ versus Dox.

4. Discussion

Dox is an anthracycline antibiotic widely used in cancer chemotherapy; however, its dose-dependent toxicity limits its clinical use. The purpose of this study was to investigate the feasibility of utilizing a Dox-bound derivative with the lymphatically absorbed antioxidant quercetin as a proof of concept linker, delivering Dox and Dox–quercetin to the systemic circulation via intestinal lymphatics after oral dosing. In addition, the flavonoid–Dox conjugate may lead to sustained release of the anti-cancer agent after IV dosing, resulting in lower peak serum concentration, which may be associated with the dose-limiting cardiotoxicity of the drug. Furthermore, the protective antioxidant effects of quercetin in DoxQ, when intact or when released, may further limit the cardiac and renal toxicity induced by Dox.

Various liposome-encapsulated formulations of Dox are currently available in human studies with the advantage of reduced acute cardiotoxicity compared to IV Dox and improved pharmacokinetics [53]. However, pegylated liposomal Dox is associated with an additional side effect of palmar plantar erythrodysesthesia [7]. In this study, we sought to examine the performance of a controlled-release Dox–quercetin conjugate with reduced side effects in vitro, which may have better tolerability compared to conventional Dox–HCl and liposomal Dox treatments.

The Dox–quercertin conjugate was synthesized using a glycine linker, resulting in a new derivative with increased lipophilicity and improved in vitro pharmacological activities. Our previous in vitro study demonstrated a controlled release of both Dox and quercetin released from DoxQ over four days [14]. Furthermore, DoxQ was less cardiotoxic than Dox to both rat and human cardiomyocytes and the mechanism of cardioprotection involved a reduction in the levels of ROS and oxidative stress markers as well as inhibitory effects on the expression and catalytic activity of CYP1B1. Additionally, DoxQ mitigated the therapeutic barriers contributing to the low oral bioavailability of Dox as it inhibited CYP3A4 and demonstrated higher cellular uptake by P–gp-positive cells (MDCK–MDR) in vitro.

In this study, our intestinal lymphatic delivery strategy was applied to the DoxQ delivery system, increasing the serum concentrations of Dox at all time points, with an overall increase in AUC_{last} of Dox after oral DoxQ administration compared to after Dox, reflecting an overall increase in the systemic exposure of Dox. In addition, only free Dox was released from oral DoxQ and detected analytically, thus it was analyzed for systemic exposure. Given that DoxQ was not detected as the intact conjugate after oral dosing of DoxQ, calculating the F of DoxQ intact was not possible; however, it was appropriate to calculate the fraction of DoxQ metabolized to Dox, as described in Section 2.9.

Therefore, the extent of systemic exposure of Dox after oral Dox and DoxQ was assessed by comparing the AUCs of Dox (Table 3).

After IV administration DoxQ was detected intact, which we have shown to be a pharmacologically active form as it retained anti-cancer activity in a triple-negative murine breast cancer cell line [14]. The actual total concentration of DoxQ intact in the serum after an equimolar dose of Dox was 5-fold higher than the concentration of Dox after Dox, allowing a greater AUC compared to the standard Dox treatment. This could result in a lower dose of DoxQ being required to achieve the same effective serum concentrations. DoxQ injections could conceivably be as effective as Dox with reduced toxicity. With regard to its pharmacokinetics, the difference in the volume of distribution between the IV Dox after Dox group and the IV DoxQ intact group was possibly due to the change in physicochemical properties and inhibition of P–gp by quercetin. Dox with a log P value of 1.3, pKa of 8.4, and a molecular weight of 543.53 g/mol rapidly crosses the lipid membrane and binds to tissues, resulting in a larger V_{SS}. On the other hand, DoxQ with a smaller V_{ss} (0.08) indicates that it is should mainly reside in the vascular compartment with much lower affinity to distribute across biological membranes compared to Dox, regardless of its higher lipophilicity (logP 2.60–3.8). This could be due to the large molecular weight of 982 g/mol and the presence of multiple potential ionization sites, which may impede its distribution across biological membranes while intact. Similar effects were observed for clozapine nano-formulation, where tissue distribution of clozapine incorporated in solid lipid nanoparticles was lower than clozapine solution because free clozapine could only be distributed after its release from nanoparticles [54]. Therefore, it is possible that DoxQ intact will distribute to a lower extent than when it is released from the conjugate or when Dox alone is administered. Examination of the total cumulative amounts of Dox and DoxQ excreted unchanged after IV dosing revealed lower cumulative amounts of DoxQ intact after DoxQ than of Dox after Dox. This could be due to the large molecular weight of DoxQ (928.8 g/mole) to be filtered at the glomerulus and also its high lipophilicity (LogP 2.6–3.8, Table 2), as opposed to Dox with a smaller size and lower lipophilicity.

With regard to intestinal lymphatic absorption of DoxQ, our results show that cumulative amounts of Dox following DoxQ oral dosing were twice as high after Dox in a mesenteric lymph cannulated rat model. This observation is likely due to the presence of quercetin in DoxQ, intact or when released, acting as a lymphatically targeted carrier to facilitate the transport of Dox into lymphatics, as quercetin has been reported to be transported via intestinal lymphatics following intragastric or intraduodenal administration [16–18]. Additionally, compounds with high lipophilicity, high logP, and large molecular size favor association with chylomicrons in the intestine, facilitating their uptake by lymphatic capillaries into the mesenteric lymph duct [19,21]. The new derivative is more lipophilic (LogP 2.6–3.8) and larger in size (molecular weight 928.8 g/mole) compared to Dox (LogP 1.3, 543.53 g/mol), both of which may in part facilitate DoxQ's lymphatic intestinal absorption. Furthermore, formulation effects of PEG-400 on the intestinal absorption and pharmacokinetics of DoxQ and even Dox are possible. PEG-400 is often utilized in dosing of rodent species [45,55] and was used as a vehicle in this study for both oral and IV administration of DoxQ and Dox because DoxQ has poor water solubility and reconstitution in 0.9% NaCl is not feasible. The diverse effects of PEG-400 on solubility, permeability, drug metabolizing enzymes, transporters, and gastrointestinal transit time may have influences on the intestinal absorption and systemic exposure of oral drugs [56–58].

In spite of the efficacy of Dox chemotherapy, its clinical use is limited due to its dose-limiting cardiac toxicity along with its renal toxicity, caused in part by the generation of oxygen species in the conversion from Dox to semiquinone, yielding very reactive hydroxyl radicals. The free radical may also cause damage to various membrane lipids and other cellular components [59]. Following a large single-dose injection of Dox (10 mg/kg IV), there was an increase in cTnI released from cardiac tissues at the 12, 24, and 48 h time points, consistent with the literature. In parallel, rats that received DoxQ (equimolar dose of Dox) also had an increase in cTnI at each time point. The significant 4–5-fold increase of circulating intact DoxQ as compared to Dox and its overall increase in systemic exposure, as well as the metabolism of DoxQ to Dox, did not result in higher cTnI compared to rats that received

Dox as no statistically significant difference in cardiac toxicity was observed between the two treatment groups (Figures 7 and 8). The in vivo cardiac effects of DoxQ in this study are different from our in vitro observations, where DoxQ formulation greatly reduced the cardiac toxicity induced by Dox in both rat and human cardiomyocytes [14]. This observation is also different from a reported study in which the combination of Dox with resveratrol and quercetin polymeric micelles was shown to mitigate Dox-induced cardiotoxicity both in vitro and in vivo [60]. The in vivo cardioprotective effects of this combination strategy were assessed by measuring levels of AST, ALT, and CK in mice and showed a significant reduction in all three biochemical markers as opposed to Dox administered alone. The observations from the later reported study [60] and our in vitro study [14] demonstrate the protective effects of quercetin on Dox-induced cardiotoxicity. The cardioprotective effects reported in [60] were attributed to the synergistic action of resveratrol and quercetin micelles when co-administered with Dox at a ratio of 10:10:1 resveratrol:quercetin:Dox, whereas our DoxQ conjugate is designed to release Dox and quercetin at a ratio of 1:1, which may have not been enough to show cardioprotection in vivo after one dose. Additionally, the use of two antioxidants, namely resveratrol and quercetin, together could have provided a greater ability to scavenge reactive oxygen species and attenuate the cardiotoxicity induced by Dox as opposed to only quercetin in the DoxQ formulation.

Urine analysis following a single acute dose of Dox showed higher cumulative amounts of β-N-acetylglucosaminidase (NAG), a lysosomal enzyme in the epithelial cells of the proximal tubules and a sensitive marker of renal damage, compared to DoxQ. This is likely due to the antioxidant protective effects of quercetin in DoxQ on Dox-induced renal toxicity and is consistent with similar studies reported in the literature [61,62].

DoxQ by injection could have greater benefits over standard dosing regimens in terms of tolerance and potential improved toxicity. Further translational efforts will focus on optimizing dose frequency, completing preclinical proof of concept in chronic studies, and examining other natural lymphatic carriers for oral delivery.

5. Conclusions

DoxQ alters the pharmacokinetic disposition of Dox both orally and intravenously and is in part transported through intestinal lymphatics. DoxQ may increase therapeutic safety compared to Dox in a rodent model and further long-term studies are warranted.

Acknowledgments: The authors would like to acknowledge Kuwait University, Faculty of Health Sciences, College of Pharmacy for the graduate scholarship awarded to Samaa Alrushaid. Sanjeewa N. Senadheera was funded by a grant from the U.S. National Cancer Institute (NCI) R01CA173292 to M. Laird Forrest.

Author Contributions: Samaa Alrushaid, Neal M. Davies, Casey L. Sayre, and M. Laird Forrest conceived and designed the experiments; Samaa Alrushaid and Sanjeewa N. Senadheera performed the experiments; Samaa Alrushaid., Neal M. Davies, Casey L. Sayre, M. Laird Forrest, Sanjeewa N. Senadheera, Jaime A. Yáñez, Frank J. Burczynski, and Raimar Löbenberg analyzed the data; Neal M. Davies, Casey L. Sayre, Jaime A. Yáñez, M. Laird Forrest, Frank J. Burczynski, and Raimar Löbenberg contributed reagents/materials/analysis tools; Samaa Alrushaid, Neal M. Davies, Casey L. Sayre, Jaime A. Yáñez, M. Laird Forrest, Sanjeewa N. Senadheera, Frank J. Burczynski, and Raimar Löbenberg wrote the paper.

References

1. Minotti, G.; Menna, P.; Salvatorelli, E.; Cairo, G.; Gianni, L. Anthracyclines: Molecular advances and pharmacologic developments in antitumor activity and cardiotoxicity. *Pharmacol. Rev.* **2004**, *56*, 185–229. [CrossRef] [PubMed]
2. Cortés-Funes, H.; Coronado, C. Role of anthracyclines in the era of targeted therapy. *Cardiovasc. Toxicol.* **2007**, *7*, 56–60. [CrossRef] [PubMed]
3. Gibbs, D.D.; Pyle, L.; Allen, M.; Vaughan, M.; Webb, A.; Johnston, S.R.; Gore, M.E. A phase I dose-finding study of a combination of pegylated liposomal doxorubicin (Doxil), carboplatin and paclitaxel in ovarian cancer. *Br. J. Cancer* **2002**, *86*, 1379–1384. [CrossRef] [PubMed]

4. Gianni, L.; Dombernowsky, P.; Sledge, G.; Martin, M.; Amadori, D.; Arbuck, S.G.; Ravdin, P.; Brown, M.; Messina, M.; Tuck, D.; et al. Cardiac function following combination therapy with paclitaxel and doxorubicin: An analysis of 657 women with advanced breast cancer. *Ann. Oncol.* **2001**, *12*, 1067–1073. [CrossRef] [PubMed]
5. McBride, N.C.; Cavenagh, J.D.; Ward, M.C.; Grant, I.; Schey, S.; Gray, A.; Hughes, A.; Mills, M.J.; Cervi, P.; Newland, A.C.; et al. Liposomal daunorubicin (DaunoXome) in combination with cyclophosphamide, vincristine and prednisolone (COP-X) as salvage therapy in poor-prognosis non-Hodgkins lymphoma. *Leuk. Lymphoma* **2001**, *42*, 89–98. [CrossRef] [PubMed]
6. Soloman, R.; Gabizon, A.A. Clinical pharmacology of liposomal anthracyclines: Focus on pegylated liposomal Doxorubicin. *Clin. Lymphoma Myeloma* **2008**, *8*, 21–32. [CrossRef] [PubMed]
7. Lorusso, D.; Stefano, A.D.; Carone, V.; Fagotti, A.; Pisconti, S.; Scambia, G. Pegylated liposomal doxorubicin-related palmar-plantar erythrodysesthesia ('hand-foot' syndrome). *Ann. Oncol.* **2007**, *18*, 1159–1164. [CrossRef] [PubMed]
8. Cai, S.; Thati, S.; Bagby, T.R.; Diab, H.M.; Davies, N.M.; Cohen, M.S.; Forrest, M.L. Localized doxorubicin chemotherapy with a biopolymeric nanocarrier improves survival and reduces toxicity in xenografts of human breast cancer. *J. Control Release* **2010**, *146*, 212–218. [CrossRef] [PubMed]
9. Matsumura, Y.; Hamaguchi, T.; Ura, T.; Muro, K.; Yamada, Y.; Shimada, Y.; Shirao, K.; Okusaka, T.; Ueno, H.; Ikeda, M.; et al. Phase I clinical trial and pharmacokinetic evaluation of NK911, a micelle-encapsulated doxorubicin. *Br. J. Cancer* **2004**, *91*, 1775–1781. [CrossRef] [PubMed]
10. Ríhová, B.; Strohalm, J.; Prausová, J.; Kubácková, K.; Jelínková, M.; Rozprimová, L.; Sírová, M.; Plocová, D.; Etrych, T.; Subr, V.; et al. Cytostatic and immunomobilizing activities of polymer-bound drugs: Experimental and first clinical data. *J. Control Release* **2003**, *91*, 1–16. [PubMed]
11. Tolcher, A.W.; Sugarman, S.; Gelmon, K.A.; Cohen, R.; Saleh, M.; Isaacs, C.; Young, L.; Healey, D.; Onetto, N.; Slichenmyer, W. Randomized phase II study of BR96-doxorubicin conjugate in patients with metastatic breast cancer. *J. Clin. Oncol.* **1999**, *17*, 478–484. [CrossRef] [PubMed]
12. Gustafson, D.L.; Merz, A.L.; Long, M.E. Pharmacokinetics of combined doxorubicin and paclitaxel in mice. *Cancer Lett.* **2005**, *220*, 161–169. [CrossRef] [PubMed]
13. Lee, H.J.; Lee, M.G. Effects of dexamethasone on the pharmacokinetics of adriamycin after intravenous administration to rats. *Res. Commun. Mol. Pathol. Pharmacol.* **1999**, *105*, 87–96. [PubMed]
14. Alrushaid, S.; Zhao, Y.; Sayre, C.L.; Maayah, Z.H.; Forrest, M.L.; Senadheera, S.N.; Chaboyer, K.; Anderson, H.D.; El-Kadi, A.; Davies, N.M. Mechanistically Elucidating the In Vitro Safety and Efficacy of a Novel Doxorubicin Derivative. *Drug Deliv. Transl. Res.* **2017**, *7*, 582–597. [CrossRef] [PubMed]
15. Choi, J.S.; Piao, Y.J.; Kang, K.W. Effects of quercetin on the bioavailability of doxorubicin in rats: Role of CYP3A4 and P-gp inhibition by quercetin. *Arch Pharm. Res.* **2011**, *34*, 607–613. [CrossRef] [PubMed]
16. Chen, I.L.; Tsai, Y.J.; Huang, C.M.; Tsai, T.H. Lymphatic absorption of quercetin and rutin in rat and their pharmacokinetics in systemic plasma. *J. Agric. Food Chem.* **2010**, *58*, 546–551. [CrossRef] [PubMed]
17. Murota, K.; Cermak, R.; Terao, J.; Wolffram, S. Influence of fatty acid patterns on the intestinal absorption pathway of quercetin in thoracic lymph duct-cannulated rats. *Br. J. Nutr.* **2013**, *109*, 2147–2153. [CrossRef] [PubMed]
18. Murota, K.; Terao, J. Quercetin appears in the lymph of unanesthetized rats as its phase II metabolites after administered into the stomach. *FEBS Lett.* **2005**, *579*, 5343–5346. [CrossRef] [PubMed]
19. Trevaskis, N.L.; Kaminskas, L.M.; Porter, C.J. From sewer to saviour—Targeting the lymphatic system to promote drug exposure and activity. *Nat. Rev. Drug Discov.* **2015**, *14*, 781–803. [CrossRef] [PubMed]
20. Trevaskis, N.L.; Hu, L.; Caliph, S.M.; Han, S.; Porter, C.J. The mesenteric lymph duct cannulated rat model: Application to the assessment of intestinal lymphatic drug transport. *J. Vis. Exp.* **2015**. [CrossRef] [PubMed]
21. Yáñez, J.A.; Wang, S.W.; Knemeyer, I.W.; Wirth, M.A.; Alton, K.B. Intestinal lymphatic transport for drug delivery. *Adv. Drug Deliv. Rev.* **2011**, *63*, 923–942. [CrossRef] [PubMed]
22. Porter, C.J.; Trevaskis, N.L.; Charman, W.N. Lipids and lipid-based formulations: Optimizing the oral delivery of lipophilic drugs. *Nat. Rev. Drug Discov.* **2007**, *6*, 231–248. [CrossRef] [PubMed]
23. Tetko, I.V.; Gasteiger, J.; Todeschini, R.; Mauri, A.; Livingstone, D.; Ertl, P.; Palyulin, V.A.; Radchenko, E.V.; Zefirov, N.S.; Makarenko, A.S.; et al. Virtual computational chemistry laboratory—Design and description. *J. Comput. Aid. Mol. Des.* **2005**, *19*, 453–463. [CrossRef] [PubMed]
24. Virtual Computational Chemistry Laboratory. Available online: http://www.vcclab.org (accessed on 24 August 2017).

25. Daeihamed, M.; Haeri, A.; Dadashzadeh, S. A Simple and Sensitive HPLC Method for Fluorescence Quantitation of Doxorubicin in Micro-volume Plasma: Applications to Pharmacokinetic Studies in Rats. *Iran J. Pharm. Res.* **2015**, *14* (Suppl. 1), 33–42. [PubMed]
26. Dahan, A.; Hoffman, A. Evaluation of a chylomicron flow blocking to investigate the intestinal lymphatic transport of lipophilic drugs. *Eur. J. Pharm. Sci.* **2005**, *24*, 381–388. [CrossRef] [PubMed]
27. Bhalekar, M.R.; Upadhaya, P.G.; Madgulkar, A.R.; Kshirsagar, S.J.; Dube, A.; Bartakke, U.S. In-Vivo bioavailability and lymphatic uptake evaluation of lipid nanoparticulates of darunavir. *Drug Deliv.* **2016**, *23*, 2581–2586. [PubMed]
28. Fu, Q.; Sun, J.; Ai, X.; Zhang, P.; Li, M.; Wang, Y.; Liu, X.; Sun, Y.; Sui, X.; Sun, L.; et al. Nimodipine nanocrystals for oral bioavailability improvement: Role of mesenteric lymph transport in the oral absorption. *Int. J. Pharm.* **2013**, *448*, 290–297. [CrossRef] [PubMed]
29. Attili-Qadri, S.; Karra, N.; Nemirovski, A.; Schwob, O.; Talmon, Y.; Nassar, T.; Benita, S. Oral delivery system prolongs blood circulation of docetaxel nanocapsules via lymphatic absorption. *Proc. Natl. Acad. Sci. USA* **2013**, *110*, 17498–17503. [CrossRef] [PubMed]
30. Sun, M.; Zhai, X.; Xue, K.; Hu, L.; Yang, X.; Li, G.; Si, L. Intestinal absorption and intestinal lymphatic transport of sirolimus from self-microemulsifying drug delivery systems assessed using the single-passintestinal perfusion (SPIP) technique and a chylomicron flow blocking approach: Linear correlation with oral bioavailabilities in rats. *Eur. J. Pharm. Sci.* **2011**, *43*, 132–140. [PubMed]
31. Lind, M.L.; Jacobsen, J.; Holm, R.; Müllertz, A. Intestinal lymphatic transport of halofantrine in rats assessed using a chylomicron flow blocking approach: The influence of polysorbate 60 and 80. *Eur. J. Pharm. Sci.* **2008**, *35*, 211–218. [CrossRef] [PubMed]
32. Gao, F.; Zhang, Z.; Bu, H.; Huang, Y.; Gao, Z.; Shen, J.; Zhao, C.; Li, Y. Nanoemulsion improves the oral absorption of candesartan cilexetil in rats:Performance and mechanism. *J. Control Release* **2011**, *149*, 168–174. [CrossRef] [PubMed]
33. Mishra, A.; Vuddanda, P.R.; Singh, S. Intestinal Lymphatic Delivery of Praziquantel by Solid Lipid Nanoparticles: Formulation Design, In Vitro and In Vivo Studies. *J. Nanotechnol. vol.* **2014**, *2014*, 1–12. [CrossRef]
34. Makwana, V.; Jain, R.; Patel, K.; Nivsarkar, M.; Joshi, A. Solid lipid nanoparticles (SLN) of Efavirenz as lymph targeting drug delivery system: Elucidation of mechanism of uptake using chylomicron flow blocking approach. *Int. J. Pharm.* **2015**, *495*, 439–446. [CrossRef] [PubMed]
35. Tsai, Y.J.; Tsai, T.H. Mesenteric lymphatic absorption and the pharmacokinetics of naringin and naringenin in the rat. *J. Agric. Food Chem.* **2012**, *60*, 12435–12442. [CrossRef] [PubMed]
36. Rowland, M.; Tozer, T.N. Metabolites and drug response. In *Clinical Pharmacokinetics and Pharmacodynamics: Concepts and applications*, 4th ed.; Tozer, R.M., Thomas, N., Eds.; Lippincott Williams & Wilkins: Baltimore, MD, USA, 2011; pp. 603–631.
37. Mehvar, R.; Jamali, F.; Watson, M.W.; Skelton, D. Pharmacokinetics of tetrabenazine and its major metabolite in man and rat. Bioavailability and dose dependency studies. *Drug Metab. Dispos.* **1987**, *15*, 250–255. [PubMed]
38. Hanafy, S.; Dagenais, N.J.; Dryden, W.F.; Jamali, F. Effects of angiotensin II blockade on inflammation-induced alterations of pharmacokinetics and pharmacodynamics of calcium channel blockers. *Br. J. Pharmacol.* **2008**, *153*, 90–99. [CrossRef] [PubMed]
39. Sattari, S.; Dryden, W.F.; Eliot, L.A.; Jamali, F. Despite increased plasma concentration, inflammation reduces potency of calcium channel antagonists due to lower binding to the rat heart. *Br. J. Pharmacol.* **2003**, *139*, 945–954. [CrossRef] [PubMed]
40. Singh, N.P.; Ganguli, A.; Prakash, A. Drug-induced kidney diseases. *J. Assoc. Physic. India* **2003**, *51*, 970–979.
41. Naughton, C.A. Drug-induced nephrotoxicity. *Am. Fam. Physic.* **2008**, *78*, 743–750.
42. Okuda, S.; Oh, Y.; Tsuruda, H.; Onoyama, K.; Fujimi, S.; Fujishima, M. Adriamycin-induced nephropathy as a model of chronic progressive glomerular disease. *Kidney Int.* **1986**, *29*, 502–510. [CrossRef] [PubMed]
43. Le, J.M.; Han, Y.H.; Choi, S.J.; Park, J.S.; Jang, J.J.; Bae, R.J.; Lee, M.J.; Kim, M.J.; Lee, Y.H.; Kim, D.; et al. Variation of nephrotoxicity biomarkers by urinary storage condition in rats. *Toxicol. Res.* **2014**, *30*, 305–309. [CrossRef] [PubMed]
44. Martinez, S.E.; Davies, N.M. Enantiospecific pharmacokinetics of isoxanthohumol and its metabolite 8-prenylnaringenin in the rat. *Mol. Nutr. Food Res.* **2015**, *59*, 1674–1689. [CrossRef] [PubMed]

45. Oliveira, A.L.; Martinez, S.E.; Nagabushnam, K.; Majeed, M.; Alrushaid, S.; Sayre, C.L.; Davies, N.M. Calebin A: Analytical Development for Pharmacokinetics Study, Elucidation of Pharmacological Activities and Content Analysis of Natural Health Products. *J. Pharm. Pharm. Sci.* **2015**, *18*, 494–514. [CrossRef] [PubMed]
46. PubChem. Available online: https://pubchem.ncbi.nlm.nih.gov/compound/5280343#section=Entrez-Crosslink (accessed on 24 August 2017).
47. Tian, S.; Hirshfield, K.M.; Jabbour, S.K.; Toppmeyer, D.; Haffty, B.G.; Khan, A.J.; Goyal, S. Serum biomarkers for the detection of cardiac toxicity after chemotherapy and radiation therapy in breast cancer patients. *Front. Oncol.* **2014**, *4*, 277. [CrossRef] [PubMed]
48. Hadi, N.; Yousif, N.G.; Al-amran, F.G.; Huntei, N.K.; Mohammad, B.I.; Ali, S.J. Vitamin E and telmisartan attenuates doxorubicin induced cardiac injury in rat through down regulation of inflammatory response. *BMC Cardiovasc. Disord.* **2012**, *12*, 63. [CrossRef] [PubMed]
49. Adamcova, M.; Sterba, M.; Simunek, T.; Potacova, A.; Popelova, O.; Mazurova, Y.; Gersl, V. Troponin as a marker of myocardiac damage in drug-induced cardiotoxicity. *Expert Opin. Drug Saf.* **2005**, *4*, 457–472. [CrossRef] [PubMed]
50. Babuin, L.; Jaffe, A.S. Troponin: The biomarker of choice for the detection of cardiac injury. *CMAJ* **2005**, *173*, 1191–1202. [CrossRef] [PubMed]
51. Teng, X.W.; Abu-Mellal, A.K.; Davies, N.M. Formulation dependent pharmacokinetics, bioavailability and renal toxicity of a selective cyclooxygenase-1 inhibitor SC-560 in the rat. *J. Pharm. Pharm. Sci.* **2003**, *6*, 205–210. [PubMed]
52. Burke, J.F.; Laucius, J.F.; Brodovsky, H.S.; Soriano, R.Z. Doxorubicin Hydrochloride-Associated Renal Failure. *Arch Int. Med.* **1977**, *137*, 385–388. [CrossRef]
53. Luo, R.; Li, Y.; He, M.; Zhang, H.; Yuan, H.; Johnson, M.; Palmisano, M.; Zhou, S.; Sun, D. Distinct biodistribution of doxorubicin and the altered dispositions mediated by different liposomal formulations. *Int. J. Pharm.* **2017**, *519*, 1–10. [CrossRef] [PubMed]
54. Manjunath, K.; Venkateswarlu, V. Pharmacokinetics, tissue distribution and bioavailability of clozapine solid nanoparticles after intravenous and intraduodenal administration. *J. Control Release* **2005**, *107*, 215–228. [CrossRef] [PubMed]
55. Martinez, S.E.; Sayre, C.L.; Davies, N.M. Pharmacometrics of 3-Methoxypterostilbene: A Component of Traditional Chinese Medicinal Plants. *Evid.-Based Complement. Altern. Med.* **2013**. [CrossRef] [PubMed]
56. Schulze, J.D.; Waddington, W.A.; Eli, P.J.; Parsons, G.E.; Coffin, M.D.; Basit, A.W. Concentration-dependent effects of polyethylene glycol 400 on gastrointestinal transit and drug absorption. *Pharm. Res.* **2003**, *20*, 1984–1988. [CrossRef] [PubMed]
57. Basit, A.W.; Newton, J.M.; Short, M.D.; Waddington, W.A.; Ell, P.J.; Lacey, L.F. The effect of polyethylene glycol 400 on gastrointestinal transit: Implications for the formulation of poorly-water soluble drugs. *Pharm. Res.* **2001**, *18*, 1146–1150. [CrossRef] [PubMed]
58. Ma, B.L.; Yang, Y.; Dai, Y.; Li, Q.; Lin, G.; Ma, Y.M. Polyethylene glycol 400 (PEG400) affects the systemic exposure of oral drugs based on multiple mechanisms: Taking berberine as an example. *RSC Adv.* **2017**, *7*, 2435–2442. [CrossRef]
59. Olson, R.D.; Mushlin, P.S. Doxorubicin cardiotoxicity: Analysis of prevailing hypotheses. *FASEB J.* **1990**, *4*, 3076–3086. [PubMed]
60. Cote, B.; Carlson, L.J.; Rao, D.A.; Alani, A.W.G. Combinatorial resveratrol and quercetin polymeric micelles mitigate doxorubicin induced cardiotoxicity in vitro and in vivo. *J. Control Release* **2015**, *213*, 128–133. [CrossRef] [PubMed]
61. Yagmurca, M.; Yasar, Z.; Bas, O. Effects of quercetin on kidney injury induced by doxorubicin. *Bratisl. Lekárske Listy* **2015**, *116*, 486–489. [CrossRef]
62. Heeba, G.H.; Mahmoud, M.E. Dual effects of quercetin in doxorubicin-induced nephrotoxicity in rats and its modulation of the cytotoxic activity of doxorubicin on human carcinoma cells. *Environ. Toxicol.* **2016**, *31*, 624–636. [CrossRef] [PubMed]

9

Qualification and Application of a Liquid Chromatography-Quadrupole Time-of-Flight Mass Spectrometric Method for the Determination of Adalimumab in Rat Plasma

Yuri Park, Nahye Kim, Jangmi Choi, Min-Ho Park, Byeong ill Lee, Seok-Ho Shin, Jin-Ju Byeon and Young G. Shin

College of Pharmacy and Institute of Drug Research and Development, Chungnam National University, Daejeon 34134, Korea; yuri.park.cnu@gmail.com (Y.P.); nahye.kim.cnu@gmail.com (N.K.); jangmi.choi.cnu@gmail.com (J.C.); minho.park.cnu@gmail.com (M.-H.P.); byungill.lee.cnu@gmail.com (B.i.L.); seokho.shin.cnu@gmail.com (S.-H.S.); jinju.byeon.cnu@gmail.com (J.-J.B.)

* Correspondence: yshin@cnu.ac.kr

Abstract: A liquid chromatography–quadrupole time-of-flight (Q-TOF) mass spectrometric method was developed for early-stage research on adalimumab in rats. The method consisted of immunoprecipitation followed by tryptic digestion for sample preparation and LC-QTOF-MS/MS analysis of specific signature peptides of adalimumab in the positive ion mode using electrospray ionization. This specific signature peptide is derived from the complementarity-determining region (CDR) of adalimumab. A quadratic regression (weighted 1/concentration), with an equation $y = ax^2 + bx + c$, was used to fit calibration curves over the concentration range of 1–100 μg/mL for adalimumab. The qualification run met the acceptance criteria of ±25% accuracy and precision values for quality control (QC) samples. This qualified LC-QTOF-MS/MS method was successfully applied to a pharmacokinetic study of adalimumab in rats as a case study. This LC-QTOF-MS/MS approach would be useful as a complementary method for adalimumab or its biosimilars at an early stage of research.

Keywords: adalimumab; immunoprecipitation; liquid chromatography-quadrupole TOF MS; bioanalysis

---

1. Introduction

Since humanized and fully human monoclonal antibodies (mAbs) were approved as therapeutic pharmaceutical products, the attention for monoclonal antibody products has been growing significantly in the global pharmaceutical market [1,2].

Therapeutic mAbs offer many advantages when compared to small-molecule drugs [3]. In general, mAbs have three main characteristics: (i) target-specific binding ability to increase or decrease an important biological effect, (ii) interaction of the constant domain with cell surface receptors that causes immune-mediated effector functions, including antibody-dependent cell-mediated cytotoxicity (ADCC), complement dependent cytotoxicity (CDC) or antibody-dependent phagocytosis; and (iii) deposition of complement on multimeric immune complexes between the mAb and the target and subsequent activation of complement-dependent cytotoxicity [2,4].

Tumor necrosis factor α (TNF-α) is an inflammatory cytokine produced by activated monocytes or macrophages [5]. Therefore, TNF-α antagonist (anti-TNF) is one of the agents that has the highest affinity for TNF-α molecules and suppresses the biological activity of TNF-α [6]. One of the well-known anti-TNF drugs is adalimumab, which consists of a fully humanized monoclonal antibody and was approved by the FDA in 2002 [7]. Adalimumab is a tetramer composed of two heavy immunoglobulin G1 (IgG1) chains and two light IgG1 chains [7]. It is currently used to treat rheumatoid arthritis, psoriasis, psoriatic arthritis, ankylosing spondylitis and Crohn's disease [8].

Traditionally, pharmacokinetic evaluation of mAbs has been mainly performed by immunoassays such as enzyme-linked immunosorbent assays (ELISA), radioimmunoassay immunofluorescence assay and etc. [9]. Immunoassays have several advantages in terms of high sensitivity, robust performance and high throughput [2,10]. However, these methods also have several disadvantages such as non-specific binding as well as time-consuming and labor-intensive reagent development [8]. Immunoassays also often show cross-reactions with precursors of the target protein or with smaller metabolized fragments that are not suitable for early-stage mAbs bioanalysis [11].

Liquid chromatographic mass spectrometry (LC-MS/MS) is a complementary technique that can quantify not only small molecules or peptides but also proteins [12]. LC-MS/MS is accurate and precise and enables throughput analysis because this combines a robust separation technique with identification and quantification based on the molecular weights of the analytes [10]. In addition, LC-MS/MS is less matrix-dependent than ELISA [13].

The purpose of this paper is to explore an adalimumab quantification method using LC-QTOF-MS/MS and employing adalimumab's specific signature peptides that are involved in variable regions and produced by tryptic digestion.

2. Materials and Methods

2.1. Materials

Adalimumab was purchased from Dongwon Pharmaceutical Wholesale (Deajeon, Korea). Protein A magnetic beads were purchased from Millipore Corp (Billerica, MA, USA). RapiGest surfactant was purchased from Waters Korea (Seoul, Korea). 1,4-Dithiothreitol (DTT) was purchased from Carl Roth (Karlsruhe, Germany). Iodoacetic acid (IAA) was purchased from Wako (Osaka, Japan). The sequencing grade modified trypsin was purchased from Promega (Madison, WI, USA). All other chemicals were commercial products of analytical or reagent grade and were used without further purification.

2.2. Preparation of Stocks, Standard (STD) and Quality Control (QC) Samples

Stock solution of adalimumab was prepared at a concentration of 5000 μg/mL in a phosphate buffer solution (PBS) containing 0.1% tween 20. The stock solution was stored at 4 °C. Stock solution of adalimumab was further diluted at a concentration 500 μg/mL in PBS containing 0.1% tween 20 as sub-stock solution. Calibration working solution was prepared by serial dilution of the sub-stock solution with PBS containing 0.1% tween 20. Then, the working solution was spiked into rat plasma to yield calibration standard concentrations of 1.0, 2.0, 5.0, 10, 20, 40, 80 and 100 μg/mL. The quality control (QC) samples with final concentrations of 2.5, 25 and 50 μg/mL were also prepared in the same manner.

2.3. Preparation of Sample Digests for Quantification

Each 24 μL aliquot of plasma study samples, QCs and standards (STDs) were separately mixed with 370 μL of PBS containing 0.1% tween 20 and 30 μL of magnetic bead suspension. After gentle shaking at room temperature overnight, the magnetic bead was washed using 600 μL PBS containing 0.1% tween 20 and then was washed again using 600 μL PBS. Seventy-five microliters of RapiGest and 10 μL of DTT were added to the mixture, which was incubated for 50 min at 60 °C to denature and reduce the adalimumab bound to the magnetic beads. After a 10-min incubation at room temperature (RT), 25 μL of IAA was added and the sample was incubated in dark conditions for 30 min at RT. Ten microliters of the sequencing grade-modified trypsin were added to the sample to digest the antibody. After 1 min of shaking, the sample was incubated at 37 °C overnight. Fifteen microliters of

2 N HCl were added to the sample for quenching purposes and the sample was incubated for another 30 min at 37 °C to stop the digestion. The resulting sample was centrifuged at 7000 rpm for 5 min at 4 °C and transferred into a HPLC vial.

2.4. Liquid Chromatography–Mass Spectrometry

The liquid chromatography–mass spectrometry system consisted of a Shimadzu CBM-20A HPLC pump controller (Shimadzu Corporation, Columbia, MD, USA), two Shimadzu LC-20AD pumps, a CTC HTS PAL autosampler (CEAP Technologies, Carrboro, NC, USA) and a quadrupole time-of-flight (Q-TOF) TripleTOF™ 5600 mass spectrometer (Sciex, Foster City, CA, USA). The analytical column used for this assay was a Phenomenex Kinetex Phenyl-hexyl column (50 × 2.1 mm, 2.6 μm). The mobile phase consisted of: mobile phase A, distilled and deionized water containing 0.1% formic acid; and mobile phase B, acetonitrile containing 0.1% formic acid. The gradient was as follows: from 0 min to 0.6 min, 5% B; from 0.5 min to 1.6 min by a linear gradient from 5% B to 95% B; 95% B was maintained for 0.2 min; from 1.8 min to 1.9 min by a linear gradient from 95% B to 5% B and then 5% B was maintained for 1.5 min for column re-equilibrium. The gradient was delivered at a flow rate of 0.4 mL/min and the injection volume was 10 μL.

The TOF-MS scan mass spectra and TOF-MS/MS scan mass spectra were recorded in the positive ion mode. For TOF-MS scan, m/z 100~950 with 0.2 s accumulation time was used. For TOF-MS/MS scan, the scan range was m/z 500~1000. For the quantification, doubly charged $[M + 2H]^{2+}$ ion for the specific signature peptide APYTFGQGTK (m/z 535.4) was selected and its product ion at m/z 901.8 was used for the quantitative analysis of adalimumab. High-purity nitrogen gas was used for the nebulizer/Duospray™ and curtain gases. The ESI spray voltage was set at 5500 V. The source temperature was 500 °C. The curtain gas (CUR) was 30 L/min; the auxiliary gas setting (GS1 and GS2) was 50 L/min.

2.5. Method Qualification and Sample Analysis Procedure

2.5.1. Calibration Curve, Accuracy and Precision

Method qualification was carried out with a 'fit-for-purpose' approach. Quality control (QC) samples as well as standards (STDs) were used for batch acceptance. The qualification run contained duplicate calibration curves at eight concentrations and QCs at three concentrations (low, medium and high concentrations). The acceptance criterion for STDs and QCs in the qualification run was within ±25% of precision and accuracy, which is acceptable for early-stage drug discovery. Calibration curve was done by establishing a quadratic regression function, with an equation $y = ax^2 + bx + c$ after 1/concentration weighting. In addition, two blank plasma samples were in the set. QC samples (2.5, 25 and 50 μg/mL) were processed and analyzed three times in the same run (precision). The accuracy was calculated at each QC concentration as the ratio of the measured concentration to the nominal concentration multiplied by 100%.

2.5.2. Species-Dependent Matrix Effect

For species-dependent matrix effect test, three levels of QC samples were prepared in mouse and monkey plasma. Samples were quantitated with a calibration curve prepared in rat plasma. Mean accuracy and precision were also calculated.

2.5.3. Freeze and Thaw Stability

The freeze and thaw stability in rat, mouse and monkey plasma was assessed using low, medium and high QC samples ($n = 3$ at each concentration). For this study, the samples were subjected to three freeze and thaw cycles at −80 °C.

2.6. Software

Analyst® TF Version 1.6 (Sciex, Foster City, CA, USA) operated with Windows® (Microsoft) was used for instrument control and data acquisition. Peak integrations were operated by MultiQuant® Version 2.1.1 (Sciex, Foster City, CA, USA). Calculations including peak area ratios, standard curve regressions, sample concentration values and descriptive statistics were calculated with MultiQuant® Version 2.1.1. Pharmacokinetic calculations were performed using WinNonLin® version 6.4 (Pharsight Corporation, Mountain View, CA, USA).

2.7. Application for a Pharmacokinetic Study in Rat

Four adult male Sprague–Dawley rats (SD, 250–300 g) were purchased from the Samtako Biokorea Co. (Gyeonggi, Korea). The animals were housed in laminar flow cages that were maintained at 22 ± 2 °C and 50–60% relative humidity. The animals were kept in these facilities for at least a week prior to the experiment and were fasted for at least 24 h before the commencement of the experiments. Rats were cared for and treated in accordance with the Guiding Principles for the Use of Animals in Toxicology adopted by the Society of Toxicology (Reston, VA, USA) and the experimental protocols were approved by the Animal Care Committee of Chungnam National University (protocol No. CNU-00560).

Plasma samples were collected from the Sprague-Dawley rats ($n = 4$) after dosing intravenously with adalimumab at 1 mg/kg. The sampling times were 0.0014, 0.0417, 0.1667, 0.25, 1, 2, 3, 4, 7, 15, 21 and 28 days. The same set of pharmacokinetic study samples was analyzed by LC-QTOF-MS/MS.

3. Results

3.1. Method Development

3.1.1. Sample Preparation Method

In general, biological matrices such as plasma have highly abundant endogenous proteins such as albumin and immunoglobulins [14]. These endogenous proteins often interfere with the analysis of target mAb and decrease the sensitivity of the analyte. Therefore, a sample preparation method with minimal endogenous protein interference was necessary. To solve this problem, several approaches have been considered, such as albumin depletion kit, solid phase Protein A, and specific immunocapture [2,10,15]. In this study, the immunocapture using protein A magnetic beads was considered to be acceptable due to its selectivity as well as specificity. Plasma IgG and mAb were captured by a protein A magnetic bead and then washed out to remove other endogenous interference. After that, plasma IgG and mAb, bound to a protein A magnetic bead, were digested on-bead by the sequencing grade-modified trypsin. Trypsin-cleaved lysine and arginine residues in the amino acid sequence and various digested peptides from plasma IgG and mAbs were released into the supernatants. The supernatants were then analyzed by LC-QTOF-MS/MS for the target-specific signature peptide of adalimumab.

Generally, it would be ideal if trypsin digestion was carried out after acid dissociation and elution. However, one big challenge of this approach would be recovery from the protein A bead after binding. In addition, trypsin digestion efficiency is another challenge to consider due to lower pH after acid dissociation. Other matrix interference from endogenous immunoglobulins and etc. is another factor to carefully evaluate from this conventional trypsin digestion after acid dissociation followed by elution. Our approach, using on-bead digestion with trypsin, could have some disadvantages such as a large excess of tryptic peptide matrices derived from the protein A ligand, which might interfere with our assay. However, this method is very fast and robust and the interference from these endogenous matrix peptides could be minimized by selecting a specific signature peptide as well as its unique parent ion-product ion transition combination in the next section.

3.1.2. Selection of Target-Specific Signature Peptide

A couple of specific signature peptides were sought that would be applicable and specific to adalimumab using freeware software 'Skyline' (MacCoss Lab Software, https://skyline.ms/). As a result, three peptides out of various digested peptides were selected from the complementarity-determining region (CDR) of adalimumab. The three specific peptide sequences are as follows: NYLAWYQQKPGK, APYTFGQGTK and GLEWVSAITWNSGHIDYADSVEGR.

During the LC-QTOF-MS/MS analysis, two out of three peptides were detected (APYTFGQGTK and NYLAWYQQKPGK), while the GLEWVSAITWNSGHIDYADSVEGR peptide was not, possibly due to poor ionization. Although both APYTFGQGTK and NYLAWYQQKPGK peptides looks acceptable, APYTFGQGTK showed better peak intensity and better signal-to-noise ratio than NYLAWYQQKPGK in our experimental conditions (Figure 1). APYTFGQGTK was not detected in rat blank plasma or any other source during sample preparation and therefore was proven to be quite a unique signature peptide representing adalimumab. Therefore, APYTFGQGTK was chosen as the specific signature peptide for the quantitation of adalimumab in our experiment.

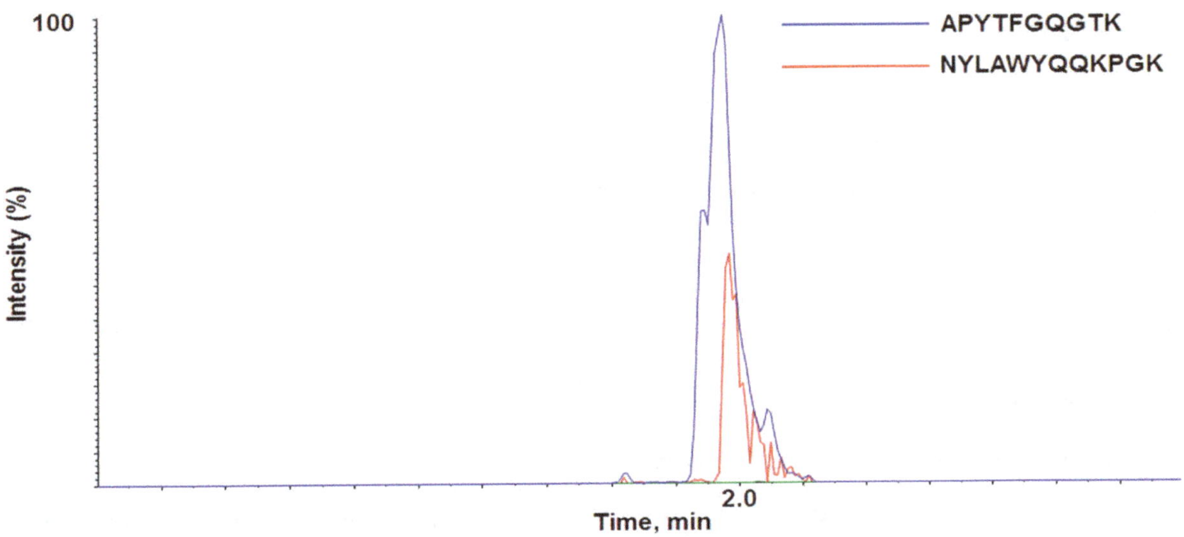

Figure 1. LC-QTOF-MS/MS chromatogram of the two proposed signature peptides.

Figure 2 shows the MS/MS spectrum of the adalimumab-specific signature peptide (APYTFGQGTK). From the doubly charged parent ion observed at m/z 535.27, several product ions were observed and the ion at m/z 901.45 showed the best sensitivity and selectivity.

3.1.3. Liquid Chromatography–Mass Spectrometry Analysis Using Quadrupole Time-of-Flight mass spectrometer

Conventionally, triple quadrupole mass spectrometers (low-resolution instrument) have been used for the quantitative analysis of small molecules. Recently, a Q-TOF mass spectrometer has been introduced to quantify large molecules such as proteins for pharmacokinetic studies [16]. In the past, Q-TOF had drawbacks in terms of sensitivity, linear dynamic range and speed, which meant it was unlikely to fill the need for reliable quantification in bioanalysis when compared to triple quadrupole mass spectrometer. However, the latest Q-TOF is good enough to overcome these shortcomings and shows good sensitivity and selectivity for the analysis of large molecules or peptides in single injection. In this study, the lower limit of quantification (LLOQ), accuracy, precision and linear dynamic range using LC-QTOF-MS/MS were good enough for our discovery non-GLP PK studies in rats.

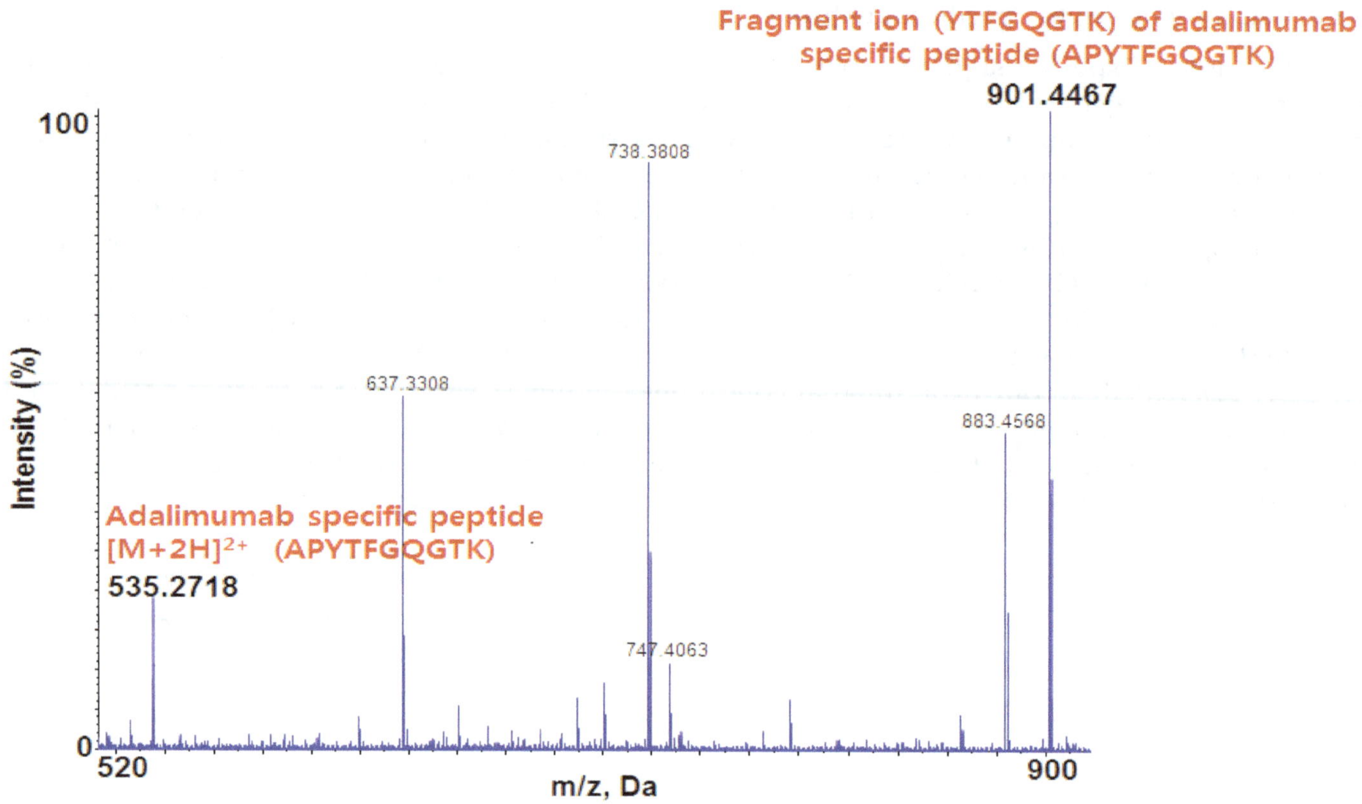

Figure 2. MS/MS spectrum of adalimumab specific peptide $[M + 2H]^{2+}$ and its fragment peptide.

3.2. *Method Qualification*

3.2.1. Calibration Curve, Linearity and Sensitivity

LC-QTOF-MS/MS analysis using the specific signature peptide in high-resolution mode was used for the quantitation of adalimumab. Calibration curves consisting of eight points in duplicate were prepared fresh for all datasets in rat plasma. The calibration curve range was 1–100 µg/mL. A representative chromatogram at the LLOQ (signal-to-noise ratio: ~9) is shown in Figure 3. This sensitivity was significant enough for most preclinical studies with a dose level ≥1 mg/kg to cover the expected concentration range throughout the PK time course. With a larger volume (~40 µL) of sample (or trypsin), more optimized conditions of LC-QTOF-MS/MS or a more sensitive mass spectrometer, we were also able to improve the LLOQ below 1 µg/mL in the preclinical species plasma, if needed (data not shown). The quadratic regression of the curves using peak area versus concentrations was weighted by 1/concentration. The calculated correlation coefficient value (r) for calibration curve was used to evaluate the linearity of the curve. The correlation coefficient of the calibration curve was ≥0.9931 and the LLOQ of 1 µg/mL was easily achieved in this method.

3.2.2. Accuracy, Precision and Species-Dependent Matrix Effect

Assay performance was determined by assessing inter/intra-day accuracy (%) and precision (%CV) of the QC samples (Table 1). Inter/intra-day accuracy and precision for rat plasma were performed using QC samples ($n = 9$) at low, medium and high QC levels. Accuracy (%) was defined as the calculated concentration, expressed as a percent deviation from nominal concentration. Precision was expressed as the percent coefficient of variation (%CV). The qualification run met the acceptance criteria of ±25% accuracy and precision for all QC samples.

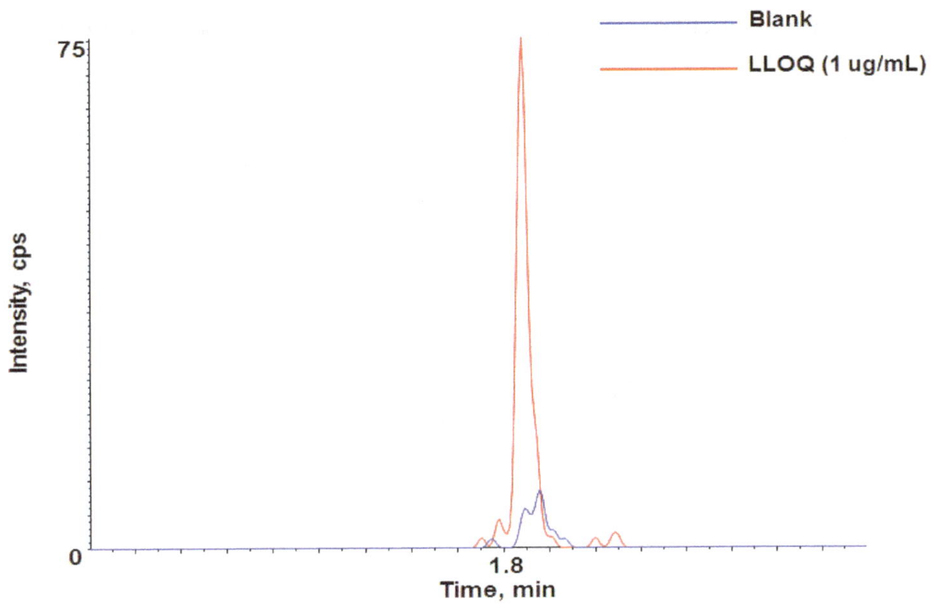

Figure 3. Representative chromatogram of lower limit of quantification (LLOQ, 1 μg/mL) for adalimumab-specific signature peptide in rat plasma.

Table 1. Inter/intra-day accuracy and precision of adalimumab in quality control samples.

Run No.	Statistics	QC Low (2.5 μg/mL)	QC Med (25 μg/mL)	QC High (50 μg/mL)
1	Mean	2.53	25.3	52.3
	Precision (%CV)	13.1	1.76	3.54
	n	3	3	3
	Accuracy (%)	101	101	105
2	Mean	2.73	23.9	56.3
	Precision (%CV)	2.6	11.13	11.55
	n	3	3	3
	Accuracy (%)	109	95	113
3	Mean	2.57	25.1	47.3
	Precision (%CV)	17.3	10.54	4.44
	n	3	3	3
	Accuracy (%)	103	100	95
Inter-day	Mean	2.61	24.77	51.97
	Precision (%CV)	11	7.81	6.51
	n	9	9	9
	Accuracy (%)	104	99	104

This assay developed for rat plasma samples was also evaluated for plasma samples from other species (mouse and monkey). If there are no/few species-dependent matrix effects between species, the rat plasma calibration curve should be able to quantitate adalimumab in other preclinical species as well. Table 2 shows no significant species-dependent matrix effects between rat plasma and other species. Also, Figure 4 shows that the selected signature peptides are unique in the plasma of several preclinical species. Although all three levels of the QC samples were passed, the interference from the blank monkey plasma appeared to be slightly higher than in rat or mouse blank plasma. Therefore, if this method was to be applied to monkey plasma PK samples, a slightly higher LLOQ (e.g., 2 μg/mL) would be helpful for the calibration curve in monkey plasma. Overall, the rat plasma calibration curve should be applicable to analyze adalimumab in mouse and monkey plasma samples if needed.

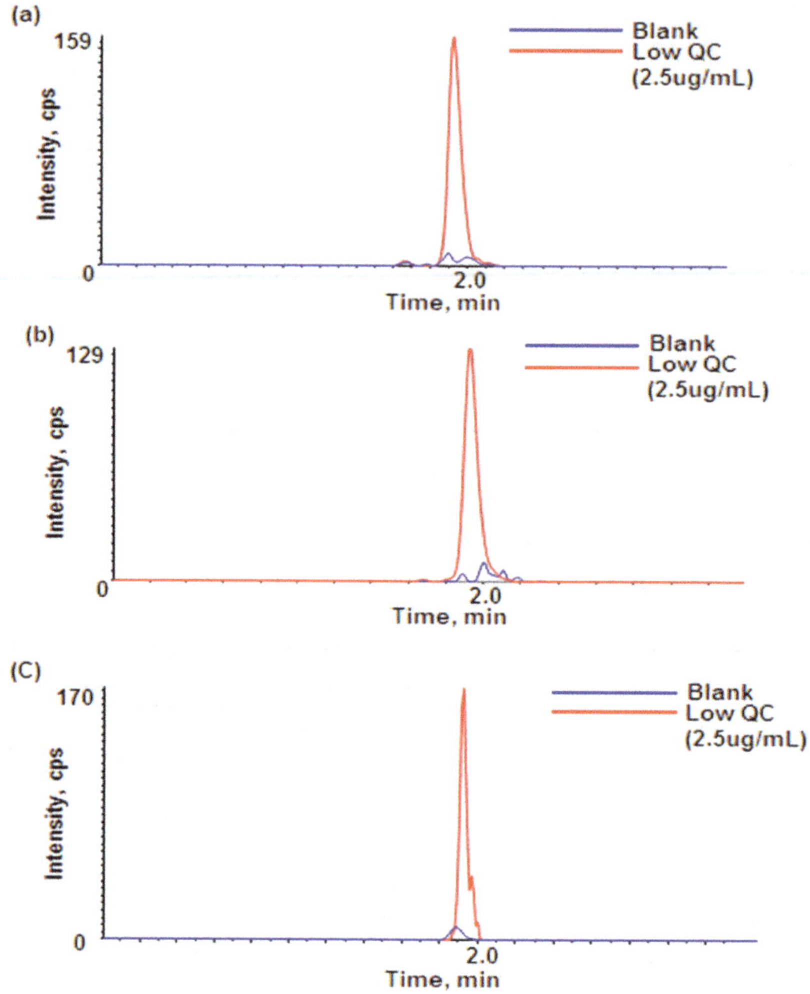

Figure 4. Comparison of peak intensities between blank and QC low in plasma: (**a**) blank and QC low in rat plasma; (**b**) blank and QC low in mouse plasma; (**c**) blank and QC low in monkey plasma.

Table 2. Various species-dependent matrix effects in mouse and monkey plasma. (a) Quality control result in mouse plasma; (b) quality control result in monkey plasma.

(a)

Mouse	Theoretical Concentration (μg/mL)	Mean Concentration (μg/mL)	Precision (%CV)	n	Accuracy (%)
QC low	2.5	2.85	13.2	3	114
QC medium	25	29.4	5.74	3	118
QC high	50	57	1.43	3	114

(b)

Monkey	Theoretical Concentration (μg/mL)	Mean Concentration (μg/mL)	Precision (%CV)	n	Accuracy (%)
QC low	2.5	2.09	4.9	3	84
QC medium	25	23.4	11.19	3	94
QC high	50	48.1	5.12	3	96

3.2.3. Freeze and Thaw Stability

Freeze and thaw stability assessments were carried out to demonstrate that adalimumab in plasma samples was stable under freeze and thaw conditions. The freeze and thaw stability experiments for rat, mouse and monkey plasma were performed using QC samples (n = 3) at low, medium and high QC levels. The mean values of the freeze and thaw stability QC samples at each level were compared with the nominal concentrations. The results are summarized in Table 3. The acceptance criterion for the freeze and thaw stability samples was within ± 25% precision and accuracy, which is acceptable for early drug discovery studies, and the results all met the acceptance criteria. As a result, adalimumab in rat, mouse and monkey plasma QC samples was stable through three freeze and thaw cycles.

Table 3. Freeze and thaw stability assessment in preclinical species (three cycles) (**a**) Freeze and thaw stability in rat plasma; (**b**) freeze and thaw stability in mouse plasma; (**c**) freeze and thaw stability in monkey plasma.

(a)

Rat	Theoretical Concentration (μg/mL)	Mean Concentration (μg/mL)	Precision (%)	n	Accuracy (%)
QC low	2.5	2.58	10.5	3	103
QC medium	25	25.6	13.67	3	102
QC high	50	57.3	8.73	3	115

(b)

Mouse	Theoretical Concentration (μg/mL)	Mean Concentration (μg/mL)	Precision (%)	n	Accuracy (%)
QC low	2.5	2.62	16.7	3	105
QC medium	25	28	3.26	3	112
QC high	50	60.2	0.94	3	120

(c)

Monkey	Theoretical Concentration (μg/mL)	Mean Concentration (μg/mL)	Precision (%)	n	Accuracy (%)
QC low	2.5	2.26	2.8	3	91
QC medium	25	19.5	12.42	3	78
QC high	50	40.3	8.52	3	81

3.2.4. Application to a Pharmacokinetic Study in Rats

The qualified LC-QTOF-MS/MS method was successfully applied to a pharmacokinetic study of adalimumab in Sprague–Dawley (SD) rats. Plasma samples obtained after intravenous administration of 1 mg/kg were analyzed by LC-QTOF-MS/MS for the quantification of adalimumab concentrations. To assure acceptance of study sample analytical runs, at least two-thirds of the QC samples had to be within ±25% accuracy, with at least half of the QC samples at each concentration meeting these criteria. When 1 mg/kg of adalimumab was administered to the rats, the drug concentrations in rat plasma were all within the calibration curve range. The time–concentration profile is shown in Figure 5. Although no head-to-head comparison for the PK profiles was carried out between this LC-QTOF-MS/MS method and other conventional methods, the PK profile produced by LC-QTOF-MS/MS looked comparable to the reference adalimumab human PK profile published in studies using conventional methods. Unlike the PK profiles of small molecules, most monoclonal antibody drugs typically show bi-phase elimination PK profiles, which consist of a short half-life alpha-phase distribution followed by a beta-phase elimination with a long half-life. Therefore, a two-compartment model was used for the PK parameters of adalimumab in this experiment. (Table 4) [17]. The time-concentration graph of adalimumab in Figure 5 also showed typical two-compartment monoclonal antibody PK characteristics with a short alpha-phase and a long beta-phase half-life (~10 days).

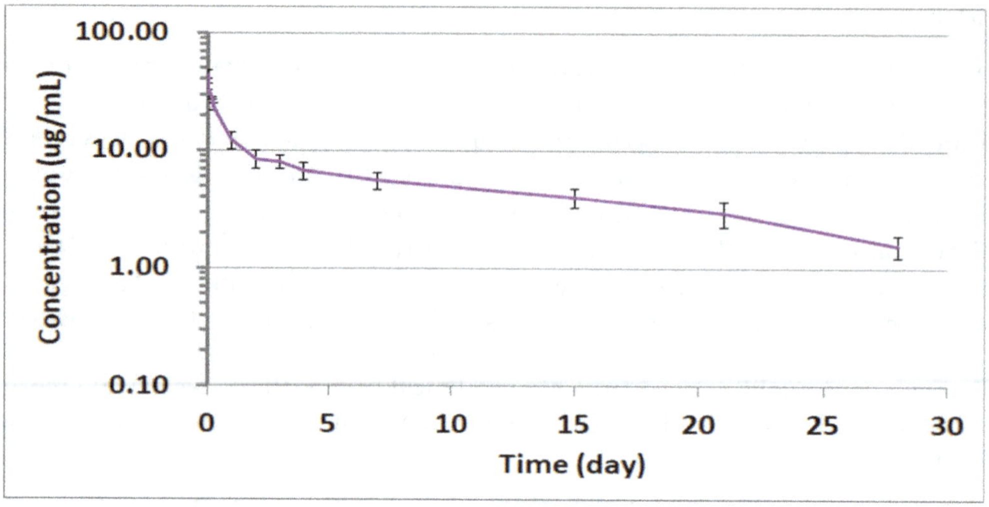

Figure 5. Time-concentration profile of adalimumab in rat plasma from the study subjects receiving 1 mg/kg adalimumab by intravenous administration. The data represent the mean ± standard deviation (SD, n = 4).

Table 4. Pharmacokinetic parameters of adalimumab after 1 mg/kg intravenous injection in rats.

	PK parameters							
Compound	AUC (μg·Day/mL)	Cl (mL/Day/kg)	Alpha Half Life (Day)	Beta Half Life (Day)	C_{max} (μg/mL)	V_1 (mL/kg)	V_{ss} (mL/kg)	Compartment Model
Adalimumab	155.29	6.68	0.2	9.82	41.64	24.1	85.83	2

4. Discussion

Immunoassay has been used for over 50 years and has traditionally been used to quantify large molecules. However, this method has some disadvantages [18]. The main disadvantages are that it is time-consuming and requires labor-intensive reagent development [8]. Immunoassays also often show cross-reaction with precursors of the target protein or with smaller metabolized fragments that are not suitable for early-stage mAbs bioanalysis [11]. LC-MS/MS can overcome the disadvantages of immunoassay. Compared to traditional immunoassay, LC-MS/MS technique does not require the preparation of time-consuming and high-cost reagents for specific antibody detection. Combined with LC-MS/MS and immunocapture methods, analytes can be selectively extracted without interferences such as anti-drug antibodies (ADA), which interfere with protein drug targets in the biological matrix [19].

Adalimumab is a recombinant human IgG1 monoclonal antibody [20]. Therefore, human IgG1 is also detected when quantifying adalimumab in the human matrix, making it difficult to distinguish it from the target drug. Therefore, the specific signature peptide of adalimumab was selected because it was distinguishable from human IgG1.

A LC-QTOF-MS/MS method was developed for the determination of adalimumab in rat plasma using a specific signature peptide (APYTFGQGTK) to demonstrate the feasibility of this method for adalimumab or its biosimilars. The calibration curve was acceptable over a concentration range from 1 to 100 μg/mL for adalimumab using quadratic regression with 1/concentration weighting. This LC-QTOF-MS/MS method was sensitive, selective, accurate and reproducible for the determination of adalimumab concentration and has been applied successfully to an adalimumab rat PK study. There was no significant species-dependent matrix effect between rats and other preclinical species, which means this method would be applicable to other preclinical sample analyses without developing new reagents for sample preparation. In conclusion, this method was useful for the analysis of adalimumab and could also be used as a complementary method for adalimumab or its biosimilars in early-stage research and development.

Author Contributions: Y.P., M.-H.P. and Y.G.S. designed the experiment; Y.P., N.K., J.C., M.-H.P., B.i.L., S.-H.S. and J.-J.B. performed the experiments; Y.P., N.K. and J.C. analyzed the data; Y.P. wrote the paper; Y.G.S. reviewed and revised the paper.

Acknowledgments: This research was supported by a research fund of Chungnam National University.

References

1. Ecker, D.M.; Jones, S.D.; Levine, H.L. The therapeutic monoclonal antibody market. *MAbs* **2015**, *7*, 9–14. [CrossRef] [PubMed]
2. Park, M.H.; Lee, M.W.; Shin, Y.G. Qualification and application of a liquid chromatography-quadrupole time-of-flight mass spectrometric method for the determination of trastuzumab in rat plasma. *Biomed. Chromatogr.* **2016**, *30*, 625–631. [CrossRef] [PubMed]
3. Breedveld, F.C. Therapeutic monoclonal antibodies. *Lancet* **2000**, *355*, 735–740. [CrossRef]
4. Catapano, A.L.; Papadopoulos, N. The safety of therapeutic monoclonal antibodies: Implications for cardiovascular disease and targeting the pcsk9 pathway. *Atherosclerosis* **2013**, *228*, 18–28. [CrossRef] [PubMed]
5. Voller, A.; Bartlett, A.; Bidwell, D.E. Enzyme immunoassays with special reference to elisa techniques. *J. Clin. Pathol.* **1978**, *31*, 507–520. [CrossRef] [PubMed]
6. Balkwill, F. Tnf-alpha in promotion and progression of cancer. *Cancer Metastasis Rev.* **2006**, *25*, 409–416. [CrossRef] [PubMed]
7. Azevedo, V.F.; Troiano, L.D.C.; Galli, N.B.; Kleinfelder, A.; Catolino, N.M.; Martins, P.C.U. Adalimumab: A review of the reference product and biosimilars. *Biosimilars* **2016**, *6*, 29–44. [CrossRef]
8. Sandborn, W.J.; Hanauer, S.B.; Rutgeerts, P.; Fedorak, R.N.; Lukas, M.; MacIntosh, D.G.; Panaccione, R.; Wolf, D.; Kent, J.D.; Bittle, B.; et al. Adalimumab for maintenance treatment of crohn's disease: Results of the classic ii trial. *Gut* **2007**, *56*, 1232–1239. [CrossRef] [PubMed]
9. Darwish, I.A. Immunoassay methods and their applications in pharmaceutical analysis: Basic methodology and recent advances. *Int. J. Biomed. Sci.* **2006**, *2*, 217–235. [PubMed]
10. Liu, H.; Manuilov, A.V.; Chumsae, C.; Babineau, M.L.; Tarcsa, E. Quantitation of a recombinant monoclonal antibody in monkey serum by liquid chromatography-mass spectrometry. *Anal. Biochem.* **2011**, *414*, 147–153. [CrossRef] [PubMed]
11. Becher, F.; Pruvost, A.; Clement, G.; Tabet, J.C.; Ezan, E. Quantification of small therapeutic proteins in plasma by liquid chromatography-tandem mass spectrometry: Application to an elastase inhibitor epi-hne4. *Anal. Chem.* **2006**, *78*, 2306–2313. [CrossRef] [PubMed]
12. Domon, B.; Aebersold, R. Mass spectrometry and protein analysis. *Science* **2006**, *312*, 212–217. [CrossRef] [PubMed]
13. Heudi, O.; Barteau, S.; Zimmer, D.; Schmidt, J.; Bill, K.; Lehmann, N.; Bauer, C.; Kretz, O. Towards absolute quantification of therapeutic monoclonal antibody in serum by lc-ms/ms using isotope-labeled antibody standard and protein cleavage isotope dilution mass spectrometry. *Anal. Chem.* **2008**, *80*, 4200–4207. [CrossRef] [PubMed]
14. Roopenian, D.C.; Akilesh, S. Fcrn: The neonatal fc receptor comes of age. *Nat. Rev. Immunol.* **2007**, *7*, 715–725. [CrossRef] [PubMed]
15. Li, H.; Ortiz, R.; Tran, L.; Hall, M.; Spahr, C.; Walker, K.; Laudemann, J.; Miller, S.; Salimi-Moosavi, H.; Lee, J.W. General lc-ms/ms method approach to quantify therapeutic monoclonal antibodies using a common whole antibody internal standard with application to preclinical studies. *Anal. Chem.* **2012**, *84*, 1267–1273. [CrossRef] [PubMed]
16. Shen, H.W.; Yu, A.M. Conference report: New analytical technologies for biological discovery. *Bioanalysis* **2010**, *2*, 181–184. [CrossRef] [PubMed]
17. Ferri, N.; Bellosta, S.; Baldessin, L.; Boccia, D.; Racagni, G.; Corsini, A. Pharmacokinetics interactions of monoclonal antibodies. *Pharmacol. Res.* **2016**, *111*, 592–599. [CrossRef] [PubMed]
18. Cross, T.G.; Hornshaw, M.P. Can lc and lc-ms ever replace immunoassays? *J. Appl. Bioanal.* **2016**, *2*, 108–116. [CrossRef]

19. Wilffert, D.; Bischoff, R.; van de Merbel, N.C. Antibody-free workflows for protein quantification by lc-ms/ms. *Bioanalysis* **2015**, *7*, 763–779. [CrossRef] [PubMed]
20. Kaymakcalan, Z.; Sakorafas, P.; Bose, S.; Scesney, S.; Xiong, L.; Hanzatian, D.K.; Salfeld, J.; Sasso, E.H. Comparisons of affinities, avidities, and complement activation of adalimumab, infliximab, and etanercept in binding to soluble and membrane tumor necrosis factor. *Clin. Immunol.* **2009**, *131*, 308–316. [CrossRef] [PubMed]

10

An Overview of Chitosan Nanoparticles and its Application in Non-Parenteral Drug Delivery

Munawar A. Mohammed, Jaweria T. M. Syeda, Kishor M. Wasan and Ellen K. Wasan *

College of Pharmacy and Nutrition, University of Saskatchewan, Saskatoon, SK S7N 2Z4, Canada; mum495@mail.usask.ca (M.A.M.); jaweria.syeda@usask.ca (J.T.M.S.); kishor.wasan@usask.ca (K.M.W.)

* Correspondence: ellen.wasan@usask.ca

Abstract: The focus of this review is to provide an overview of the chitosan based nanoparticles for various non-parenteral applications and also to put a spotlight on current research including sustained release and mucoadhesive chitosan dosage forms. Chitosan is a biodegradable, biocompatible polymer regarded as safe for human dietary use and approved for wound dressing applications. Chitosan has been used as a carrier in polymeric nanoparticles for drug delivery through various routes of administration. Chitosan has chemical functional groups that can be modified to achieve specific goals, making it a polymer with a tremendous range of potential applications. Nanoparticles (NP) prepared with chitosan and chitosan derivatives typically possess a positive surface charge and mucoadhesive properties such that can adhere to mucus membranes and release the drug payload in a sustained release manner. Chitosan-based NP have various applications in non-parenteral drug delivery for the treatment of cancer, gastrointestinal diseases, pulmonary diseases, drug delivery to the brain and ocular infections which will be exemplified in this review. Chitosan shows low toxicity both in vitro and some in vivo models. This review explores recent research on chitosan based NP for non-parenteral drug delivery, chitosan properties, modification, toxicity, pharmacokinetics and preclinical studies.

Keywords: chitosan; mucoadhesive; polymeric nanoparticles; sustained release; oral drug delivery

1. Introduction

The mucosal route is gaining attention for noninvasive drug delivery via the oral, nasal, pulmonary or vaginal routes [1]. At the same time, nanoparticle technology has also come to the forefront as a viable drug delivery strategy, presenting opportunities for controlled release, protection of active components from enzymatic or environmental degradation and localized retention. Nanoparticle fabrication methods are readily scalable and applicable to a broad range of drugs. Of all the nanoparticle drug delivery approaches, polymeric nanoparticles have gained significant importance as they are biodegradable, biocompatible and because formulation methods are more widely available; the range of applications has been expanding to include a variety of chemical drug classes and dosage forms [2]. Chitosan-based NP are particularly appropriate for the mucosal route, with their low toxicity, mucoadhesion and tunable physical properties. Examples will be given of chitosan-based nanoparticles used for the treatment of cancer, gastrointestinal diseases, pulmonary diseases, drug delivery to the brain and ocular infections. Recent research on chitosan-based NP for nonparenteral drug delivery is based on the field's expanding understanding of chitosan properties and methods of chemical or physical modification, which are applied to the optimization of nanoparticle drug loading and release features. We will also discuss the current understanding of in vitro and in vivo toxicity and the effect of chitosan nanoparticle formulation on drug pharmacokinetics in preclinical studies.

Chitosan

Chitosan is the most important derivative of chitin, produced by removing the acetate moiety from chitin as shown in Figure 1.

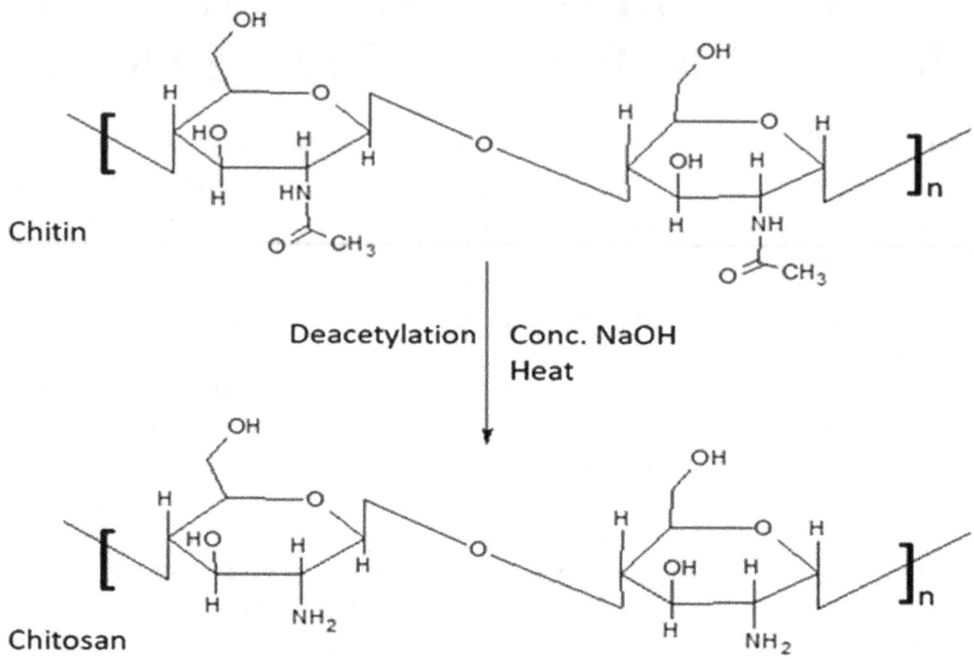

Figure 1. Deacetylation of chitin to chitosan.

It is derived from crustacean shells such as those from prawns or crabs, as well as from the cell walls of fungi. It is a naturally occurring polysaccharide, cationic, highly basic, mucoadhesive biocompatible polymer and approved by the U.S. FDA for tissue engineering and drug delivery. Chitin from natural sources is found bound to proteins and minerals, which must be removed prior to preparation of chitosan, though processes of acidification and alkalization. Purified chitin is then *N*-deacetylated to chitosan. This process can be modified to control the end product properties [including molecular weight and pKa (6–7.5)] [3,4] by controlling the degree of deacetylation with factors such as reaction conditions (concentration, ratios of chitin to alkali, temperature), chitin source and extent of the reaction, for example. While these chemical processes are well in hand for industrial processors, research is ongoing to more fully develop scalable biological, enzymatic or hybrid methods such as those using microorganisms [5]. It will be interesting to see how these approaches will be used to manufacture specific types of deacetylated chitosan and whether these bioprocesses will have any environmental advantage in the future.

Chitosan acts a penetration enhancer by opening the tight junctions of the epithelium. Chitosan facilitates both paracellular and transcellular transport of drugs as indicated in Figure 2. Chitosan interacts with mucus (negatively charged) to form a complex by ionic or hydrogen bonding as well as though hydrophobic interactions. The pKa of the primary amine of chitosan is ~6.5, depending on the degree of *N*-deacetylation. This group also contributes to the solubility of chitosan in acidic pH environments and the partial neutralization of this primary amine may also explain why chitosan has been reported to aggregate at neutral to high pH [6]. However, it should be noted that while this may be the tendency for chitosan with fraction of acetylated units <0.4 and medium/high molecular weight, chitosan with acetylation degrees in the range 40–60% are well known as being soluble even at physiological pH [4]. Thus, the nanoparticle formulator must carefully match the desired chemical and physical properties of the chitosan, as well as the anticipated biological environment, with the chitosan processing method.

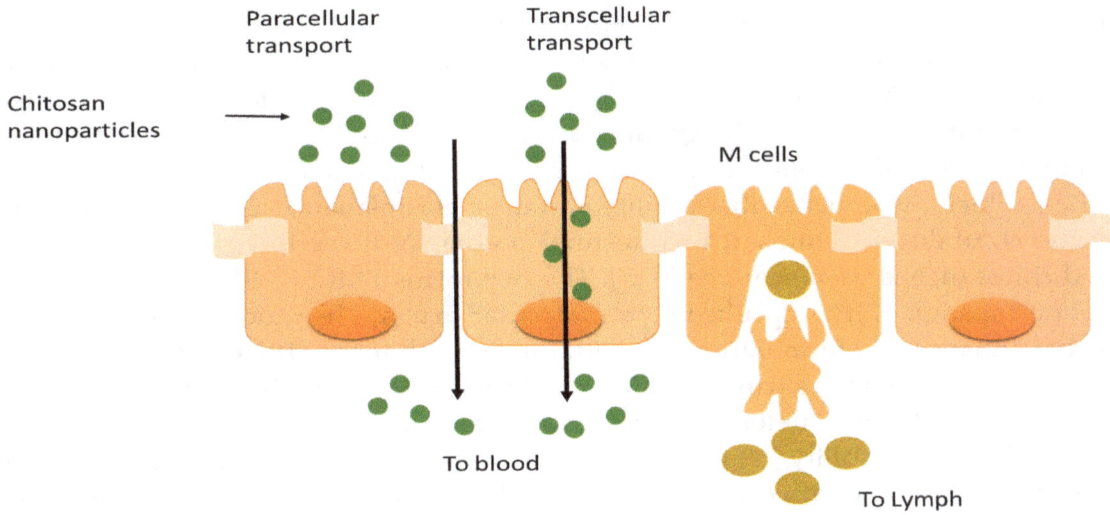

Figure 2. Schematic illustration of the presumed mechanism of transcellular and paracellular transport of chitosan NP across the epithelium.

2. Modification of Chitosan

The chitosan backbone can be modified to alter properties such as solubility, mucoadhesion and stability as discussed throughout this paper for specific applications. Both the -NH_2 and -OH groups of chitosan are the active sites for modification. Some of the commonly used techniques described below for preparing chitosan polymers are: blending, graft co-polymerization and curing [7]. Blending involves the simple mixing of two or more polymers. Graft co-polymerization involves the covalent bonding of polymers, while curing converts the polymers into a solidified mass by formation of three-dimensional bonds within the polymer mass by means of thermal, electrochemical or ultraviolet radiation processing methods.

2.1. Physical Modification

Physical modification is achieved by blending, which involves the physical mixing of two or more polymers. It is one of the oldest and easiest ways of modifying polymers. The quality and performance of the blend can be modified depending on the ratios of the polymers which are being mixed. Blending is the most economical technique by which the polymer properties can be tailored for specific applications [8].

Some of the common hydrophilic polymers that can be blended with chitosan to achieve oral drug delivery are poly (vinyl alcohol) (PVA), poly (vinyl pyrrolidone) (PVP) and poly (ethyl oxide) (PEO). Blending of chitosan and PVA improves the mechanical (tensile strength) and barrier properties (water vapor permeability) of chitosan films [9]. The intermolecular interactions between chitosan and PVA result in blends of PVA-chitosan that show improved mechanical properties (tensile strength) of chitosan films for controlled drug delivery [10]. An example of physical modification in controlled drug delivery is represented by amoxicillin formulated with a crosslinked chitosan/PVP blend with glutaraldehyde to form a semi-interpenetrating polymer (semi-IPN) [11]. The semi-IPN is formed because of the protonation of the amino group of chitosan, as confirmed by Fourier transform infrared spectroscopy (FTIR). Additional methods used for characterization of chitosan blends other than FTIR are: differential scanning calorimetry (DSC) [12], X-ray diffraction (XRD) [13], FTIR spectroscopy and rheology [14], enabling an understanding of the effects of processing on bonding and flow properties.

2.2. Chemical Modification

Chemical modification is achieved by altering the functional groups in a compound. Chemical modification can be done by several ways which include: chemical, radiation, photochemical, plasma-induced and enzymatic grafting methods [7]. Chemical modification of chitosan results in the formation of several derivatives such as quaternized chitosan, thiolated chitosan, carboxylated chitosan, amphiphilic chitosan, chitosan with chelating agents, PEGylated chitosan and lactose-modified chitosan. The primary amine (-NH_2) groups of chitosan provide a reaction site for chemical modification to achieve various pharmaceutical applications [7], reacting with sulphates, citrates and phosphates [15], which can enhance the stability and drug encapsulation efficiency [16]. For example, to improve the solubility of chitosan in intestinal media, *N*-trimethyl chitosan chloride (TMC), a quaternized chitosan, has been produced [17]. The two forms TMC, TMC 40 and TMC 60, enhance the intestinal permeation of hydrophilic macromolecular drugs. The mucoadhesiveness of chitosan has been further enhanced by formulating NP with thiolated chitosan [18]. Quaternization of chitosan forms several derivatives such as trimethyl (TMC), dimethylethyl (DMEC), diethylmethyl (DEMC) and triethyl chitosan (TEC). Quaternization of chitosan aids in the opening of tight junctions and improving the permeability of insulin across Caco-2 cells [19]. Chitosan-thioglycolic acid, chitosan-cysteine, chitosan-glutathione, chitosan-thioethylamidine are some of the thiolated chitosan derivatives presently in use. TMC-cysteine based NPs have shown significantly higher mucoadhesion and permeation compared to TMC NPs [20]. Grafting carboxylated chitosan with poly (methyl methacrylate) helps achieve pH-sensitive properties. The NPs made with the grafted polymer and insulin have shown very minimal drug release in simulated gastric fluid and an instant release in simulated intestinal fluid [21]. A pH sensitive polymer gel can be prepared by chemically linking D,L-lactic acid with -NH_2 groups of the chitosan for an application in the drug delivery to the different regions of the gastrointestinal tract (GIT) [22]. Lactose modification of the chitosan backbone (1-deoxylactit-1-yl chitosan) has been used in combination with the polyvalent ion tripolyphosphate (TPP) to form colloidal coacervates though polyionic interactions, forming highly uniform and small (200 nm diameter) nanoparticles [23,24].

3. Drug Release from Chitosan Nanoparticles

There are several mechanisms which govern drug release from chitosan nanoparticles such as: swelling of the polymer [25], diffusion of the adsorbed drug, drug diffusion through the polymeric matrix, polymer erosion or degradation and a combination of both erosion and degradation [26] as represented in Figure 3. The initial burst release from the chitosan nanoparticles is either because of swelling of the polymer, creating pores, or diffusion of the drug from the surface of the polymer [27]. Chitosan nanoparticles also exhibit a pH-dependent drug release because of the solubility of chitosan [28]. Chitosan derivatives alter the release of drug from the NP, affording tunable drug release [29] and impacting the pharmacokinetic profile of the loaded drug.

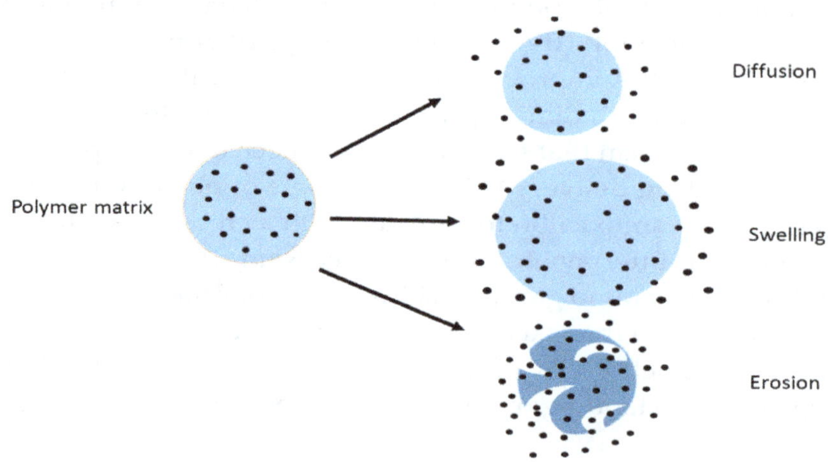

Figure 3. Diagram representing the possible mechanisms of drug release by diffusion, swelling and erosion of polymer (chitosan) matrix.

In diffusion-controlled release, the drug permeates through the interior of the polymeric matrix to the surrounding medium. Polymer chains form the diffusion barrier making it difficult for the drug to pass through and this barrier serves as the rate-limiting membrane for drug release. Diffusion may also be associated with polymer swelling or erosion. The mathematical representation of diffusion is given by Fick's law of diffusion.

$$F = -D\frac{\partial c}{\partial x} \tag{1}$$

where, F is the rate of transfer per unit area of section (flux), c is the concentration of the drug and D is the diffusion coefficient (diffusivity). To derive the parameters of Fick's law, there are few assumptions to be made such as: pseudo-steady state is maintained during drug release, the diameter of the drug particles is less than the average distance of drug diffusion through the polymeric matrix and sink conditions are always provided by the medium surrounding the nanoparticles [30].

The swelling of the polymer is characterized by the imbibition of water into the polymer until the polymer dissolves. This drug release mechanism is characterized by the solubility of the polymer in water, or the surrounding biological medium. When the polymer encounters the surrounding medium and swelling commences, the polymer chains detangle. This is followed by drug release from that region of the polymer matrix. Generally, the hydrophilicity of the polymer, the polymer swelling rate and the density of the polymer chains play a key role in the drug release profile [31]. Subsequently, this will affect the rate of drug absorption from the site of delivery in vivo, as it will affect the rate at which drug is available for membrane transport or cellular uptake.

Erosion and degradation of polymers are interrelated features. Sometimes, degradation of the polymer may cause subsequent physical erosion as bonds break. Erosion of polymers is a complex phenomenon as it involves swelling, diffusion and dissolution. Erosion occurs in two ways: homogenous and heterogeneous. Homogenous erosion is erosion of the polymer at the same rate throughout the matrix whereas heterogeneous erosion is erosion of the polymer from the surface towards the inner core. Polymer degradation may be due to the surrounding media or the presence of enzymes. The degradation of the polymer also depends on the pH of the surrounding media, the copolymer composition and water uptake by the polymer. Drug release depends on the type of polymer and internal bonding, any additives (chitosan derivatives), as well as the shape and size of the nanoparticles as this reflects surface area and free energy [32].

Generally, drug release from the chitosan nanoparticles is similar to that of PLGA (Poly(D,L-lactide-*co*-glycolide)) nanoparticles [33] but the drug release from chitosan nanoparticles is more pH-dependent [34]. As an example, exendin-4 loaded PLGA and chitosan-PLGA nanoparticles have been studied. Exendin-4 is generally used for the treatment of type-2 diabetes. The NPs were evaluated for transmembrane permeability studies in MDCK (Madin-Darby Canine Kidney) cells and in an in vivo study in male Wistar rats. The in vitro transmembrane permeability studies revealed that exendin-4 was transported across the cell layer by active transport when formulated as PLGA or chitosan-PLGA NP compared to the free drug solution. The permeability coefficient (P_{app}) with PLGA and chitosan-PLGA NP was 1.52×10^{-6} and $2.5–3.0 \times 10^{-6}$, respectively, significantly greater than exendin-4 solution alone. Some of the PLGA NPs that enter the cell are trafficked into endosomes and suffer degradation while some reach the basolateral membrane via the trans-Golgi pathway. Similar mechanisms occur with chitosan-PLGA NPs, however, due to their positive charge electrostatic interactions occur with the negatively charged cell membrane resulting in a higher P_{app}. The in vivo study revealed higher plasma drug levels and longer retention times of exendin-4 when administered as chitosan-PLGA NP compared to PLGA NP [35].

4. Chitosan in Oral Drug Delivery

Oral drug delivery certainly is the most convenient route of drug administration because of the ease of administration. But there are several challenges in achieving oral delivery such as varying pH (highly acidic stomach), the presence of enzymes, first-pass effect in the liver and the intestinal barrier to drug absorption. The above challenges limit the drug from entering the systemic circulation thereby reducing oral bioavailability [36]. Nanoparticle technology is an increasingly exploited formulation technique to overcome the limitations of oral drug delivery [7,37]. NPs have several advantages such as small particle size, large surface area and potentially a modifiable surface. Small particle size is well known to increase the dissolution rate of drugs. Besides these advantages, NPs can increase the gastrointestinal tract stability of acid-labile drugs compared to other drug delivery systems such as liposomes and lipid based systems [38]. Chitosan can be formulated as polymeric nanoparticles for various applications in oral drug delivery as explained below with several examples.

Catechin and epigallocatechin are flavonoids present in green tea and are strong antioxidants. These undergo degradation in intestinal fluid and are poorly absorbed across intestinal membranes. The intestinal absorption of catechin and epigallocatechin gallate can be improved by encapsulating them in chitosan nanoparticles [39]. Tamoxifen, an anti-cancer drug, is slightly water soluble and a good candidate for oral cancer drug delivery. Permeation of tamoxifen across the intestinal epithelium was increased by formulating tamoxifen into lecithin-chitosan nanoparticles [40]. The NPs are mucoadhesive and increase the permeation of tamoxifen by the paracellular pathway. Feng et al. have also reported a potential oral delivery strategy for anti-cancer drugs. They have prepared nanoparticles of doxorubicin hydrochloride (DOX) with chitosan and carboxymethyl chitosan. These nanostructures were found to enhance the intestinal absorption of DOX throughout the small intestine [41]. Alendronate sodium is used in the treatment of osteoporosis and suffers from low oral bioavailability and gastrointestinal side effects. High NP encapsulation efficiency of alendronate sodium was achieved by formulating chitosan nanoparticles via an ion gelation technique. Drug release was clearly pH-dependent; in 0.1N HCl, almost 80% of the drug was released within 60 min while in PBS (pH 6.8) a maximum of 40% of the drug was released over 4 h, suggesting that factors other than chitosan's pH solubility profile influenced drug release in this case and that optimization is multifactorial [28]. This highlights the importance of examining the degree of surface coverage of the nanoparticles with chitosan and of performing ongoing dissolution studies in biorelevant media during formulation development. For effective sustained delivery of sunitinib, a tyrosine kinase inhibitor, chitosan NPs were prepared by an ion crosslinking method. The encapsulation efficiency of the NPs was 98% and sustained drug release was achieved up to 72 h [42]. The harsh conditions of the GIT denature proteins such as insulin when administered orally, yet oral insulin is a highly desired goal. In one example of insulin-loaded chitosan NPs the chitosan was crosslinked with tripolyphosphate. The particle size was reduced by this crosslinking process and the stability of the NPs was increased by freeze drying. NP uptake was significant in the intestine epithelium; unfortunately, however, the NPs were unstable in gastric pH [43] and further efforts to fabricate stable oral insulin NP are still needed. Bay 41-4109, an active inhibitor of hepatitis B virus was formulated as chitosan NPs to improve drug solubility and oral bioavailability. The cytotoxicity of Bay 41-4109-chitosan NP was found to be negligible and drug uptake was higher from the NPs, which was attributed to the positive charge from the chitosan [44]. Table 1 provides detailed insight into the extensive range of applications of chitosan NP for oral drug delivery.

Table 1. Applications of chitosan nanoparticles in oral drug delivery.

Drug	Composition	Purpose	Research Findings	In Vivo	Reference
Tamoxifen citrate	Chitosan, soybean lecithin NP	Intestinal permeation of tamoxifen in lecithin/chitosan NPs through the rat intestinal wall.	Ex vivo experiment using a jejunum chamber from the small intestine of male Wistar rats. Lecithin/chitosan nanoparticles improved the non-metabolized drug passage across the rat intestinal tissue.		[40]
Sunitinib	Chitosan	Biophysical characterization	1. In vitro biodegradation was improved in the presence of lysozyme. 2. In vitro controlled release was demonstrated with 69% released within 72 h.		[42]
Hydro phobic Bay41-4109	LMW chitosan	Solubility and bioavailability enhancement.	1. In vitro drug release studies showed a sustained release profile. 2. Low cytotoxicity was demonstrated in a liver cell line.	In vivo studies were performed in rats. The absolute bioavailability of Bay41-4109 NPs was >70%, nearly 4-fold higher than other formulations	[44]
Insulin	Chitosan, TPP	Preparation, characterization and stabilization of insulin—chitosan NPs.	1. In vitro validation-Caco2 and co-culture: Caco-2 cells internalized the NPs effectively.	In vivo studies where decreased glycaemia was observed in diabetic rats after insulin NP administration.	[43]
Cyclosporin-A	Chitosan HCl, Poloxamer 188, sodium glycolate, gelatin, soya lecithin	To develop and characterize Cy-A as positive charge NPs to improve GI uptake, bioavailability	Cy-A encapsulation efficiency was very high at 88–94%.	In vivo studies in beagle dogs showed relative bioavailability of Cy-A was significantly increased by NPs.	[45]
Extra cellular products (ECPs) of *Vibrio anguillarum* (Protein carrier)	Chitosan carboxymethyl chitosan	To study the efficacy of chitosan NPs as a vehicle for oral antigen delivery in fish vaccination.	In vitro release study was performed in Tris-buffer (pH 2.0, 4.5) & PBS (pH 7.4); the highest cumulative release was 58% at pH 7.4 followed by 37% at pH 2.0.	Biodistribution showed NP uptake in spleen and kidney. Lysozyme and complement evaluation. It showed elevated specific antibody and higher concentrations of lysozyme activity and complement	[46]
Alendro-nate sodium	Chitosan LMW, sodium tripolyphosphate (TPP), fluorenyl-methyloxycarbonyl chloride (FMOC)	To study the influence of physical parameters on drug encapsulation efficiency	In vitro drug release was performed in 0.1N HCl and PBS (pH 6.8). The NPs released alendronate faster in 0.1N HCl compared to PBS. Encapsulation efficiency was ~80%.		[28]
Catechins (+) catechin (C) and (−) epigallocatechingallate (EGCg)	Chitosan LMW, sodium tripolyphos-phate, tris[2-carboxyethyl] phosphine hydrochloride (TCEP)	To enhance the intestinal absorption by encapsulation of C, EGCg in chitosan NPs	Ex vivo study using a jejunum chamber from mice. The cumulative amounts transported after encapsulation were significantly higher for C and EGCg, respectively.		[39]

Table 1. *Cont.*

Drug	Composition	Purpose	Research Findings	In Vivo	Reference
Enoxaparin	Chitosan, STPP, sodium alginate	Alginate coated chitosan-NPs containing enoxaparin for oral controlled release	In vitro drug release showed only 2% drug release in SGF (pH 1.2) but 60% in SIF (pH 6.5).	In vivo studies were performed in albino rats: the oral bioavailability of enoxaparin in Alg-CS-NPs bioavailability was significantly higher compared to enoxaparin solution. A 60% reduction was seen in thrombus formation in rat venous thrombosis model.	[47]
Scutellarin	Chitosan, deoxycholic acid, vitamin B12	Enhancement of scutellarin oral delivery efficacy by Vit B12 modified amphiphilic chitosan derivatives to treat type II diabetes-induced retinopathy	Cytotoxicity study of Chit-DC and Chit-DC-VB12 displayed low cytotoxicity in Caco-2 cells.	In vivo studies: 1. Zebra fish embryo: development of the embryo was unaffected 2. Sprague-Dawleys rats: the AUC of scutellarin NP was 2–3 fold higher than free scutellarin and efficacy was achieved	[48]
Fucoidan	Chitosan, Tc-methylene di-phosphonate	To prepare and evaluate pH sensitivity of CS/F NPs	In vitro drug release of Tc-MDP from CS/F NPs rose as the pH levels changed from 2.5 to 7.4. CS/F NPs was stable into the stomach and decompose in the intestine.		[49]
Tolbut-amide	Chitosan, PLGA, streptozotocin	To prepare PLGA NPs modified with chitosan to form TOL-CS-PLGA NPs to improve bioavailability and reduce dose frequency.	In vitro drug release of TOL-CS-PLGA NPs showed sustained release in PBS, pH 7.4. Cytotoxicity study of TOL-CS-PLGA NPs were non-toxic in HePG2 cells.	In vivo study was performed in adult Sprague-Dawley rats: the TOL-CS-PLGA NPS showed a long-acting hypoglycemic effect over 8 h, significantly longer than metformin tablets.	[50]
Gemcita-bine	Chitosan LMW, penta sodium tripolyphos-phate	To prepare gemcitabine-loaded chitosan NPs (Gem-CS-NP) for oral bio-availability enhancement	1. In vitro drug release of Gem-CS-NPs showed controlled release by a two-phase process. 2. Absorption studies in an intestinal sac model: the absorption of Gem-CS-NPs intestinal transport increased 3–5-fold compared to free drug.		[51]
Naringenin	Sodium alginate, chitosan, streptozotocin	To prepare alginate coated chitosan core shell NPs for effective oral delivery	In vitro drug release from NPs was 15% in SGF (pH 1.2) and 90% in pH 7.4 in slow, sustained fashion.	In vivo study in rats showed lack of toxicity; and an anti-diabetic effect: naringenin NPs have better efficacy in lowering blood glucose levels compare to free drug.	[52]
Epigallocatechin gallate (EGCG)	*N*-carboxymethyl chitosan (MW = 61 kDa), chitosan hydrochloride	To develop EGCG-chitosan/β-Lg NPs to achieve a prolong release for oral administration in the GI tract	In vitro drug release and degradation of EGCG-chitosan/β-Lg NPs was slower in simulated stomach condition compare to control particles		[53]
Quercetin	Chitosan, sodium alginate, sodium pyruvate, L-glutamine	To develop and evaluate quercetin-chitosan/alginate NPs to preserve its antioxidant property without causing systemic toxicity.	In vitro cytotoxicity of both empty NPs and quercetin NPs exhibited nontoxic behavior in HepG2 liver cells when exposed for a period up to 72 h.	In vivo toxicity study in Wistar rats displayed no change in body weight, rat liver weight, histology, hematology and biochemical parameters after oral administration of empty NPs and quercetin loaded NPs.	[54]

Oral delivery of vaccines is critical as the antigens degrade in GIT hindering their reaching Peyer's patches, the gastrointestinal lymphoid tissue. Moreover, vaccines containing chitosan NP can only be prepared by methods that avoid organic solvents as the organic solvents may alter the immunogenicity of antigens if the peptide secondary structure is disturbed [55]. Chitosan and carboxymethyl chitosan NP were found to be excellent carriers for oral vaccine delivery of extracellular products of *V. anguillarum* (pathogenic bacteria). The NP prepared were stable in the gastric pH, had sustained release and protected the antigenic protein from entering spleen and kidney which is critical for immune response [46].

5. Chitosan in Nasal Drug Delivery

Nasal delivery is a non-invasive technique of delivering drugs to reach the respiratory system, the brain and/or systemic circulation. A significant challenge with the delivery of drugs through the nasal route is the mucociliary clearance of drugs. Moreover, hydrophilic drugs, proteins and peptides, nucleic acids and polysaccharides present difficulties because of their low permeability across the nasal epithelium. Nasal absorption is critical for the drugs to exhibit their action. The physical characteristics of drugs that govern nasal absorption include molecular weight, lipophilicity and charge. The drugs that do not cross the nasal membrane undergo mucociliary clearance. This limitation can be overcome by developing a mucoadhesive system. Chitosan is biodegradable, biocompatible, exhibits low toxicity, adheres to mucus and opens the tight junctions of nasal membrane. Owing to these properties, chitosan has applications in nasal delivery [56]. The three ways of nasal absorption is by transcellular pathway, paracellular pathway and via trigeminal nerves [57]. Several specific examples are given below.

Carbamazepine is used in the treatment of epilepsy and it is very important for the drug to cross the blood brain barrier (BBB). Carboxymethyl chitosan NPs of carbamazepine have found to enhance the bioavailability and brain targeting via the nasal route. The brain-to-plasma exposure ratio was 150% when carbamazepine was administered as chitosan NPs intranasally [25]. In Alzheimer's disease (AD), a person's sex is a risk factor and in women with AD, the levels of 17β-estradiol are found to be relatively low. Estradiol, a potent sex hormone, has been used in the prevention and treatment of AD. It is important for estradiol to achieve a sufficient tissue concentration in the brain to exhibit it effect. When estradiol is given orally, the cerebrospinal levels are very low. The cerebrospinal fluid levels of estradiol were found to be high compared to plasma levels when estradiol was administered intranasally as chitosan NPs. These results suggest that estradiol is transported to the brain directly when given through the nasal route as chitosan NPs. As another example, the bioavailability of leuprolide, used in the treatment of prostate cancer and hormone-dependent diseases, was found to be increased when formulated as thiolated-chitosan NPs [57]. Chitosan NPs and thiolated-chitosan NPs of leuprolide were prepared. There was a 2–5-fold increase in drug transport across porcine nasal mucosa when leuprolide was formulated as chitosan NPs or thiolated-chitosan NP, respectively, compared to leuprolide solution. The drug exposure, as measured by area under the plasma concentration vs. time curve AUC, increased by 6.9-fold with thiolated-chitosan NP [58].

6. Chitosan in Pulmonary Drug Delivery

Both local and systemic effects can be achieved by drug delivery to the lungs. There are several advantages to delivering drug to the lungs compared to other routes such as rapid and sustained drug delivery, high efficacy and no hepatic first-pass effect. The factors that enhance drug delivery via the lungs are the large surface area of the lungs, high tissue vascularity and the thin absorption barrier [59].

The barriers for drug delivery via the lungs include the bronchial mucus layer, the alveolar lining fluid, epithelial cells, macrophage clearance and proteolytic degradation [60]. In the recent review published by Islam and Ferro [61], drug delivery to the lungs with the help of chitosan based nanoparticles can be achieved. The authors claimed it to be beneficial that for pulmonary drug delivery, the positive charge on the surface of chitosan provides mucoadhesive properties. This adherence to the lung mucosa increases the potential for drug absorption; the positive charge on chitosan has been previously shown to open the intercellular tight junctions of the lung epithelium thereby increasing uptake. Interestingly, chitosan possesses antibacterial activity by binding to phosphoryl groups and lipopolysaccharides on bacterial cell membranes, which is an additional benefit in fighting pulmonary bacterial infections.

A NP dry powder inhalation (DPI) of rifampicin, an antitubercular drug, was formulated with chitosan as the polymer. This NP formulation has shown sustained drug release until 24 h and no toxicity at both cell and organ. An in vivo study of this formulation showed that rifampicin exhibited increased maximal plasma concentration (C_{max}), AUC and extended mean residence time (MRT) with the NP formulation [62]. Itraconazole is an anti-fungal drug which, when administered orally, suffers from low solubility. To treat pulmonary infections effectively, itraconazole has to be administered via the pulmonary route. Aerosolization would be an advantage for antifungal agents as it can provide a high drug concentration at the site of action, passive targeting and reduced systemic toxicity. The aerosolization properties of itraconazole can be significantly improved by formulating the drug in spray-dried chitosan NP with lactose, mannitol and leucine. The pulmonary deposition of itraconazole was shown to be increased when formulated as spray-dried microparticles containing itraconazole loaded chitosan NP [63]. Some of the other applications of chitosan in pulmonary drug delivery as depicted in Table 2.

Table 2. Applications of chitosan nanoparticles in pulmonary drug delivery.

Drug	Composition	Purpose	Research Findings	In Vivo	Reference
Rifampicin	TPP, lactose, Tween 80	Preparing CS-NPs dry powder to achieve local and sustained targeting of anti-tubercular drugs in order to reduce dosage and frequency	1. In vitro release showed 90% release of RFM from CS-NPs within 24 h. 2. Cell viability of J774 macrophage cells showed negligible toxicity of RFM-NPs up to 12 h exposure at concentrations up to 0.5 mg/mL	In vivo study—male Wistar rats. A marked increase in Cmax, t1/2 and AUC was seen in RFM-NPs compared to other formulations.	[62]
Itraconazole	Hydroxypropyl-beta-cyclodextrin (HPβCD), mannitol, lactose, TPP, L-leucine	To develop chitosan NPs for pulmonary delivery of itraconazole as a dry powder formulation	1. Encapsulation efficiency of 55% was obtained in 1:3 ratio of chitosan:TPP. 2. In vitro drug release was ~80% during the first 4 h and the remaining encapsulated drug was released over 48 h.		[63]
Baclofen and siRNA	*N,N,N*-tri-methyl chitosan, TPP	To prepare and evaluate baclofen-trimethyl chitosan/TPP NPs (Bac-TMC/TPP NPs) in a dry powder formulation	1. Low in vitro cytotoxicity of TMC and Bac-TMC in A549 cells when treated with four different polymers for 48 h. 2. Cellular uptake of Bac-TMC3/TPP/siRNA NPs was greatly enhanced by clathrin -mediated cellular uptake pathway.		[64]
Heparin (LMWH)	Chitosan, lipoid S100, glycol chitosan	To prepare and evaluate LMWH chitosan and glycol chitosan NPs for enhancing the pulmonary absorption of LMW heparin.	In vitro drug release of lipoid S100-LMWH GCS NPs in SLF showed progressive LMWH release up to 6 h, followed by a plateau for 24 h.	In vivo studies were performed in mice: the aerosol-type administration of free LMWH and Lipoid S100-LMWH GCS NPs led to a significant elongation of the coagulation time	[65]
Theo-phylline	Chitosan thioglycolic acid, TPP	To develop and evaluate whether theophylline-thiolated chitosan NPs can enhance theophylline's capacity to alleviate allergic asthma	In vitro mucoadhesive study of TCNs exhibited a gradual increase in mucin binding and adsorption for 12 h compared to unmodified chitosan	In vivo study was performed in mice and the anti-inflammatory effects of theophylline were markedly enhanced when the drug was delivered by TCNs compared to unmodified chitosan or theophylline alone.	[66]
Leuprolide	Thiolated chitosan	To prepare and evaluate leuprolide thiolated-CS-NPs to enhance the half-life and bioavailability of leuprolide via nasal administration	In vitro drug release of leuprolide from thiolated chitosan showed slow and sustained release of drug about 43% in 2 h.	In vivo study was performed in male Sprague-Dawley rats showed improved nasal bioavailability of leuprolide thiolated NPs calculated based on AUC (0–6) was about 19.6% as compared to leuprolide solution alone 2.8%.	[60]
Estradiol (E2)	Chitosan, methylated β-cyclodextrin, TPP	To prepare estradiol-chitosan NPs for improving nasal absorption and brain targeting		In vivo study was performed in male Wister rats: The plasma concentration of E2 from E2-CS-NPs was significantly lower in intranasal administration compare to IV but CSF concentrations of E2 from E2-CS-NPs was significantly higher for intranasal administration compare to IV.	[67]
Tetanus toxoid (TT)	LMW Chitosan, TPP, trehalose	To prepare tetanus toxoid chitosan nanoparticles (TT-CS NPs) as a new long-term nasal vaccine delivery vehicle	In vitro drug release of the TT from CS-NPs showed a rapid release over first 2 h followed by slow release for up to 16 days.	Intranasal immunization with two doses of TT-CS NPs in mice: The results showed the titers were significantly higher for the TT-loaded particles than for the free toxoid and at post-administration of TT-CS NPs IgA levels were significantly higher than the fluid vaccine.	[68]

7. Mucoadhesion

One of the major drawbacks of delivering proteins/peptides or macromolecules through a non-injection route is the limited absorption at mucosal sites. For local delivery in the GI tract or nasal/buccal cavity or to the vaginal, urethral or pulmonary sites, the drug delivery system should be mucoadhesive and release the drug. Mucoadhesive nanoparticles/microparticles can adhere to the mucus membrane and release the drug over time (Figure 4), with the potential to reduce dosing frequency. Uptake of drugs into the systemic circulation can be achieved by transient and reversible opening of tight junctions in between epithelial cells by certain polymers and chitosan is one such polymer [69]. Some of the other mucoadhesive polymers apart from chitosan are alginate, guar gum, pectin, carrageenan K type II, gelatin, poly (vinyl pyrrolidone), poly (vinyl amine), poly (ethylene glycol) and poly (ethylene oxide) and its copolymers and poly (acrylic acid) and poly (methacrylic acid) derivatives [70].

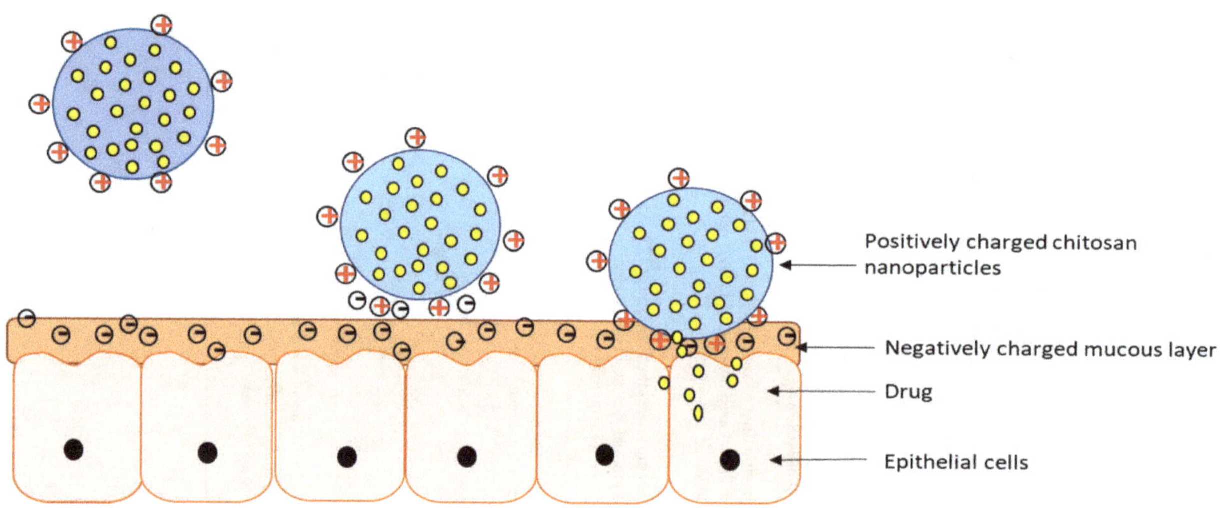

Figure 4. Schematic representation of chitosan loaded nanoparticles (CS-NP) structure and interaction with the mucus layer. From left to right: CS-NP upon reaching the mucosal layer bind to the negatively charged mucus by virtue of electrostatic attraction and release the drug over time.

As discussed earlier, the mucoadhesive property of the chitosan is attributed to its strong positive charge which helps in forming a bond with negatively charged mucus. Mucus is present in the organs of the GIT and the respiratory tract. The GIT is characterized by varying pH and an enzyme environment which makes it difficult for oral delivery of protein/peptide drugs and DNA. Chitosan is an excellent carrier for such drugs as it is mucoadhesive, permeation enhancer and forms a protective barrier for the drug [71]. Particle size also plays a role in the case of chitosan nanoparticles, as smaller particles may be more able to penetrate the mucous layer. Table 3 provides examples where the mucoadhesive property of chitosan is utilized.

Table 3. Applications of chitosan nanoparticles in mucoadhesive drug delivery.

Drug	Composition	Purpose	Research Findings	In Vivo	Reference
Doxorubicin HCL (DOX)	Chitosan (MW = 400 kDa), 4-CBS, TPP, 1-ethyl-3-(3-dimethylaminopropyl) carbodiimide HCl (EDAC)	Preparation, characterization, in vitro drug release, Topo II inhibitor activity and evaluation of DOX-loaded 4-CBS-chitosan/PLA nanoparticles.	1. In vitro drug release of DOX loaded 4-CBS-chitosan/PLA nanoparticles showed sustained release up to 26 days. 2. Cytotoxic study (MTT) of DOX loaded nanoparticles showed the lowest effect on the cell viability of HepG2 compared to SW620, KAT03 and CHAGO cell lines. 3. Over 72% inhibition of Topo II.		[72]
Alpha-mangostin (AP)	Chitosan (MW = 600 kDa), methane-sulfonic acid, oleoyl chloride, sodium bicarbonate, glycidyl-trimethyl ammonium chloride	To develop a mucoadhesive oleoyl-quaternized chitosan coated nanostructure lipid carrier (NLC) for potential oral administration with enhanced mucoadhesion	In vitro cytotoxicity of AP-NLC and CS-AP-NLC exhibited higher toxicity against Caco-2 than Hela cells.	In vivo toxicology study was performed in zebrafish embryos.	[73]
Cetirizine	Chitosan, 1-ethyl-3-(3-dimethylaminopropyl) carbodiimide hydrochloride (EDC. HCl), *N*-hydroxyl succinimide	Preparation and characterization of mucosal adhesion and drug release of cetirizine-chitosan NP	1. In vitro, the cumulative release of cedH from cedH:CS-NPs and cedH:CTZ-CS-1-NPs were 71% & 76% in absence of lysozyme and increased to 77% & 84% in presence of lysozyme. Burst release and lysozyme induced sustained release was achieved. 2. In vitro cytotoxicity of cedH:CTZ-CS-1 NPs showed non-toxicity in L929 cells and biocompatibility with RBCs.	[74]	
5-amino levulinic acid	Chitosan, lactic acid.	To develop and characterize chitosan-based 5-ALA mucoadhesive film to enhance its retention in oral mucosa	In vitro permeation and retention of 5-ALA (1.0% or 10%) were increased. However, 10% 5-ALA exhibited highest values 4 and 17 times, respectively, compared to propylene glycol vehicle.		[75]
Curcumin	Chitosan Low (CLS 50,000–190,000 Da), medium (CSM 190,000–310,00 Da), high (CSH 310,000 to >375,000 Da), polycaprolactone, glycerol	Preparation of mucoadhesive films containing curcumin-loaded NPs to prolong the residence time of the dosage form in the oral cavity and to increase drug absorption through the buccal mucosa	1. Swelling studies for mucoadhesive films containing curcumin loaded NPs showed good hydration in simulated saliva. 2. In vitro release of CSHG5-NP and CSMG5-NP exhibited high release rate approximately 3.4% and 2.8% curcumin respectively, over 24 h.	[76]	
Propranolol HCl	Chitosan, TPP, Carbopol 940, poloxamer 407.	To develop a propranolol-chitosan NPs transdermal gels to improve the systemic bioavailability of the drug.	1. In vitro drug release was performed in buffer solution, only 7% and 11% of propranolol was released in 24 h from nanoparticle suspension and gel. 2. Ex vivo drug release was performed in pig ear, skin showed a slow permeation rate from nanoparticles in gel over 24 h.	[77]	
C-glycosyl flavonoid enriched fractions of cecropia glaziovii (EFF-Cg)	Resomer PLGA, ploxamer 188, sorbitan monoaleate, chitosan	To develop and characterize EFF-Cg nanocomposites chitosan film containing PLGA NPs.	In vitro cytotoxicity study was performed in Vero cell line: chitosan film and nanocomposite film exhibited low toxicity.	[78]	
Alginate and pectin	Chitosan, TPP, Triton X-100	Preparation of alginate and pectin chitosan NPs for oral drug delivery	1. Cytotoxicity was performed in TR146 cells: Chit-NP showed cytocompatibility while Alg-NP, Pec-NP exhibited cytotoxicity at some concentrations. 2. Stability of NP in simulated salivary fluid: The Alg-NP were the most stable (a > 2 h), while Pec-NP and especially Chit-NP were unstable.	[79]	
Insulin	Chitosan MMW, PEG, PVP, trehalose	To develop and characterize chitosan films with insulin loaded PEG-b-PLA NPs	In vitro drug release of both insulin NPs showed pH dependent classic biphasic sustained release of protein over 5 weeks and insulin encapsulation efficiency of 30–70%.	[80]	

7.1. *Buccal Drug Delivery*

Buccal drug delivery involves drug delivery to the buccal cavity and to the systemic circulation. The advantages by delivering drug through buccal route include; increased bioavailability, less amount of drug required and bypassing the hepatic first pass effect. Moreover, the drug need not be exposed to the harsh GI environment [81]. The high permeability of buccal mucosa is a suitable target for novel formulations [82].

Giovino and co-workers have investigated chitosan buccal films of insulin loaded poly (ethylene glycol) methyl ether-block-polylactide (PEG-b-PLA) NP [83]. The NP showed excellent mucoadhesive properties and insulin release from the NP was slow and sustained (70%). Ex vivo studies reveal 1.8-fold enhancement in insulin permeation from NP compared to pure drug. Polysaccharide-based NP of alginate, chitosan and pectin for buccal delivery were prepared and compared. Chitosan NP were not stable in the saliva compared to alginate and pectin NP. Contrary to this, chitosan NP were cytocompatible while alginate and pectin NP have shown cytotoxicity [80]. As another example of buccal delivery, curcumin prepared as polycaprolactone nanoparticles coated with chitosan. As a third example, we can consider the NP encapsulation ofthe enriched flavonoid fraction (EFF-Cg) obtained from *Cecropia glaziovii*. EFF-Cg is used for several purposes such as controlling blood pressure and as a diuretic, antiasthmatic and hypoglycemic agent but it suffers from low bioavailability. EFF-Cg loaded PLGA nanoparticles were prepared for buccal delivery in the form of chitosan films. The bioavailability of EFF-Cg was improved and no signs of cytotoxicity were seen [84]. Thus, addition of chitosan in this hybrid approach has enabled both a high NP encapsulation efficiency and a stronger interaction with mucus [84]. Although the above-mentioned applications of chitosan are promising, chitosan NP suffers from stability issues in oral environment.

7.2. *Site Specific Delivery in the GIT*

Due to its properties of mucoadhesivity, permeation enhancement, biocompatibility, biodegradability and efflux pump inhibition, chitosan is one of the most suitable polymers for oral drug delivery [81]. In the above section on oral drug delivery with chitosan formulations, there are a few examples of mucoadhesive drug delivery systems there were formulated to release drug in the small intestine [40,41]. Alternatively, Suvannasara et al. attempted to enhance the mucoadhesive property of chitosan in the acidic environment (stomach) by conjugating C2-N position of chitosan with aromatic sulfonamide, 4-carboxybenzenesulfonamide-chitosan (4-CBS-chitosan) [85]. The 4-CBS-chitosan has shown higher mucoadhesion compared to pure chitosan. Moreover, the swelling ratio was higher than the pure chitosan suggesting that the polymer can tolerate acidic stomach conditions. The authors here recommend using 4-CBS-chitosan for delivering drugs specifically to the stomach (drugs with absorption window in stomach).

For the treatment of colonic diseases such as ulcerative colitis, Chron's disease, irritable bowel disease and colon infection, colon specific drug delivery is more appropriate. Several polymers have been investigated for colon specific drug delivery [86]. Of the several natural polymers available, chitosan is best suited for colon specific delivery owing to the properties of biodegradability by enzymes in colon, chelating ability and biocompatibility [87]. Chitosan-vancomycin NPs for colon delivery were prepared by two different methods; ion gelation and spray drying. The NPs prepared by spray drying have shown high encapsulation efficiency and better drug release compared to the NPs made by ion gelation [83]. Coco et al. have compared the ability of NPs made with chitosan to other polymers for inflamed colon drug delivery [88]. Several batches of NPs were prepared by entrapping ovalbumin (OVA) into Eudragit S 100, trimethylchitosan, PLGA, PEG-PLGA and PEG-PCL, separately. Of all the NPs made, NPs with trimethyl chitosan have shown the highest permeability of OVA. However, a high permeability was also seen with PEG-PLGA NPs as they were coated with mannose for active targeting of the area of inflammation. As another example, chitosan-carboxymethyl starch nanoparticles of 5-aminosalicylic acid, another drug for inflammatory bowel disease, have been prepared which achieved high entrapment efficiency as well as controlled drug release [89].

Although chitosan has shown its ability to deliver drug to the colon, there are a few issues to be addressed such as toxicity studies in humans, the impact of the GI tract inflammation characteristic of these disorders on mucoadhesion and drug absorption, the stability of these compounds in that biological environment and achieving a manufacturing scale of fabrication [90]. Demonstration of superiority to the Eudragit polymers currently in use for colon specific drug delivery of specific drugs will also be required [91].

Some of the other drug delivery routes have been explored for mucosal delivery with chitosan are vaginal, nasal, pulmonary and ocular. Systemic absorption of insulin has been demonstrated by formulationin chitosan NPs and administration by the nasal route. Insulin loading up to 55% was achieved and nasal absorption of insulin was greater from chitosan NP [92]. Rosmarinic acid loaded chitosan NP have been prepared by an ion gelation method for ocular delivery. The NPs showed no cytotoxicity against the retinal pigment epithelium (ARPE-19) nor the human cornea cell line (HCE-T). The permeability of rosmarinic acid facilitated by the NP formulation was found to be significantly higher compared to free solution. Mucoadhesion studies reveal that the NPs interact with the ocular mucosa [93]. Imiquimod was formulated as both chitosan coated PCL nanocapsules embedded in hydroethylcellulose gel and PCL nanocapsules embedded in chitosan hydrogel for vaginal delivery to treat human papillomavirus infection [94]. The former was found to show higher mucoadhesion while the latter has shown high drug permeation. Balancing the considerations of mucoadhesion, permeation and drug retention, the latter was selected as the best delivery system [94].

8. Pharmacokinetics (PK) of Chitosan Based Formulations

The pharmacokinetics of chitosan-based NPs is similar to those of other polymeric NPs because the same principles of drug release apply as discussed above. The most important property of chitosan to be exploited is its mucoadhesion. In the following section, we explore the pharmacokinetic (PK) features of chitosan-based NP. A PK study was done in beagle dogs to assess the bioavailability of cyclosporin-A (Cy-A) encapsulated into NPs comprised of chitosan, gelatin-A or sodium glycocholate (SGC). A control group received the standard oral micro-emulsion formulation (Neoral®). The C_{max} was markedly increased in the case of both the chitosan and gelatin NP formulations while the C_{max} decreased with SGC NPs as compared to Neoral. There was a 2.6-fold increase in the AUC of Cy-A from chitosan NPs compared to SGC NPs and 1.8-fold increase in AUC from gelatin NPs compared to SGC NPs. The relative bioavailability of Cy-A from SGC NPs was decreased by 36% when compared to marketed formulation. This could be due to the negative charge of the SGC NPs which could have hindered the NPs from adhering to the intestinal mucus and thus may have reduced the drug absorption across the intestinal epithelium. This supports the idea that a positive charge on chitosan NPs can help in mucoadhesion and increase in relative bioavailability, improved by 73% in this case [45].

Chitosan based NPs of Bay 41-4109 were developed with the primary goal of prolonging circulation time of the drug in blood. A PK study in rats demonstrated a 3.3-fold increase in C_{max}, increased AUC and 4-fold increase in absolute bioavailability of chitosan NPs compared to the Bay 41-4109 suspension. The enhanced intestinal absorption of Bay 41-4109 can be attributed to either increased interaction between the positive charge of chitosan with the negative charge of cell membranes or the mucoadhesive character of chitosan NPs, enabling them to release drug over time in the small intestine [44]. Enoxaparin has little to no oral bioavailability. In order to facilitate oral bioavailability, enoxaparin-loaded alginate-coated chitosan NPs (Enx-Alg-CS-NPs) were formulated, resulting in a 3-fold increase in AUC for oral enoxaparin (50 mg/kg in rats) and representing 20% of the AUC achieved with intravenous dosing (1 mg/kg). The increased intestinal permeation of enoxaparin in rats could be due to enhanced paracellular transport of the drug across intestinal epithelium owing to the mucoadhesive property of chitosan [47]. Chitosan NPs have many applications in increasing the oral bioavailability and the in vivo efficiency, illustrated in the following schematic representation (Figure 5).

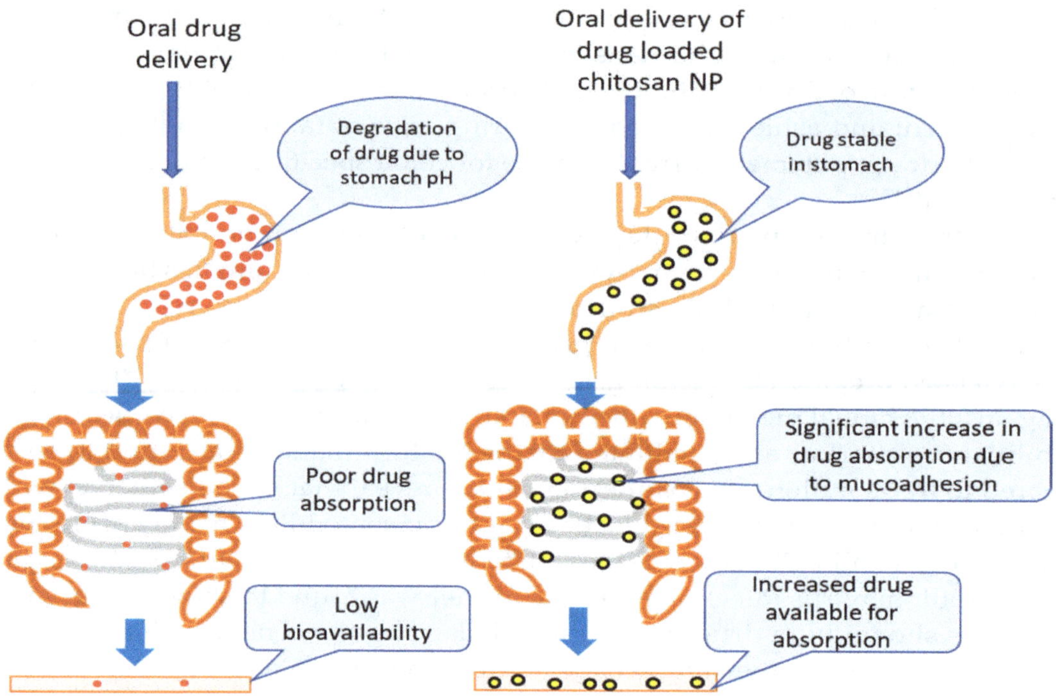

Figure 5. In vivo efficiency of drug loaded chitosan NPs in enhancing the drug absorption via the intestinal epithelium thereby increasing the drug available for absorption.

9. Toxicity and Safety of Chitosan

Chitosan is biodegradable and the process occurs either by chemical or enzyme catalysis. Degradation of chitosan is dependent on the degree of deacetylation and the availability of amino groups. Additionally, chitosan is approved as safe by US-FDA and EU for dietary use and wound dressing applications. However, the toxicity of chitosan increases by increasing charge density and degree of deacetylation [37]. As of this writing, we have not found any published data showing human toxicity of chitosan based formulations or questioning the safety of chitosan for human use. However, there are several animal toxicity studies reporting good safety in vivo and in vitro.

Aluani et al. have reported an in vivo toxicity study of two types of quercetin-loaded chitosan NPs (QR-NP1, QR-NP2) in male Wistar albino rats [56]. Briefly, the rats were divided into six groups and treated with saline, quercetin, empty NP or quercetin NPs in two related formulations. The rats were sacrificed, livers were collected, antioxidant defense marker (malondialdehyde (MDA) and glutathione (GSH)) levels were assessed. Oral administration of empty and quercetin loaded chitosan NPs indicated no change in body weight, relative rat liver weights, liver histology and hematology and biochemical parameters. There was no increase in MDA levels with both empty and quercetin loaded chitosan NP. GSH levels in animals with one of the NP formulations were slightly decreased. This data was also supported by in vitro cytotoxicity study which concludes chitosan NPs as safe carrier for quercetin in oxidative stress associated injuries.

Several airway-based cell culture models such as bronchial Calu-3 and alveolar 549 cells are in use to demonstrate the safety and toxicity of chitosan-based formulations for pulmonary drug delivery [61]. Lung toxicity of these biodegradable NPs was evaluated in mice in vivo [95]. Three NP formulations, PLGA NPs coated with chitosan, poloxamer 188 NPs and PVA NPs, were analyzed for biodistribution and inflammatory potential after a single dose administration in mice. Analysis of brancheoalveolar lavage cell population, protein secretion, cytokine release and histopathology were carried out. Chitosan-coated PLGA NPs showed better biodistribution and lower toxicity compared to non-coated NPs. Low levels of cytokine release indicate that chitosan coated PLGA NPs did not induce an inflammatory response. Chitosan-coated PLGA NPs showed a favorable biodistrbution as well [91]. Grenha et al. 2007 reported absence of toxicity in vitro with Calu-3 cells and A549 epithelial cells with NP concentrations up to 1.3 mg/mL [96].

In vitro cytotoxicity of chitosan based NP against buccal cells (TR146) was evaluated by Pistone et al. [79]. Three types of NP were prepared; alginate, Zn^{+2}—crosslinked pectin NP and chitosan NP crosslinked with TPP. An in vitro cytotoxicity test showed favorably that chitosan NPs were less cytotoxic compared to the alginate and pectin NPs. Moreover, chitosan alone was found to be more cytotoxic than the chitosan NP which could be due to the linker attached to chitosan NP or the intracellular processing response differential to free material vs NPs. The cytotoxicity of chitosan NP was shown to be further reduced either by increasing the concentration of the linker (TPP) or using chitosan with lesser degree of deacetylation.

10. Clinical Vaccine Trials of Chitosan Based Formulations

While clinical use of oral or mucoadhesive drug formulations containing chitosan remain on the horizon, there are already human vaccines in development which use chitosan as an adjuvant. CRM_{197}, a diphtheria toxoid antigen formulated as a chitosan-glutamate intranasal system, was evaluated in healthy human volunteers for the safety and immunostimulatory effects. Three groups of volunteers received intranasal diphtheria vaccine (500 μg of CRM_{197} with 9.5 mg of chitosan glutamate 213 and 2.5 mg mannitol), antigen alone (Day 0 and 28) and alum-adsorbed diphtheria toxoid vaccine via IM injection (Day 0). Serum IgG and IgA were collected on Days 27 and 42. Results suggest that chitosan was well tolerated with only minor adverse effects such as nasal discharge, blockage and discomfort. Antibody levels of the group receiving CRM_{197} and chitosan intranasally increased after the second (booster) vaccination [97].

An intranasal vaccine (NV-VLP) was formulated as spray dried powder composed of chitosan and norovirus VLP antigen with monophosphoryl lipid (MPL) as immune enhancer. This was tested in Phase 1 clinical studies, two randomized, double blinded, controlled studies with healthy volunteers. In one study, 5, 15 and 50 μg of antigen and chitosan alone were evaluated. In another trial, four groups of healthy volunteers were given MPL/chitosan (500 or 100 μg VLP per dose), chitosan only and placebo. Symptoms were recorded for a week after vaccination and safety evaluation up to 180 days. No vaccine related adverse effects were seen and significant immune response was seen with 100 μg dose. These results reveal that intranasal administration of vaccine may induce IgA secretion from intestinal mucosal tissues [98]. Similar such work has been done in healthy volunteers which provide further evidence of the efficacy of this vaccine approach [99].

11. Preparation of Chitosan Nanoparticles

Ionotropic gelation, microemulsion, emulsification solvent diffusion and emulsion based solvent evaporation are the most common methods to prepare chitosan-based nanoparticles. Usage of less organic solvent and lesser force are some of the main advantages most of these methods offer. The key characteristics that are found to affect the particle size and surface charge of chitosan NPs prepared by these methods are molecular weight and the degree of acetylation of the chitosan. Some of the mechanisms by which drugs are entrapped within the polymeric matrix are electrostatic interaction, hydrogen bonding and hydrophobic interactions. Drug loading and release are not the only key features, however. The intended use of the nanoparticles and the physiological environment at the site of administration must be taken into account, e.g. not only ionic strength, or the presence of salts, enzymes and proteins but also pH stability (consider the milieu of the eye vs. the GI tract). Fortunately, we now have multiple formulation methods to choose from.

11.1. Ionotropic Gelation

This is a simple technique where the chitosan solution (positively charged) is dissolved in acetic acid or any polyanionic solution (negatively charged) with or without a stabilizing agent such as poloxamer. Nanoparticles are readily formed due to complexation between positive and negative charged species during mechanical stirring at room temperature, resulting in separation of chitosan in spherical particles of different sizes and surface charges. Generally, the reported particle size ranges from 20 to 200 and 550 to 900 nm. Chitosan-TPP/vitamin C nanoparticles were prepared via ionotropic gelation between the positively charged amino groups of chitosan-TPP and the vitamin C, with constant stirring at room temperature for just 1 h [100,101]. A few advantages of ionotropic gelation include: the processing conditions are mild and it uses an aqueous environment, low toxicity and little chance of altering the chemistry of the drug to be encapsulated. The main disadvantages of this method are its poor stability in acidic conditions and difficulty in entrapping high molecular weight drugs [2,102].

11.2. Complex Coacervation Method

Coacervation is a technique of separating spherical particles by mixing electrostatically driven liquids. DNA-chitosan nanoparticles are formed by coacervation of the positively charged amine groups of chitosan and the negatively charged DNA phosphate groups [103,104]. Entrapment efficiency and drug release are governed by the molecular weight of the two polymers [105,106]. An advantage of complex coacervation is that the process can be entirely performed in an aqueous solution at low temperature. This provides a better chance of preserving the activity of the encapsulated substances. The main disadvantages of this method are the poor stability of the NPs, low drug loading and crosslinking of the complex by a chemical reagent such as toxic glutaraldehyde is necessary [101,107,108]. In the polyelectrolyte complex (PEC) method, an anionic solution (for example, dextran sulfate DNA solution) is added to the cationic polymer (e.g., chitosan solution dissolved in acetic acid, gelatin and polyethylenimine), under mechanical stirring at room temperature followed by charge neutralization. Advantages include: the method is simple, there is an absence of harsh conditions and the nanoparticles form spontaneously [2,101]. Low molecular weight water-soluble chitosan (LMWSC) nanocarriers were developed by the PEC method for insulin, resulting in insulin-loaded chitosan NPs with a reported mean diameter of ~200 nm and sustained release profile in vitro [101].

11.3. Coprecipitation Method

The addition of a chitosan solution, prepared in low pH acetic acid solution, to a high pH 8.5–9.0 solution, such as ammonium hydroxide, results in coprecipitation and the formation of a highly monodisperse nanoparticle population. Nanoparticles of diameters as low as 10 nm can be prepared with high encapsulation efficiency [101,107]. The wide range of particle size is seen with this method which could be a disadvantage. A coprecipitation method was used to prepare lactic acid-grafted chitosan (LA-g-chitosan) nanoparticles where ammonium hydroxide was used to form coacervate drops. This method yielded spherical and uniformly distributed nanoparticles [109].

11.4. Microemulsion Method

In this method, chitosan in acetic acid solution and glutaraldehyde are added to a surfactant in an organic solvent such as hexane. This mixture is kept on continuous stirring at room temperature, allowing the nanoparticles to form overnight as the cross-linking process is completed. Organic solvent is then removed by evaporating under low pressure. The product at this point has excess surfactant which can be removed by precipitating with calcium chloride followed by centrifugation. The final nanoparticle suspension is then dialyzed and then lyophilized [110]. A very narrow size distribution is seen with this method and the size can be controlled by the concentration of glutaraldehyde in the preparation of the NPs. This method results in formation of small sized nanoparticles [111]. Some disadvantages with this method include usage of organic solvent, a lengthy process and a complex washing step [2].

11.5. Emulsification Solvent Diffusion Method

An o/w emulsion is prepared by mixing organic solvent into a solution of chitosan with stabilizer under mechanical stirring followed by high pressure homogenization [45,112]. Size range of 300–500 nm could be achieved with this method. Polymer precipitation occurs when a large amount of water is added to the emulsion, forming nanoparticles. This method is best suited for entrapment of hydrophobic drugs, for which the entrapment efficiency is found to be high. The major disadvantage of the method includes usage of high shear forces.

11.6. Emulsion Based Solvent Evaporation Method

This method is a slight modification of the above method but avoids high shear forces. Particle size of below 300 nm can be achieved with this method. An emulsion is prepared by adding organic solvent to a solution of chitosan with surfactant followed by ultrasonication. The emulsion formed is then added to a surfactant solution and allowed to stir until the organic solvent is evaporated, forming nanoparticles. The NP are then washed and centrifuged multiple times to remove excess surfactant followed, by lyophilization to achieve freeze-dried nanoparticles [113,114].

11.7. Reverse Micellar Method

The surfactant is dissolved in an organic solvent followed by the addition of chitosan, drug and crosslinking agent, under constant overnight vortex mixing. The organic solvent is evaporated results in formation of transparent dry mass, then the latter is dispersed in water and then a suitable salt is added for precipitating the surfactant [115,116]. A very narrow size range nanoparticle is seen and organic solvents are used [117]. Doxorubicin-dextran conjugate loaded chitosan nanoparticles were prepared by reverse micellar method. The surfactant used in this method was sodium bis (ethyl hexyl) sulfosuccinate (AOT) was dissolved in n-hexane. The NP are formed by adding liquid ammonia and 0.01% glutaraldehyde to AOT solution, 0.1% chitosan in acetic acid, doxorubicin–dextran conjugate upon continuous stirring at room temperature [118,119].

12. Limitations

Chitosan has low solubility in neutral and alkaline pH. For GI applications, its mucoadhesion and permeation enhancer properties are strongest in the duodenal area, which can be modulated with chitosan derivatives. The toxicological profile of chitosan derivatives is still under investigation. There are multiple preparation methods now available for chitosan nanoparticles but formulators will have to adapt methods to suit the physicochemical properties of the specific drug to be encapsulated, with a careful choice of a specific chitosan in terms of its molecular weight and degree of acetylation and consideration of chemical modification. To date, chitosan has shown little or no toxicity in animal models and there have been no reports of major adverse effects in healthy human volunteers but clinical data are lacking. Even though chitosan is approved in dietary use, wound dressing applications and cartilage formulations, as of this writing there is not yet a chitosan-based drug formulation approved for mass marketing [120]. Issues regarding scale up of fabrication methods will likely be informed by that of other polymeric formulations.

13. Conclusions and Future Work

Based on the versatility of chitosan, it has many potential applications in drug delivery via the GIT, nasal, pulmonary routes as explained in this review. Chitosan NP can effectively deliver drug at specific sites by retaining the drug locally to permit an extended time for drug absorption. Mucoadhesion and absorption enhancement of chitosan makes it possible to deliver drugs directly from the nose to the brain. Similarly, lung infections and colon diseases can be effectively targeted locally with chitosan NP. A chitosan-based nasal formulation of morphine (Rylomine™) is currently in Phase 2 clinical trials (UK and EU) and Phase 3 clinical trials in the U.S. We anticipate that when it reaches the market it will pave way for similar products in the near future as well as assist in discerning any unanticipated effects in humans [120]. And, while not specifically addressed herein, we look forward to additional advances in the use of chitosan nanoparticles in targeted cancer theranostics, dermatologic applications and targeted parenteral drug delivery systems [121–124]. With the advent of new strategies in overcoming the limitations of chitosan by improved formulation methods for a wider variety of drugs and even macromolecules, we expect to see more chitosan research work in near future, especially in nasal and pulmonary drug delivery. We hope that future work on chitosan nanoparticles prepared by chitosan or chitosan derivatives will also focus on toxicity studies in humans.

Author Contributions: Munawar A. Mohammed was the primary author of this manuscript. Jaweria T.M. Syeda prepared the tables and figures and contributed to part of the text. Kishor M. Wasan provided guidance regarding article scope and pharmacokinetics. Ellen K. Wasan conceived the design of the article, supervised its writing and had editorial responsibility.

References

1. Rampino, A.; Borgogna, M.; Blasi, P.; Bellich, B.; Cesàro, A. Chitosan nanoparticles: Preparation, size evolution and stability. *Int. J. Pharm.* **2013**, *455*, 219–228. [CrossRef] [PubMed]
2. Nagpal, K.; Singh, S.K.; Mishra, D.N. Chitosan Nanoparticles: A Promising System in Novel Drug Delivery. *Chem. Pharm. Bull.* **2010**, *58*, 1423–1430. [CrossRef] [PubMed]
3. Sorlier, P.; Denuzière, A.; Viton, C.; Domard, A. Relation between the Degree of Acetylation and the Electrostatic Properties of Chitin and Chitosan. *Biomacromolecules* **2001**, *2*, 765–772. [CrossRef] [PubMed]
4. Vårum, K.M.; Ottøy, M.H.; Smidsrød, O. Water-solubility of partially *N*-acetylated chitosans as a function of pH: Effect of chemical composition and depolymerisation. *Carbohydr. Polym.* **1994**, *25*, 65–70. [CrossRef]
5. Van den Broek, L.A.M.; Knoop, R.J.I.; Kappen, F.H.J.; Boeriu, C.G. Chitosan films and blends for packaging material. *Carbohydr. Polym.* **2015**, *116* (Suppl. C), 237–242. [CrossRef] [PubMed]
6. Chen, M.C.; Mi, F.L.; Liao, Z.X.; Hsiao, C.W.; Sonaje, K.; Chung, M.F.; Hsu, L.W.; Sung, H.W. Recent advances in chitosan-based nanoparticles for oral delivery of macromolecules. *Adv. Drug Deliv. Rev.* **2013**, *65*, 865–879. [CrossRef] [PubMed]
7. Shukla, S.K.; Mishra, A.K.; Arotiba, O.A.; Mamba, B.B. Chitosan-based nanomaterials: A state-of-the-art review. *Int. J. Biol. Macromol.* **2013**, *59*, 46–58. [CrossRef] [PubMed]
8. Strobl, G.R. *The Physics of Polymers*; Springer: Berlin/Heidelberg, Germany, 2007; ISBN 978-3-540-25278-8.
9. Park, S.Y.; Jun, S.T.; Marsh, K.S. Physical properties of PVOH/chitosan-blended films cast from different solvents. *Food Hydrocoll.* **2001**, *15*, 499–502. [CrossRef]
10. Mima, S.; Miya, M.; Iwamoto, R.; Yoshikawa, S. Highly deacetylated chitosan and its properties. *J. Appl. Polym. Sci.* **1983**, *28*, 1909–1917. [CrossRef]
11. Risbud, M.V.; Hardikar, A.A.; Bhat, S.V.; Bhonde, R.R. pH-sensitive freeze-dried chitosan–polyvinyl pyrrolidone hydrogels as controlled release system for antibiotic delivery. *J. Control. Release* **2000**, *68*, 23–30. [CrossRef]
12. Kolhe, P.; Kannan, R.M. Improvement in Ductility of Chitosan through Blending and Copolymerization with PEG: FTIR Investigation of Molecular Interactions. *Biomacromolecules* **2003**, *4*, 173–180. [CrossRef] [PubMed]
13. Koul, V.; Mohamed, R.; Kuckling, D.; Adler, H.-J.P.; Choudhary, V. Interpenetrating polymer network (IPN) nanogels based on gelatin and poly(acrylic acid) by inverse miniemulsion technique: Synthesis and characterization. *Colloids Surf. B Biointerfaces* **2011**, *83*, 204–213. [CrossRef] [PubMed]
14. El-Hefian, E.A.; Yahaya, A.H. Rheological study of chitosan and its blends: An overview. *Maejo Int. J. Sci. Technol.* **2010**, *4*, 210–220.
15. Dambies, L.; Vincent, T.; Domard, A.; Guibal, E. Preparation of Chitosan Gel Beads by Ionotropic Molybdate Gelation. *Biomacromolecules* **2001**, *2*, 1198–1205. [CrossRef] [PubMed]
16. Al-Qadi, S.; Grenha, A.; Carrión-Recio, D.; Seijo, B.; Remuñán-López, C. Microencapsulated chitosan nanoparticles for pulmonary protein delivery: In vivo evaluation of insulin-loaded formulations. *J. Control. Release* **2012**, *157*, 383–390. [CrossRef] [PubMed]
17. Thanou, M.M.; Kotze, A.F.; Scharringhausen, T.; Lueßen, H.L.; De Boer, A.G.; Verhoef, J.C.; Junginger, H.E. Effect of degree of quaternization of *N*-trimethyl chitosan chloride for enhanced transport of hydrophilic compounds across intestinal Caco-2 cell monolayers. *J. Control. Release* **2000**, *64*, 15–25. [CrossRef]

18. Bernkop-Schnürch, A.; Hornof, M.; Zoidl, T. Thiolated polymers—Thiomers: Synthesis and in vitro evaluation of chitosan–2-iminothiolane conjugates. *Int. J. Pharm.* **2003**, *260*, 229–237. [CrossRef]
19. Sadeghi, A.M.M.; Dorkoosh, F.A.; Avadi, M.R.; Weinhold, M.; Bayat, A.; Delie, F.; Gurny, R.; Larijani, B.; Rafiee-Tehrani, M.; Junginger, H.E. Permeation enhancer effect of chitosan and chitosan derivatives: Comparison of formulations as soluble polymers and nanoparticulate systems on insulin absorption in Caco-2 cells. *Eur. J. Pharm. Biopharm.* **2008**, *70*, 270–278. [CrossRef] [PubMed]
20. Yin, L.; Ding, J.; He, C.; Cui, L.; Tang, C.; Yin, C. Biomaterials Drug permeability and mucoadhesion properties of thiolated trimethyl chitosan nanoparticles in oral insulin delivery. *Biomaterials* **2009**, *30*, 5691–5700. [CrossRef] [PubMed]
21. Cui, F.; Qian, F.; Zhao, Z.; Yin, L.; Tang, C.; Yin, C. Preparation, Characterization and Oral Delivery of Insulin Loaded Carboxylated Chitosan Grafted Poly (methyl methacrylate) Nanoparticles. *Biomacromolecules* **2009**, *10*, 1253–1258. [CrossRef] [PubMed]
22. Kurita, K.; Hashimoto, S.; Yoshino, H.; Ishii, S.; Nishimura, S.-I. Preparation of Chitin/Polystyrene Hybrid Materials by Efficient Graft Copolymerization Based on Mercaptochitin. *Macromolecules* **1996**, *29*, 1939–1942. [CrossRef]
23. Furlani, F.; Sacco, P.; Marsich, E.; Donati, I.; Paoletti, S. Highly monodisperse colloidal coacervates based on a bioactive lactose-modified chitosan: From synthesis to characterization. *Carbohydr. Polym.* **2017**, *174* (Suppl. C), 360–368. [CrossRef] [PubMed]
24. Sacco, S.; Paoletti, M.; Cok, F.; Asaro, M.; Abrami, M.; Grassi, I. Donati Insight into the ionotropic gelation of chitosan using tripolyphosphate and pyrophosphate as cross-linkers. *Int. J. Biol. Macromol.* **2016**, *92*, 476–483. [CrossRef] [PubMed]
25. Liu, S.; Yang, S.; Ho, P.C. Intranasal administration of carbamazepine-loaded carboxymethyl chitosan nanoparticles for drug delivery to the brain. *Asian J. Pharm. Sci.* **2017**. [CrossRef]
26. Singh, R.; Lillard, J.W., Jr. Nanoparticle-based targeted drug delivery. *Exp. Mol. Pathol.* **2009**, *86*, 215–223. [CrossRef] [PubMed]
27. Yuan, Z.; Ye, Y.; Gao, F.; Yuan, H.; Lan, M.; Lou, K.; Wang, W. Chitosan-graft-β-cyclodextrin nanoparticles as a carrier for controlled drug release. *Int. J. Pharm.* **2013**, *446*, 191–198. [CrossRef] [PubMed]
28. Miladi, K.; Sfar, S.; Fessi, H.; Elaissari, A. Enhancement of alendronate encapsulation in chitosan nanoparticles. *J. Drug Deliv. Sci. Technol.* **2015**, *30*, 391–396. [CrossRef]
29. Siafaka, P.I.; Titopoulou, A.; Koukaras, E.N.; Kostoglou, M.; Koutris, E.; Karavas, E.; Bikiaris, D.N. Chitosan derivatives as effective nanocarriers for ocular release of timolol drug. *Int. J. Pharm.* **2015**, *495*, 249–264. [CrossRef] [PubMed]
30. Siepmann, J.; Siepmann, F. Modeling of diffusion controlled drug delivery. *J. Control. Release* **2012**, *161*, 351–362. [CrossRef] [PubMed]
31. Fonseca-Santos, B.; Chorilli, M. An overview of carboxymethyl derivatives of chitosan: Their use as biomaterials and drug delivery systems. *Mater. Sci. Eng. C* **2017**, *77*, 1349–1362. [CrossRef] [PubMed]
32. Göpferich, A. Mechanisms of polymer degradation and erosion. *Biomaterials* **1996**, *17*, 103–114. [CrossRef]
33. Pawar, D.; Mangal, S.; Goswami, R.; Jaganathan, K.S. Development and characterization of surface modified PLGA nanoparticles for nasal vaccine delivery: Effect of mucoadhesive coating on antigen uptake and immune adjuvant activity. *Eur. J. Pharm. Biopharm.* **2013**, *85*, 550–559. [CrossRef] [PubMed]
34. Manca, M.L.; Loy, G.; Zaru, M.; Fadda, A.M.; Antimisiaris, S.G. Release of rifampicin from chitosan, PLGA and chitosan-coated PLGA microparticles. *Colloids Surf. B Biointerfaces* **2008**, *67*, 166–170. [CrossRef] [PubMed]
35. Wang, M.; Zhang, Y.; Feng, J.; Gu, T.; Dong, Q.; Yang, X.; Sun, Y.; Wu, Y.; Chen, Y.; Kong, W. Preparation, characterization and in vitro and in vivo investigation of chitosan-coated poly (D,L-lactide-co-glycolide) nanoparticles for intestinal delivery of exendin-4. *Int. J. Nanomed.* **2013**, *8*, 1141–1154. [CrossRef]
36. Bowman, K.; Leong, K.W. Chitosan Nanoparticles for Oral Drug and Gene Delivery. *Int. J. Nanomed.* **2006**, *1*, 117–128. [CrossRef]
37. Wang, J.J.; Zeng, Z.W.; Xiao, R.Z.; Xie, T.; Zhou, G.L.; Zhan, X.R.; Wang, S.L. Recent advances of chitosan nanoparticles as drug carriers. *Int. J. Nanomed.* **2011**, *6*, 765–774. [CrossRef]
38. Palacio, J.; Agudelo, N.A.; Lopez, B.L. PEGylation of PLA nanoparticles to improve mucus-penetration and colloidal stability for oral delivery systems. *Curr. Opin. Chem. Eng.* **2016**, *11*, 14–19. [CrossRef]

39. Dube, A.; Nicolazzo, J.A.; Larson, I. Chitosan nanoparticles enhance the intestinal absorption of the green tea catechins (+)-catechin and (−)-epigallocatechin gallate. *Eur. J. Pharm. Sci.* **2010**, *41*, 219–225. [CrossRef] [PubMed]
40. Barbieri, S.; Buttini, F.; Rossi, A.; Bettini, R.; Colombo, P.; Ponchel, G.; Sonvico, F. Ex vivo permeation of tamoxifen and its 4-OH metabolite through rat intestine from lecithin/chitosan nanoparticles. *Int. J. Pharm.* **2015**, *491*, 99–104. [CrossRef] [PubMed]
41. Feng, C.; Wang, Z.; Jiang, C.; Kong, M.; Zhou, X.; Li, Y.; Cheng, X.; Chen, X. Chitosan/o-carboxymethyl chitosan nanoparticles for efficient and safe oral anticancer drug delivery: In vitro and in vivo evaluation. *Int. J. Pharm.* **2013**, *457*, 158–167. [CrossRef] [PubMed]
42. John, J.; Sangeetha, D.; Gomathi, T. Sunitinib loaded chitosan nanoparticles formulation and its evaluation. *Int. J. Biol. Macromol.* **2016**, *82*, 952–958. [CrossRef]
43. Diop, M.; Auberval, N.; Viciglio, A.; Langlois, A.; Bietiger, W.; Mura, C.; Peronet, C.; Bekel, A.; David, D.J.; Zhao, M.; et al. Design, characterisation and bioefficiency of insulin-chitosan nanoparticles after stabilisation by freeze-drying or cross-linking. *Int. J. Pharm.* **2015**, *491*, 402–408. [CrossRef] [PubMed]
44. Xue, M.; Hu, S.; Lu, Y.; Zhang, Y.; Jiang, X.; An, S.; Guo, Y.; Zhou, X.; Hou, H.; Jiang, C. Development of chitosan nanoparticles as drug delivery system for a prototype capsid inhibitor. *Int. J. Pharm.* **2015**, *495*, 771–782. [CrossRef] [PubMed]
45. El-Shabouri, M.H. Positively charged nanoparticles for improving the oral bioavailability of cyclosporin-A. *Int. J. Pharm.* **2002**, *249*, 101–108. [CrossRef]
46. Gao, P.; Xia, G.; Bao, Z.; Feng, C.; Cheng, X.; Kong, M.; Liu, Y.; Chen, X. Chitosan based nanoparticles as protein carriers for efficient oral antigen delivery. *Int. J. Biol. Macromol.* **2016**, *91*, 716–723. [CrossRef] [PubMed]
47. Bagre, A.P.; Jain, K.; Jain, N.K. Alginate coated chitosan core shell nanoparticles for oral delivery of enoxaparin: In vitro and in vivo assessment. *Int. J. Pharm.* **2013**, *456*, 31–40. [CrossRef] [PubMed]
48. Wang, J.; Tan, J.; Luo, J.; Huang, P.; Zhou, W.; Chen, L.; Long, L.; Zhang, L.; Zhu, B.; Yang, L.; et al. Enhancement of scutellarin oral delivery efficacy by vitamin B12-modified amphiphilic chitosan derivatives to treat type II diabetes induced-retinopathy. *J. Nanobiotechnol.* **2017**, *15*. [CrossRef] [PubMed]
49. Huang, Y.-C.; Chen, J.-K.; Lam, U.-I.; Chen, S.-Y. Preparing, characterizing and evaluating chitosan/fucoidan nanoparticles as oral delivery carriers. *J. Polym. Res.* **2014**, *21*, 415. [CrossRef]
50. Shi, Y.; Xue, J.; Jia, L.; Du, Q.; Niu, J.; Zhang, D. Surface-modified PLGA nanoparticles with chitosan for oral delivery of tolbutamide. *Colloids Surf. B Biointerfaces* **2018**, *161*, 67–72. [CrossRef] [PubMed]
51. Derakhshandeh, K.; Fathi, S. Role of chitosan nanoparticles in the oral absorption of Gemcitabine. *Int. J. Pharm.* **2012**, *437*, 172–177. [CrossRef] [PubMed]
52. Maity, S.; Mukhopadhyay, P.; Kundu, P.P.; Chakraborti, A.S. Alginate coated chitosan core-shell nanoparticles for efficient oral delivery of naringenin in diabetic animals—An in vitro and in vivo approach. *Carbohydr. Polym.* **2017**, *170*, 124–132. [CrossRef] [PubMed]
53. Liang, J.; Yan, H.; Yang, H.-J.; Kim, H.W.; Wan, X.; Lee, J.; Ko, S. Synthesis and controlled-release properties of chitosan/β-Lactoglobulin nanoparticles as carriers for oral administration of epigallocatechin gallate. *Food Sci. Biotechnol.* **2016**, *25*, 1583–1590. [CrossRef]
54. Aluani, D.; Tzankova, V.; Kondeva-Burdina, M.; Yordanov, Y.; Nikolova, E.; Odzhakov, F.; Apostolov, A.; Markova, T.; Yoncheva, K. Evaluation of biocompatibility and antioxidant efficiency of chitosan-alginate nanoparticles loaded with quercetin. *Int. J. Biol. Macromol.* **2017**, *103*, 771–782. [CrossRef] [PubMed]
55. Van der Lubben, I.M.; Verhoef, J.C.; Borchard, G.; Junginger, H.E. Chitosan for mucosal vaccination. *Adv. Drug Deliv. Rev.* **2001**, *52*, 139–144. [CrossRef]
56. Casettari, L.; Illum, L. Chitosan in nasal delivery systems for therapeutic drugs. *J. Control. Release* **2014**, *190*, 189–200. [CrossRef] [PubMed]
57. Lisbeth, I. Nasal drug delivery—Possibilities, problems and solutions. *J. Control. Release* **2003**, *87*, 187–198.
58. Shahnaz, G.; Vetter, A.; Barthelmes, J.; Rahmat, D.; Laffleur, F.; Iqbal, J.; Perera, G.; Schlocker, W.; Dünnhaput, S.; Augustijns, P.; et al. Thiolated chitosan nanoparticles for the nasal administration of leuprolide: Bioavailability and pharmacokinetic characterization. *Int. J. Pharm.* **2012**, *428*, 164–170. [CrossRef] [PubMed]

59. Ruge, C.A.; Kirch, J.; Lehr, C.-M. Pulmonary drug delivery: From generating aerosols to overcoming biological barriers—Therapeutic possibilities and technological challenges. *Lancet Respir. Med.* **2013**, *1*, 402–413. [CrossRef]
60. Lytting, E.; Nguyen, J.; Wang, X.; Kissel, T. Biodegradable polymeric nanocarriers for pulmonary drug delivery Biodegradable polymeric nanocarriers for pulmonary drug delivery. *Expert Opin. Drug Deliv.* **2008**, *56*, 629–639. [CrossRef] [PubMed]
61. Islam, N.; Ferro, V. Recent Advances in Chitosan-Based Nanoparticulate Pulmonary Drug Delivery. *Nanoscale* **2016**, 14341–14358. [CrossRef] [PubMed]
62. Rawal, T.; Parmar, R.; Tyagi, R.K.; Butani, S. Rifampicin loaded chitosan nanoparticle dry powder presents an improved therapeutic approach for alveolar tuberculosis. *Colloids Surf. B Biointerfaces* **2017**, *154*, 321–330. [CrossRef] [PubMed]
63. Jafarinejad, S.; Gilani, K.; Moazeni, E.; Ghazi-Khansari, M.; Najafabadi, A.R.; Mohajel, N. Development of chitosan-based nanoparticles for pulmonary delivery of itraconazole as dry powder formulation. *Powder Technol.* **2012**, *222*, 65–70. [CrossRef]
64. Ni, S.; Liu, Y.; Tang, Y.; Chen, J.; Li, S.; Pu, J.; Han, L. GABA B receptor ligand-directed trimethyl chitosan/tripolyphosphate nanoparticles and their pMDI formulation for survivin siRNA pulmonary delivery. *Carbohydr. Polym.* **2017**, *179*, 135–144. [CrossRef] [PubMed]
65. Trapani, A.; Di Gioia, S.; Ditaranto, N.; Cioffi, N.; Goycoolea, F.M.; Carbone, A.; Garcia-Fuentes, M.; Conese, M.; Alonso, M.J. Systemic heparin delivery by the pulmonary route using chitosan and glycol chitosan nanoparticles. *Int. J. Pharm.* **2013**, *447*, 115–123. [CrossRef] [PubMed]
66. Lee, D.-W.; Shirley, S.A.; Lockey, R.F.; Mohapatra, S.S. Thiolated chitosan nanoparticles enhance anti-inflammatory effects of intranasally delivered theophylline. *Respir. Res.* **2006**, *7*. [CrossRef] [PubMed]
67. Wang, X.; Chi, N.; Tang, X. Preparation of estradiol chitosan nanoparticles for improving nasal absorption and brain targeting. *Eur. J. Pharm. Biopharm.* **2008**, *70*, 735–740. [CrossRef] [PubMed]
68. Janes, K.; Behrens, I.; Kissel, T.; Vila, A.; Sa, A.; Vila, L. Low molecular weight chitosan nanoparticles as new carriers for nasal vaccine delivery in mice. *Eur. J. Pharm. Biopharm.* **2004**, *57*, 123–131. [CrossRef]
69. Van der Lubben, I.M.; Verhoef, J.C.; Borchard, G.; Junginger, H.E. Chitosan and its derivatives in mucosal drug and vaccine delivery. *Eur. J. Pharm. Sci.* **2001**, *14*, 201–207. [CrossRef]
70. Marguerite, R. Chitin and chitosan: Properties and applications. *Prog. Polym. Sci.* **2006**, *31*, 603–632. [CrossRef]
71. George, M.; Abraham, T.E. Polyionic hydrocolloids for the intestinal delivery of protein drugs: Alginate and chitosan—A review. *J. Control. Release* **2006**, *114*, 1–14. [CrossRef] [PubMed]
72. Soares, P.I.P.; Isabel, A.; Carvalho, J.; Ferreira, I.M.M.; Novo, C.M.M.; Paulo, J. Chitosan-based nanoparticles as drug delivery systems for doxorubicin: Optimization and modelling. *Carbohydr. Polym.* **2016**, *147*, 304–312. [CrossRef] [PubMed]
73. Yostawonkul, J.; Surassmo, S.; Iempridee, T.; Pimtong, W.; Suktham, K.; Sajomsang, W.; Gonil, P.; Ruktanonchai, U.R. Surface modification of nanostructure lipid carrier (NLC) by oleoyl-quaternized-chitosan as a mucoadhesive nanocarrier. *Colloids Surf. B Biointerfaces* **2017**, *149*, 301–311. [CrossRef] [PubMed]
74. Yu, X.; Mu, Y.; Xu, M.; Xia, G.; Wang, J.; Liu, Y.; Chen, X. Preparation and characterization of mucosal adhesive and two-step drug releasing cetirizine-chitosan nanoparticle. *Carbohydr. Polym.* **2017**, *173*, 600–609. [CrossRef] [PubMed]
75. Costa Idos, S.; Abranches, R.P.; Garcia, M.T.; Pierre, M.B. Chitosan-based mucoadhesive films containing 5-aminolevulinic acid for buccal cancer treatment. *J. Photochem. Photobiol. B Biol.* **2014**, *140*, 266–275. [CrossRef] [PubMed]
76. Icia-Mazzarino, L.; Borsali, R.; Lemos-senna, E. Mucoadhesive Films Containing Chitosan-Coated Nanoparticles: A New Strategy for Buccal Curcumin Release. *J. Pharm. Sci.* **2014**, *103*, 3764–3771. [CrossRef] [PubMed]
77. Al-Kassas, R.; Wen, J.; Cheng, A.E.; Kim, A.M.; Liu, S.S.M.; Yu, J. Transdermal delivery of propranolol hydrochloride through chitosan nanoparticles dispersed in mucoadhesive gel. *Carbohydr. Polym.* **2016**, *153*, 176–186. [CrossRef] [PubMed]
78. Santos, T.C.D.; Rescignano, N.; Boff, L.; Reginatto, F.H.; Simões, C.M.O.; de Campos, A.M.; Mijangos, C.U. Manufacture and characterization of chitosan/PLGA nanoparticles nanocomposite buccal films. *Carbohydr. Polym.* **2017**, *173*, 638–644. [CrossRef] [PubMed]

79. Pistone, S.; Goycoolea, F.M.; Young, A.; Smistad, G.; Hiorth, M. Formulation of polysaccharide-based nanoparticles for local administration into the oral cavity. *Eur. J. Pharm. Biopharm.* **2017**, *96*, 381–389. [CrossRef] [PubMed]
80. Giovino, C.; Ayensu, I.; Tetteh, J.; Boateng, J.S. Development and characterisation of chitosan films impregnated with insulin loaded PEG-b-PLA nanoparticles (NPs): A potential approach for buccal delivery of macromolecules. *Int. J. Pharm.* **2012**, *428*, 143–151. [CrossRef] [PubMed]
81. Kumar, A.; Vimal, A.; Kumar, A. Why Chitosan, From properties to perspective of mucosal drug delivery.pdf. *Int. J. Biol. Macromol.* **2016**, *91*, 615–622. [CrossRef] [PubMed]
82. Campisi, G.; Paderni, C.; Saccone, R.; Fede, O.; Wolff, A.; Giannola, L. Human Buccal Mucosa as an Innovative Site of Drug Delivery. *Curr. Pharm. Des.* **2010**, *16*, 641–652. [CrossRef] [PubMed]
83. Giovino, C.; Ayensu, I.; Tetteh, J.; Boateng, J.S. An integrated buccal delivery system combining chitosan films impregnated with peptide loaded PEG-b-PLA nanoparticles. *Colloids Surf. B Biointerfaces* **2013**, *112*, 9–15. [CrossRef] [PubMed]
84. Mazzarino, L.; Travelet, C.; Ortega-Murillo, S.; Otsuka, I.; Pignot-Paintrand, I.; Lemos-Senna, E.; Borsali, R. Elaboration of chitosan-coated nanoparticles loaded with curcumin for mucoadhesive applications. *J. Colloid Interface Sci.* **2012**, *370*, 58–66. [CrossRef] [PubMed]
85. Suvannasara, P.; Juntapram, K.; Praphairaksit, N.; Siralertmukul, K.; Muangsin, N. Mucoadhesive 4-carboxybenzenesulfonamide-chitosan with antibacterial properties.pdf. *Carbohydr. Polym.* **2013**, *94*, 244–252. [CrossRef] [PubMed]
86. Shukla, R.K.; Tiwari, A. Carbohydrate polymers: Applications and recent advances in delivering drugs to the colon. *Carbohydr. Polym.* **2012**, *88*, 399–416. [CrossRef]
87. Wang, Q.-S.; Wang, G.-F.; Zhou, J.; Gao, L.-N.; Cui, Y.-L. Colon targeted oral drug delivery system based on alginate-chitosan microspheres loaded with icariin in the treatment of ulcerative colitis. *Int. J. Pharm.* **2016**, *515*, 176–185. [CrossRef] [PubMed]
88. Cerchiara, T.; Abruzzo, A.; Di Cagno, M.; Bigucci, F.; Bauer-Brandl, A.; Parolin, C.; Vitali, B.; Gallucci, M.C.; Luppi, B. Chitosan based micro- and nanoparticles for colon-targeted delivery of vancomycin prepared by alternative processing methods. *Eur. J. Pharm. Biopharm.* **2015**, *92*, 112–119. [CrossRef] [PubMed]
89. Coco, R.; Plapied, L.; Pourcelle, V.; Jérôme, C.; Brayden, D.J.; Schneider, Y.-J.; Préat, V. Drug delivery to inflamed colon by nanoparticles: Comparison of different strategies. *Int. J. Pharm.* **2013**, *440*, 3–12. [CrossRef] [PubMed]
90. Saboktakin, M.R.; Tabatabaie, R.M.; Maharramov, A.; Ramazanov, M.A. Synthesis and in vitro evaluation of carboxymethyl starch chitosan nanoparticles as drug delivery system to the colon. *Int. J. Biol. Macromol.* **2010**, *48*, 381–385. [CrossRef] [PubMed]
91. Hua, S.; Marks, E.; Schneider, J.J.; Keely, S. Advances in oral nano-delivery systems for colon targeted drug delivery in inflammatory bowel disease: Selective targeting to diseased versus healthy tissue. *Nanomedicine* **2015**, *11*, 1117–1132. [CrossRef] [PubMed]
92. Fernandez-Urrusuno, R.; Calvo, P.; Remunan-Lopez, C.; Vila-Jato, J.L.; Alonso, M.J. Enhancement of nasal absorption of insulin using chitosan nanoparticles. *Pharm. Res.* **1999**, *16*, 1576–1581. [CrossRef] [PubMed]
93. Baptista da Silva, S.; Ferreira, D.; Pintado, M.; Sarmento, B. Chitosan-based nanoparticles for rosmarinic acid ocular delivery—In vitro tests. *Int. J. Biol. Macromol.* **2016**, *84*, 112–120. [CrossRef] [PubMed]
94. Frank, L.; Chaves, P.; D'Amore, C.; Contri, R.; Frank, A.; Beck, R.; Pohlman, A.; Buffon, A.; Guterres, S. The use of chitosan as cationic coating or gel vehicle for polymeric nanocapsules: Increasing penetration and adhesion of imiquimod in vaginal tissue. *Eur. J. Pharm. Biopharm.* **2017**, *114*, 202–212. [CrossRef] [PubMed]
95. Aragao-Santiago, L.; Hillaireau, H.; Grabowski, N.; Mura, S.; Nascimento, T.L.; Dufort, S.; Coll, J.-L.; Tsapis, N.; Fattal, E. Compared in vivo toxicity in mice of lung delivered biodegradable and non-biodegradable nanoparticles. *Nanotoxicology* **2016**, *10*, 292–302. [CrossRef] [PubMed]
96. Grenha, A.; Grainger, C.I.; Dailey, L.A.; Seijo, B.; Martin, G.P.; Remuñán-López, C.; Forbes, B. Chitosan nanoparticles are compatible with respiratory epithelial cells in vitro. *Eur. J. Pharm. Sci.* **2007**, *31*, 73–84. [CrossRef] [PubMed]
97. Mills, K.H.G.; Cosgrove, C.; McNeela, E.A.; Sexton, A.; Giemza, R.; Jabbal-Gill, I.; Church, A.; Lin, W.; Illum, L.; Podda, A.; et al. Protective levels of diphtheria-neutralizing antibody induced in healthy volunteers by unilateral priming-boosting intranasal immunization associated with restricted ipsilateral mucosal secretory immunoglobulin A. *Infect. Immun.* **2003**, *71*, 726–732. [CrossRef] [PubMed]

98. El-Kamary, S.S.; Pasetti, M.F.; Mendelman, P.M.; Frey, S.E.; Bernstein, D.I.; Treanor, J.J.; Ferreira, J.; Chen, W.H.; Sublett, R.; Richardson, C.; et al. Adjuvanted Intranasal Norwalk Virus-Like Particle Vaccine Elicits Antibodies and Antibody-Secreting Cells That Express Homing Receptors for Mucosal and Peripheral Lymphoid Tissues. *J. Infect. Dis.* **2010**, *202*, 1649–1658. [CrossRef] [PubMed]
99. Ramirez, K.; Wahid, R.; Richardson, C.; Bargatze, R.F.; El-Kamary, S.S.; Sztein, M.B.; Pasetti, M.F. Intranasal vaccination with an adjuvanted Norwalk virus-like particle vaccine elicits antigen-specific B memory responses in human adult volunteers. *Clin. Immunol.* **2012**, *144*, 98–108. [CrossRef] [PubMed]
100. Alishahi, A.; Mirvaghefi, A.; Tehrani, M.R.; Farahmand, H.; Koshio, S.; Dorkoosh, F.A.; Elsabee, M.Z. Chitosan nanoparticle to carry vitamin C through the gastrointestinal tract and induce the non-specific immunity system of rainbow trout (Oncorhynchus mykiss). *Carbohydr. Polym.* **2011**, *86*, 142–146. [CrossRef]
101. Hembram, K.C.; Prabha, S.; Chandra, R.; Ahmed, B.; Nimesh, S. Advances in preparation and characterization of chitosan nanoparticles for therapeutics. *Artif. Cells Nanomed. Biotechnol.* **2014**, *1401*, 1–10. [CrossRef]
102. Gonçalves, I.C.; Henriques, P.C.; Seabra, C.L.; Martins, M.C.L. The potential utility of chitosan micro/nanoparticles in the treatment of gastric infection. *Expert Rev. Anti. Infect. Ther.* **2014**, *12*, 981–992. [CrossRef] [PubMed]
103. Zhao, K.; Shi, X.; Zhao, Y.; Wei, H.; Sun, Q.; Huang, T.; Zhang, X.; Wang, Y. Preparation and immunological effectiveness of a swine influenza DNA vaccine encapsulated in chitosan nanoparticles. *Vaccine* **2011**, *29*, 8549–8556. [CrossRef] [PubMed]
104. Zhuo, Y.; Han, J.; Tang, L.; Liao, N.; Gui, G.-F.; Chai, Y.-Q.; Yuan, R. Quenching of the emission of peroxydisulfate system by ferrocene functionalized chitosan nanoparticles: A sensitive "signal off" electrochemiluminescence immunosensor. *Sens. Actuators B Chem.* **2014**, *192*, 791–795. [CrossRef]
105. Chen, Y.; Mohanraj, V.J.; Wang, F.; Benson, H.A.E. Designing Chitosan–Dextran Sulfate Nanoparticles Using Charge Ratios. *AAPS PharmSciTech* **2007**, *8*, E98. [CrossRef] [PubMed]
106. Leong, K.W.; Mao, H.-Q.; Truong-Le, V.L.; Roy, K.; Walsh, S.M.; August, J.T. DNA-polycation nanospheres as non-viral gene delivery vehicles. *J. Control. Release* **1998**, *53*, 183–193. [CrossRef]
107. Tiyaboonchai, W. Chitosan Nanoparticles: A Promising System for Drug Delivery. *Naresuan Univ. J.* **2003**, *11*, 51–66. [CrossRef]
108. Huang, M.; Fong, C.-W.; Khor, E.; Lim, L.-Y. Transfection efficiency of chitosan vectors: Effect of polymer molecular weight and degree of deacetylation. *J. Control. Release* **2005**, *106*, 391–406. [CrossRef] [PubMed]
109. Bhattarai, N.; Ramay, H.R.; Chou, S.-H.; Zhang, M. Chitosan and lactic acid-grafted chitosan nanoparticles as carriers for prolonged drug delivery. *Int. J. Nanomed.* **2006**, *1*, 181–187. [CrossRef]
110. Maitra, A.; Ghosh, P.K.; De, T.K.; Sahoo, S.K. Process for the Preparation of Highly Monodispersed Polymeric Hydrophilic Nanoparticles. US 5874111 A, 7 January 1999.
111. Wang, Y.; Wang, X.; Luo, G.; Dai, Y. Adsorption of bovin serum albumin (BSA) onto the magnetic chitosan nanoparticles prepared by a microemulsion system. *Bioresour. Technol.* **2008**, *99*, 3881–3884. [CrossRef] [PubMed]
112. Niwa, T.; Takeuchi, H.; Hino, T.; Kunou, N.; Kawashima, Y. Preparations of biodegradable nanospheres of water-soluble and insoluble drugs with D,L-lactide/glycolide copolymer by a novel spontaneous emulsification solvent diffusion method and the drug release behavior. *J. Control. Release* **1993**, *25*, 89–98. [CrossRef]
113. Vila, A.; Sanchez, A.; Tobío, M.; Calvo, P.; Alonso, M.J. Design of Biodegradable Partilces for Protein Delivery. *J. Control. Release* **2002**, *78*, 15–24. [CrossRef]
114. Zhang, L.; Zhao, Z.-L.; Wei, X.-H.; Liu, J.-H. Preparation and in vitro and in vivo characterization of cyclosporin A-loaded, PEGylated chitosan-modified, lipid-based nanoparticles. *Int. J. Nanomed.* **2013**, *8*, 601–610. [CrossRef]
115. Zeinab Sadat, S.; Hamed, S.-K.; Mohammad, I.; Mohammad, A.; Azizollah, N. Exploring the effect of formulation parameters on the particle size of carboxymethyl chitosan nanoparticles prepared via reverse micellar crosslinking. *J. Microencapsul.* **2017**, *34*, 270–279. [CrossRef]
116. Malmsten, M. *Surfactants and Polymers in Drug Delivery*; Marcel Dekker: New York, NY, USA, 2002; ISBN 9780824708047.
117. Banerjee, T.; Mitra, S.; Kumar-Singh, A.; Kumar-Sharma, R.; Maitra, A. Preparation, characterization and biodistribution of ultrafine chitosan nanoparticles. *Int. J. Pharm.* **2002**, *243*, 93–105. [CrossRef]

118. Liu, C.; Tan, Y.; Liu, C.; Chen, X.; Yu, L. Preparations, characterizations and applications of Chitosan-based nanoparticles. *J. Ocean Univ. China* **2007**, *6*, 237–243. [CrossRef]
119. Mitra, S.; Gaur, U.; Ghosh, P.C.; Maitra, A.N. Tumour targeted delivery of encapsulated dextran–doxorubicin conjugate using chitosan nanoparticles as carrier. *J. Control. Release* **2001**, *74*, 317–323. [CrossRef]
120. Bellich, B.; D'Agostino, I.; Semeraro, S.; Gamini, A.; Cesàro, A. "The good, the bad and the ugly" of chitosans. *Mar. Drugs* **2016**, *14*, 99. [CrossRef] [PubMed]
121. Key, J.; Park, K. Multicomponent, Tumor-Homing Chitosan Nanoparticles for Cancer Imaging and Therapy. *Int. J. Mol. Sci.* **2017**, *18*, E594. [CrossRef] [PubMed]
122. Zhang, X.; Yang, X.; Ji, J.; Liu, A.; Zhai, G. Tumor targeting strategies for chitosan-based nanoparticles. *Colloids Surf. B Biointerfaces* **2016**, *148*, 460–473. [CrossRef] [PubMed]
123. Ahmed, T.A.; Aljaeid, B.M. Preparation, characterization and potential application of chitosan, chitosan derivatives and chitosan metal nanoparticles in pharmaceutical drug delivery. *Drug Des. Devel. Ther.* **2016**, *10*, 483–507. [CrossRef] [PubMed]
124. Swierczewska, M.; Han, H.S.; Kim, K.; Park, J.H.; Lee, S. Polysaccharide-based nanoparticles for theranostic nanomedicine. *Adv. Drug Deliv. Rev.* **2016**, *99 Pt A*, 70–84. [CrossRef] [PubMed]

11

Comparative Pharmacokinetics and Pharmacodynamics of a Novel Sodium-Glucose Cotransporter 2 Inhibitor, DWP16001, with Dapagliflozin and Ipragliflozin

Min-Koo Choi [1], So Jeong Nam [2], Hye-Young Ji [3], Mi Jie Park [3], Ji-Soo Choi [3] and Im-Sook Song [2,*]

1 College of Pharmacy, Dankook University, Cheon-an 31116, Korea; minkoochoi@dankook.ac.kr
2 College of Pharmacy and Research Institute of Pharmaceutical Sciences, Kyungpook National University, Daegu 41566, Korea; goddns159@nate.com
3 Life Science Institute, Daewoong Pharmaceutical, Yongin, Gyeonggido 17028, Korea; hychi138@daewoong.co.kr (H.-Y.J.); mjpark201@daewoong.co.kr (M.J.P.); jschoi172@daewoong.co.kr (J.-S.C.)
* Correspondence: isssong@knu.ac.kr

Abstract: Since sodium-glucose cotransporter 2 (SGLT2) inhibitors reduced blood glucose level by inhibiting renal tubular glucose reabsorption mediated by SGLT2, we aimed to investigate the pharmacokinetics and kidney distribution of DWP16001, a novel SGLT2 inhibitor, and to compare these properties with those of dapagliflozin and ipragliflozin, representative SGLT2 inhibitors. The plasma exposure of DWP16001 was comparable with that of ipragliflozin but higher than that of dapagliflozin. DWP16001 showed the highest kidney distribution among three SGLT2 inhibitors when expressed as an area under curve (AUC) ratio of kidney to plasma (85.0 ± 16.1 for DWP16001, 64.6 ± 31.8 for dapagliflozin and 38.4 ± 5.3 for ipragliflozin). The organic anion transporter-mediated kidney uptake of DWP16001 could be partly attributed to the highest kidney uptake. Additionally, DWP16001 had the lowest half-maximal inhibitory concentration (IC_{50}) to SGLT2, a target transporter (0.8 ± 0.3 nM for DWP16001, 1.6 ± 0.3 nM for dapagliflozin, and 8.9 ± 1.7 nM for ipragliflozin). The inhibition mode of DWP16001 on SGLT2 was reversible and competitive, but the recovery of the SGLT2 inhibition after the removal of SGLT2 inhibitors in CHO cells overexpressing SGLT2 was retained with DWP16001, which is not the case with dapagliflozin and ipragliflozin. In conclusion, selective and competitive SGLT2 inhibition of DWP16001 could potentiate the efficacy of DWP16001 in coordination with the higher kidney distribution and retained SGLT2 inhibition of DWP16001 relative to dapagliflozin and ipragliflozin.

Keywords: sodium-glucose cotransporter 2 (SGLT2) inhibitors; DWP16001; kidney distribution; inhibition mode

1. Introduction

Achieving appropriate glycemic control for type 2 diabetes patients is a prerequisite for preventing cardiovascular and microvascular complications, and this can be guided by a combination of antidiabetic drugs with different modes of action [1].

Sodium-glucose cotransporter 2 (SGLT2) inhibitors are the latest class of antidiabetic drugs that act through the inhibition of renal tubular glucose reabsorption and a reduction of blood glucose levels without stimulating insulin release [2]. SGLT2 is expressed in the S1 segment of proximal kidney tubules and is responsible for roughly 90% of the reabsorption of filtered glucose [3]. Additionally, SGLT2 inhibitors exhibit low hypoglycemia risk and have been associated with a significant reduction in major adverse cardiovascular events in clinical trials [4], garnering SGLT2 inhibitors increased attention.

Several SGLT2 inhibitors have been approved for the treatment of type 2 diabetes, including canagliflozin (Invokana®), dapagliflozin (Farxiga®), empagliflozin (Jardiance®), ipragliflozin (Suglat®), and tofogliflozin (Apleway®) [3,5].

Additionally, there are several other similar compounds in the pipeline that may be approved in the near future. DWP16001 (Figure 1), a selective SGLT2 inhibitor, is under development by Daewoong Pharmaceutical Co. Ltd. (Yongin, Korea) and is currently undergoing phase 2 clinical trials (Registration No. NCT04014023).

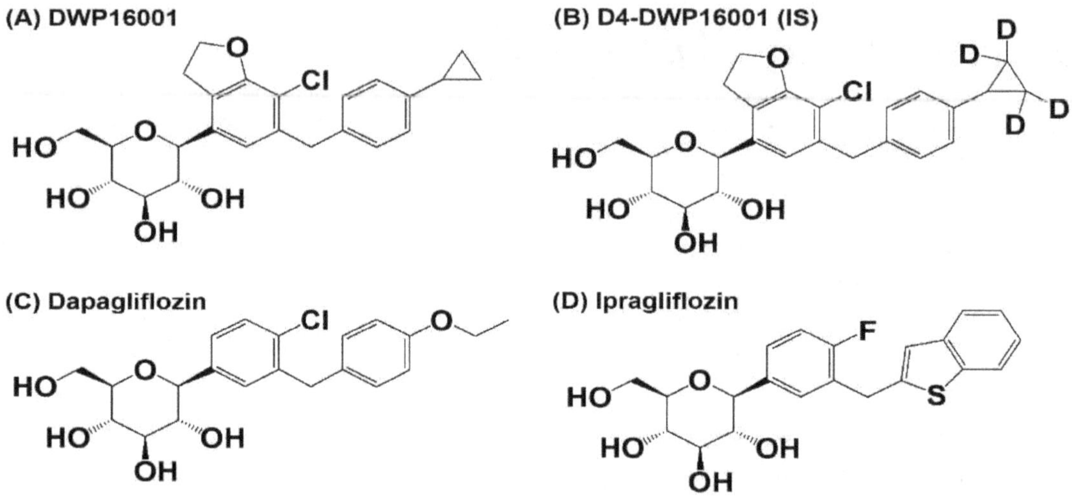

Figure 1. Structure of (**A**) DWP16001, (**B**) D4-DWP16001 (IS), (**C**) dapagliflozin, and (**D**) ipragliflozin.

Recently, Tahara et al. [5] compared the pharmacokinetics, pharmacodynamics, and pharmacological characteristics of six SGLT2 inhibitors, such as ipragliflozin, dapagliflozin, tofogliflozin, canagliflozin, empagliflozin, and luseogliflozin. The study showed that all the SGLT2 inhibitors induced urinary glucose excretion in a dose-dependent manner but the duration of action differed among the six drugs. Ipragliflozin and dapagliflozin showed persistent duration of action; these two drugs exhibited increased urinary glucose excretion even 18 h post dose but the others showed about 12 h of duration. In addition, ipragliflozin and dapagliflozind showed the lowest blood glucose and insulin level following the same daily dose (3 mg/kg) in diabetic mice. The long duration of action and glucose lowering efficacy of these two drugs closely correlated with the drug distribution and retention in the kidney and elimination half-life [5], suggesting the importance of kidney distribution and elimination profile is prerequisite in the efficacy of SGLT2 inhibitors, as well as the potent SGLT2 inhibition. Therefore, this study aimed to compare the pharmacokinetic properties and kidney distribution of DWP16001 with those of dapagliflozin and ipragliflozin, representative SGLT2 inhibitors that showed potent and long duration efficacy [5] and to compare the selectivity and mode of inhibition of DWP16001 on SGLT2 with dapagliflozin and ipragliflozin to evaluate the potency of DWP16001 over other SGLT2 inhibitors.

2. Materials and Methods

2.1. Materials

DWP16001 and D4-DWP16001 (for internal standard (IS)), were obtained from Daewoong Pharmaceutical Co. Ltd. (Yongin, Korea). Dapagliflozin and ipragliflozin were obtained from Toronto Research Chemicals Inc. (North York, ON, Canada) (Figure 1).

Para-aminohipuric acid (PAH), methyl a-D-glucopyranoside (AMG), sodium dodecyl sulfate (SDS), G418, non-essential amino acids, 4-(2-hydroxyethyl)-1-piperazineethanesulfonic acid (HEPES), and Hank's balances salts solution (HBSS, pH 7.4) were purchased from Sigma–Aldrich Chemical Co. (St. Louis, MO, USA). $[^{14}C]$Methyl-α-D-glucopyranoside (AMG) (290 mCi/mmol) was purchased from

Moravek (Brea, CA, USA). [^{3}H]Estrone-3-sulfate (ES) (2.12 TBq/mmol) and [^{3}H]para-aminohipuric acid (PAH) (0.13 TBq/mmol) were purchased from Perkin Elmer Inc. (Boston, MA, USA). Dulbecco's modified Eagle's medium (DMEM), RPMI1640 medium, fetal bovine serum (FBS), and poly-D-lysine-coated 24-well plates were purchased from Corning (Tewksbury, MA, USA). All other chemicals and solvents were reagent or analytical grade.

CHO cells overexpressing SGLT1 and SGLT2 (CHO-SGLT1 and -SGLT2, respectively) and CHO-mock cells were obtained from Daewoong Pharmaceutical Co. Ltd. (Yongin, Korea). HEK293 cells overexpressing organic anion transporter 1 (OAT1) and OAT3 (HEK293-OAT1 and -OAT3, respectively) and HEK293-mock cells were purchased from Corning (Tewksbury, MA, USA).

2.2. *Animals and Ethical Approval*

Male Institute of Cancer Research (ICR) mice (7–8-weeks-year-old, 30−35 g) were purchased from Samtako Co. (Osan, Korea). Animals were acclimatized for 1 week in an animal facility at Kyungpook National University. Food and water were available ad libitum. All animal procedures were approved by the Animal Care and Use Committee of Kyungpook National University (Approval No. 2016-0138) and carried out in accordance with the National Institutes of Health guidance for the care and use of laboratory animals.

2.3. *Pharmacokinetic Study*

ICR mice were randomly divided into three groups and were fasted for at least 12 h before the oral administration of DWP16001, dapagliflozin, and ipragliflozin but had free access to water. On the day of pharmacokinetic study, the mice received DWP16001, dapagliflozin, or ipragliflozin solution at a dose of 1 mg/kg (dissolved in a mixture of 10% DMSO and 90% saline) using oral gavage. Blood samples were collected at 0.5, 1, 2, 4, 8, 24, 48, and 72 h following the oral administration (1 mg/kg each) of DWP16001, dapagliflozin, or ipragliflozin and centrifuged at 12,000× *g* for 1 min to separate the plasma. An aliquot (30 μL) of each plasma sample was stored at −80 °C until the analysis. Kidney samples were also isolated at 8, 24, 48, and 72 h following the oral administration of DWP16001, dapagliflozin, or ipragliflozin, minced thoroughly, and homogenized with four volumes of saline using tissue grinder. An aliquot (50 μL) of each kidney homogenate sample was stored at −80 °C until the analysis.

For the analysis of SGLT2 inhibitors, aliquots of plasma (30 μL) and kidney homogenate (50 μL) were added to 100 μL of aqueous solution of D4-DWP16001 (IS, 20 ng/mL), and vigorously mixed with 500 μL methyl tert-butyl ether (MTBE) for 15 min. After centrifugation at 16,000 *g* for 5 min, samples were kept for 1 h at −80 °C to make an aqueous layer freeze. An organic upper layer was transferred to a clean tube and evaporated to dryness under a gentle stream of nitrogen. Then, the dried extract was reconstituted in 150 μL of mobile phase, and a 3 μL aliquot of the reconstituent was injected into a liquid chromatography–tandem mass spectrometry (LC–MS/MS) system.

Pharmacokinetic parameters, such as the area under plasma concentration-time curve from zero to infinity (AUC), were calculated from plasma concentration vs time curves using non-compartment analysis with WinNonlin (version 5.1; Pharsights, Cary, NC, USA). The AUC ratios (i.e., ratios of kidney AUC to plasma AUC) were calculated by dividing the AUC of the three SGLT2 inhibitors in the kidney by the plasma AUC values of the three SGLT2 inhibitors.

2.4. *Protein Binding*

The protein binding of DWP16001, dapagliflozin, and ipragliflozin (1000 ng/mL) in mouse plasma and 20% kidney homogenate was determined using a rapid equilibrium dialysis kit (ThermoFisher Scientific Korea, Seoul, Korea) according to the manufacturer's instructions. Briefly, 100 μL of mouse plasma and 20% kidney homogenate samples containing 1000 ng/mL of DWP16001, dapagliflozin, or ipragliflozin were added to the sample chamber of a semipermeable membrane (molecular weight cut-off 8000 Da) and 300 μL of phosphate buffered saline (PBS) was added to the outer buffer chamber.

Four hours after incubation at 37 °C on a shaking incubator at 300 rpm, aliquots (50 μL) were collected from both the sample and buffer chambers and treated with equal volumes of fresh PBS and blank plasma or blank kidney homogenate, respectively, to match the sample matrices. The matrix-matched sample (100 μL) was added 100 μL of aqueous solution of D4-DWP16001 (IS, 20 ng/mL), and vigorously mixed with 1000 μL MTBE for 15 min. After centrifugation at 16,000 *g* for 5 min, samples were kept for 1 h at −80 °C. An organic upper layer was transferred to a clean tube and evaporated to dryness under a gentle stream of nitrogen. Then, the dried extract was reconstituted in 300 μL of mobile phase and a 3 μL aliquot of the reconstituent was injected into the LC-MS/MS system.

Plasma protein binding was calculated using the following Equation (1) [6,7].

$$\text{Undiluted free drug fraction (fu)} = \frac{\text{Drug concentration in buffer chamber}}{\text{Drug concentration in plasma sample chamber}} \tag{1}$$

Kidney protein binding was calculated using the following equations, Equations (2) and (3), and a dilution factor (D as a value of 5) for tissue homogenates was used since we used 20% kidney homogenates [6,7].

$$\text{Diluted free drug fraction (fu}') = \frac{\text{Drug concentration in buffer chamber}}{\text{Drug concentration in kidney homogenate chamber}}, \tag{2}$$

$$\text{Undiluted free drug fraction (fu)} = \frac{1/D}{\left(\frac{1}{fu'} - 1\right) + 1/D} = \frac{fu' \times 0.2}{1 - fu' \times 0.8}. \tag{3}$$

2.5. Substrate Specificity of DWP16001, Dapagliflozin, and Ipragliflozin for OAT1 and OAT3

HEK293-mock cells and HEK293 cells overexpressing OAT1 and OAT3 transporters (HEK293-OAT1 and -OAT3, respectively) were seeded in poly-D-lysine-coated 24-well plates at a density of 4×10^5 cells/well and cultured for 24 h in DMEM supplemented with 10% FBS and 5 mM non-essential amino acids at 37 °C in 8% CO_2 condition.

For each experiment, the growth medium was discarded after 24 h, and the attached cells were washed with pre-warmed HBSS and incubated with pre-warmed HBSS for 20 min at 37 °C. To confirm the functionality of OAT1 and OAT3, we measured the uptake of 0.1 μM [^{3}H]PAH and 0.1 μM [^{3}H]ES, representative substrates for OAT1 and OAT3, respectively, into in the HEK293-mock cells and HEK293-OAT1 and -OAT3 cells, respectively, for 5 min in the presence and absence of 20 μM probenecid, a typical inhibitor for both OAT1 and OAT3 [8,9]. The cells were then washed three times with 500 μL of ice-cold HBSS immediately after placing the plates on ice. Subsequently, cells were lysed with 10% sodium dodecyl sulfate and mixed with Optiphase cocktail solution overnight. The radioactivity of the cell lysate was measured using a liquid scintillation counter (Microbeta 2; Perkin Elmer Inc., Boston, MA, USA).

The uptake of DWP16001, dapagliflozin, and ipragliflozin (2 μM each) was measured for 5 min at 37 °C in the HEK293-mock cells and HEK293-OAT1 and -OAT3 cells, respectively, in the absence and presence of 20 μM probenecid. For the concentration dependency in the uptake of DWP16001, the uptake of DWP16001 in a concentration range of 0.5–50 μM dissolved in HBSS was measured for 5 min at 37 °C in the mock cells and HEK293-OAT1 and -OAT3 cells, respectively. After 5 min, the cells were washed three times with 500 μL of ice-cold HBSS immediately after placing the plates on ice. Subsequently, the cells were scraped using a cell scraper with 100 μL of PBS, and cell suspensions were transferred to a clean tube, combined with 100 μL of aqueous solution of D4-DWP16001 (IS, 20 ng/mL), and vigorously mixed with 1000 μL MTBE for 15 min. After centrifugation at 16,000 *g* for 5 min, samples were kept for 1 h at −80 °C. An organic upper layer was transferred to a clean tube and evaporated to dryness under a gentle stream of nitrogen. Then, the dried extract was reconstituted in 300 μL of mobile phase and a 3 μL aliquot of the reconstituent was injected into the LC-MS/MS system.

In the concentration-dependent uptake studies, the transporter-mediated uptake of DWP16001 was calculated by the subtraction of the transport rates of DWP16001 into the mock cells from those of the HEK293-OAT1 and -OAT3 cells. Kinetic parameters for the OAT1- and OAT3-mediated transport of DWP16001 were determined using the Michaelis-Menten equation [$V = V_{max} \cdot S/(K_m + S)$] [10].

2.6. LC-MS/MS Analysis of DWP16001, Dapagliflozin, and Ipragliflozin

Concentrations of DWP16001, dapagliflozin, and ipragliflozin in plasma and kidney homogenate samples were analyzed using an Agilent 6470 triple quadrupole LC–MS/MS system (Agilent, Wilmington, DE, USA).

DWP16001, dapagliflozin, and ipragliflozin were separated on a Synergi Polar RP column (2.0 × 150 mm, 4 μm particle size; Phenomenex, Torrence, CA) using a mobile phase consisting of water (15%) and methanol (85%) containing 0.1% formic acid at a flow rate of 0.25 mL/min.

Quantification of a separated analyte peak was performed at m/z 464 → 131 for DWP16001 (T_R (retention time) 2.8 min), m/z 422 → 151 for ipragliflozin (T_R 2.5 min), m/z 426 → 167 for dapagliflozin (T_R 2.5 min), m/z 468 → 135 for D4-DWP16001 (T_R 2.8 min), in the positive ionization mode with a collision energy (CE) of 25 eV. The calibration standards of a mixture of DWP16001, dapagliflozin, and ipragliflozin in mouse plasma were 5–1000 ng/mL, and intraday and interday precision and accuracy were less than 14.7% in all samples. The calibration standards of a mixture of DWP16001, dapagliflozin, and ipragliflozin in mouse kidney homogenate were 5–1000 ng/mL, and intraday and interday precision and accuracy were less than 13.8% in all samples.

2.7. Inhibitory Effects of DWP16001, Dapagliflozin, and Ipragliflozin on the SGLT1 and SGLT2 Activities

CHO cells overexpressing SGLT1 and SGLT2 cells (CHO-SGLT1 and -SGLT2) and CHO-mock cells were characterized as previously described [11]. Cells were maintained in RPMI1640 medium supplemented with 10% fetal bovine serum and 200 μg/mL G418 at 37 °C in 5% CO_2 conditions. CHO-SGLT1 and -SGLT2 cells were seeded at a density of 1×10^5 cells/well in 96-well plates. After 24 h, the growth medium was discarded from the cells, and the cells were washed with pre-warmed Na^+-free buffer (10 mM HEPES, 5 mM Tris, 140 mM choline chloride, 2 mM KCl, 1 mM $CaCl_2$, 1 mM $MgCl_2$, pH7.4) and incubated for 1 h in Na^+-free buffer. After replacing Na^+-free buffer with Na^+ gradient buffer (10 mM HEPES, 5 mM Tris, 140 mM NaCl, 2 mM KCl, 1 mM $CaCl_2$, 1 mM $MgCl_2$, pH7.4) containing 10 μM [^{14}C]AMG, the uptake of [^{14}C]AMG into the CHO-mock cells and CHO-SGLT1 and -SLGT2 cells was measured for 0.5, 1, 1.5, 2, and 3 h. After a predetermined incubation time, cells were washed three times with 200 μL of ice-cold Na^+-free buffer immediately after placing the plates on ice. Then, the cells were lysed with 10% SDS, and the cell lysates were mixed with Optiphase cocktail solution. Thereafter, the radioactivity of the cell lysates was measured using a liquid scintillation counter.

The inhibitory effect of known inhibitors, such as dapagliflozin and ipragliflozin, on [^{14}C]AMG uptake in the CHO-mock cells and CHO-SGLT1 and -SLGT2 cells was measured in the presence or absence of dapagliflozin and ipragliflozin (1, 10 μM for SGLT1; 10, 100 nM for SGLT2) for 2 h. For the calculation of IC_{50} values, the uptake of 10 μM [^{14}C]AMG in the CHO-mock cells and CHO-SGLT1 and -SLGT2 cells was measured for 2 h with or without DWP16001, dapagliflozin, or ipragliflozin (1 nM–50 μM for SGLT1; 0.01 nM–1 μM for SGLT2). After 2 h, cells were washed three times with 200 μL of ice-cold Na^+-free buffer and the cells were lysed with 10% SDS (40 μL), followed by adding Optiphase cocktail solution (200 μL). The radioactivity of the cell lysates was measured using a liquid scintillation counter. The SGLT1 or SGLT2-mediated uptake of [^{14}C]AMG was calculated by the subtraction of the uptake rates of [^{14}C]AMG into the mock cells from those of the CHO-SGLT1 and -SLGT2 cells. In the inhibition studies, the percentages of the transport rate of AMG with or without SGLT2 inhibitors were calculated and the data were fitted to an inhibitory effect model. The IC_{50} (the concentration of the inhibitor to show half-maximal inhibition) values were calculated using Sigma Plot ver.10.0 (Systat Software, Inc.; San Jose, CA, USA) [12].

To investigate time dependency in the inhibition of SGLT2, CHO-mock and -SGLT2 cells were seeded at a density of 1×10^5 cells/well in 96-well plates. After 24 h, the growth medium was discarded from the cells, and the cells were washed with pre-warmed Na^+-free buffer and pre-incubated with Na^+-free buffer containing various concentrations of DWP16001, dapagliflozin, or ipragliflozin (0.001 nM–100 nM) for 1 and 2 h. Then, after replacing Na^+-free buffer with Na^+ gradient buffer containing 10 μM [^{14}C]AMG and various concentrations of DWP16001, dapagliflozin, or ipragliflozin (0.001 nM–100 nM), the uptake of [^{14}C]AMG into the CHO-mock and -SGLT2 cells was measured for 2 h. After 2 h of incubation, the radioactivity of the cell lysate was measured following the same sample preparation method described above.

To investigate the mode of inhibition of the three SGLT2 inhibitors, the inhibition experiments were initiated by replacing Na^+-free buffer with Na^+ gradient buffer containing 1, 2.5, 5, and 50 μM [^{14}C]AMG and various concentrations of DWP16001, dapagliflozin, or ipragliflozin (0.001 nM–250 nM) and the uptake of [^{14}C]AMG into the CHO-mock and -SGLT2 cells was measured for 2 h. The radioactivity of the cell lysate was measured following the same sample preparation method described above. Uptake rate of AMG and concentrations of DWP16001, dapagliflozin, or ipragliflozin were plotted to Dixon plots to identify the mode of inhibition [13,14].

To investigate the recovery of SGLT2 activity depending on the washout period after 24 h exposure of DWP16001, dapagliflozin, or ipragliflozin, CHO-SGLT2 cells were seeded at a density of 1×10^5 cells/well in 96-well plates. After 24 h, the growth medium was discarded from the cells, and the cells were treated with RPMI1640 medium containing DWP16001, dapagliflozin, or ipragliflozin (0.2, 2, 20, and 200 nM) for 24 h. After 24 h, the RPMI1640 medium was replaced with pre-warmed fresh RPMI1640 medium and incubated for 1, 2, 3, 5, and 6 h, and proceeded another pre-incubation with Na^+-free buffer for 1 h. Then, after replacing Na^+-free buffer with Na^+ gradient buffer containing 10 μM [^{14}C]AMG, the uptake of [^{14}C]AMG into the CHO-SGLT2 cells was measured for 2 h. After 2 h of incubation, the radioactivity of the cell lysate was measured following the same sample preparation method described above.

2.8. Statistics

The statistical significance was assessed by t-test using SPSS for Windows (version 24.0; IBM Corp., Armonk, NY, USA).

3. Results

3.1. LC-MS/MS Analysis of DWP16001, Dapagliflozin, and Ipragliflozin

To compare the pharmacokinetics and tissue distribution of DWP16001, dapagliflozin, ipragliflozin in mice, analyses of the three SGLT2 inhibitors using LC-MS/MS were applied. Figure 2 shows the selected precursor and product ions of DWP16001, dapagliflozin, ipragliflozin, and D4-DWP16001 (IS). The selected precursor and product ions of dapagliflozin and ipragliflozin were consistent with previously published findings [12,15].

Representative multiple reaction-monitoring (MRM) chromatograms of DWP16001, D4-DWP16001 (IS), dapagliflozin, and ipragliflozin (Figure 3) showed that all the analyte peaks obtained using the liquid-liquid extraction method using MTBE were well separated with no interfering peaks at their respective retention times.

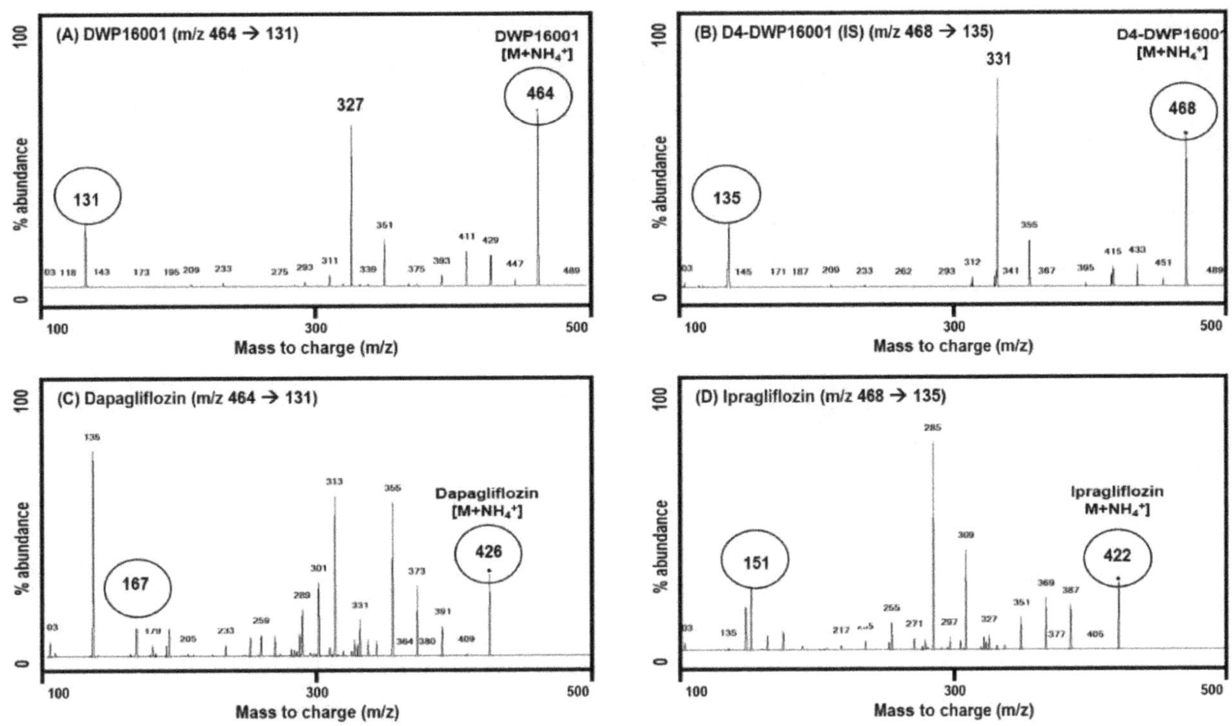

Figure 2. Product ion spectra of (**A**) DWP16001, (**B**) D4-DWP16001 (IS), (**C**) dapagliflozin, and (**D**) ipragliflozin.

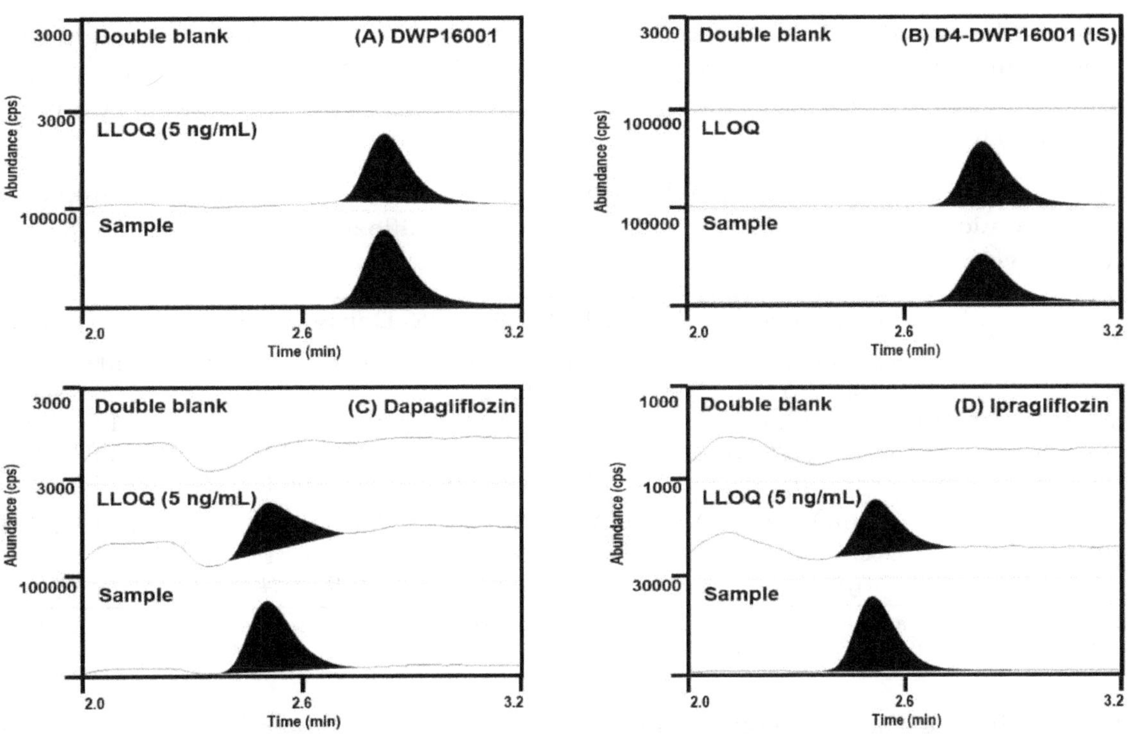

Figure 3. Representative multiple reaction-monitoring (MRM) chromatograms of (**A**) DWP16001, (**B**) D4-DWP16001 (IS), (**C**) dapagliflozin, and (**D**) ipragliflozin in mouse double-blank plasma, blank plasma spiked with DWP16001, dapagliflozin, ipragliflozin at the lower limit of quantification (LLOQ) (5 ng/mL), and plasma samples at 1 h following single oral administration of DWP16001, dapagliflozin, or ipragliflozin at a dose of 1 mg/kg.

3.2. Pharmacokinetics and Kidney Distribution of DWP16001, Dapagliflozin, and Ipragliflozin in Mice

To compare the pharmacokinetic profile of DWP16001 with those of dapagliflozin and ipragliflozin, the same dose of the three SGLT2 inhibitors was orally administered to ICR mice (1 mg/kg each), and the concentrations of DWP16001, dapagliflozin, and ipragliflozin in plasma and kidney samples were analyzed. The PK profiles of DWP16001, dapagliflozin, and ipragliflozin are shown in Figure 4 and the PK parameters were summarized in Table 1.

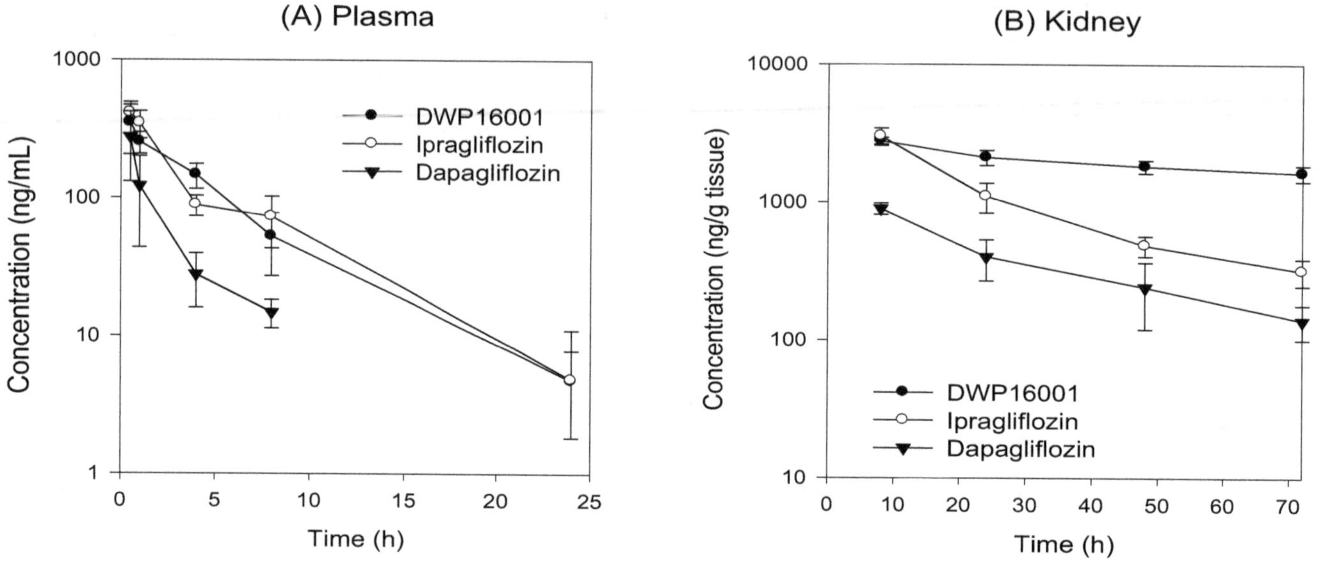

Figure 4. (**A**) Plasma and (**B**) kidney concentration vs. time profile of DWP16001 (•), dapagliflozin (▼), and ipragliflozin (○) after a single oral administrations of DWP16001, dapagliflozin, and ipragliflozin at a dose of 1 mg/kg in Institute of Cancer Research (ICR) mice, respectively. Data are expressed as mean±SD from five mice.

Table 1. Pharmacokinetic parameters of DWP16001, dapagliflozin, and ipragliflozin after a single oral administrations of DWP16001, dapagliflozin, and ipragliflozin at a dose of 1 mg/kg in ICR mice, respectively.

	Parameters	DWP16001	Dapagliflozin	Ipragliflozin
Plasma	C_{max} (ng/mL)	371.4 ± 108.6	274.8 ± 143.6	409.6 ± 59.1
	T_{max} (h)	0.7 ± 0.3	0.5 ± 0.0	0.6 ± 0.2
	AUC_{72h} (μg·h/mL)	1.69 ± 0.34	0.48 ± 0.18 *	1.96 ± 0.41
	AUC_{∞} (μg·h/mL)	1.73 ± 0.34	0.55 ± 143.8 *	1.97 ± 0.41
	$t_{1/2}$ (h)	3.8 ± 1.4	2.1 ± 0.2 *	3.1 ± 0.5
Kidney	AUC_{72h} (μg·h/g tissue)	139.2 ± 5.19	26.30 ± 3.34 *	73.65 ± 7.05 *
	AUC ratio	85.0 ± 16.1	64.6 ± 31.8	38.4 ± 5.3 *
	$t_{1/2}$ (h)	125.5 ± 80.4	24.9 ± 5.4 *	24.3 ± 5.7 *

Area under curve (AUC) ratio: Ratios of Kidney AUC to plasma AUC; Data expressed as mean ± SD from five mice; *: $p < 0.05$, compared with DWP16001 group.

As shown in Figure 4, plasma concentrations of DWP16001 were similar to those of ipragliflozin and greater than those of dapagliflozin. Consequently, the AUC and C_{max} values of DWP16001 were similar to those of ipragliflozin and higher than those of dapagliflozin. However, the concentrations of DWP16001 in the kidney were maintained at higher concentrations for 72 h compared with those of ipragliflozin and dapagliflozin, suggesting the prolonged efficacy of DWP16001 via the inhibition of SGLT2, which is located in the renal proximal tubule [3]. Because of the high and prolonged concentration of DWP16001, the AUC, AUC ratio, and $t_{1/2}$ values of DWP16001 were significantly greater than those of dapagliflozin and ipragliflozin (Table 1).

3.3. *Substrate Specificity of DWP16001, Dapagliflozin, and Ipragliflozin for OAT1 and OAT3*

The AUC ratios of these three SGLT2 inhibitors were much greater than unity, suggesting that DWP16001, dapagliflozin, and ipragliflozin are distributed in the kidney, in which tissue protein binding ability to the specific protein or drug transporters may be involved. Therefore, firstly, we measured the protein binding of DWP16001, dapagliflozin, and ipragliflozin in the plasma and kidney homogenate.

The plasma and kidney tissue protein binding of DWP16001, dapagliflozin, and ipragliflozin were high and comparable and the logP values of three compound were also comparable (i.e., in the range of 2.27–2.65) (Table 2). It suggests that the large distribution of DWP16001, dapagliflozin, and ipragliflozin in the kidney was not necessarily reliant on plasma/tissue-specific binding ability or lipophilicity of these compounds.

Table 2. Protein binding of DWP16001, dapagliflozin, and ipragliflozin in mouse plasma and kidney homogenates.

Compounds	logP [a]	Protein Binding (% Bound) [b]	
		Plasma	Kidney
DWP16001	2.65	98.50 ± 0.20	97.24 ± 0.08
Dapagliflozin	2.27	94.19 ± 1.07	95.83 ± 0.68
Ipragliflozin	2.56	96.58 ± 0.75	96.50 ± 1.01

[a] logP values were obtained from the partition coefficient of n-octanol/water; [b] Data expressed as mean ± SD of triplicate experiments.

We conducted further investigations into the tissue-specific transport of DWP16001, dapagliflozin, and ipragliflozin by using cell systems overexpressing OAT1 and OAT3 since OAT1 and OAT3 are exclusively distributed in the kidney and contribute to the drug distribution to the kidney [16]. The functionality of the OAT1 and OAT3 transport system was confirmed by the significantly greater uptake rates of the probe substrates in HEK293-OAT1 and -OAT3 cells than that in HEK293-mock cells (i.e., 14.7-fold increase in PAH uptake for OAT1 and 16.4-fold increase in ES uptake for OAT3) and by the decreased uptake rate of each probe substrate by the addition of a representative inhibitor, probenecid (Figure 5A,B) [17]. The uptake of DWP16001 in HEK293-OAT1 and OAT3 cells was significantly higher than that in HEK293-mock cells, and it was significantly decreased by the presence of probenecid (Figure 5C). However, dapagliflozin and ipragliflozin were not substrates for both OAT1 and OAT3 (Figure 5D,E). Next, we investigated the concentration dependency in the OAT1 and OAT3-mediated DWP16001 uptake. As shown in the figure, the OAT1 and OAT3-mediated uptake of DWP16001 showed saturable kinetics, and the kinetic parameters, such as K_m and V_{max}, calculated from the concentration-dependent uptake of DWP16001 in HEK293-OAT1 and –OAT3 cells are shown in Figure 6. Collectively, OAT1 and OAT3-mediated uptake of DWP16001 could contribute to the highest kidney distribution of DWP16001 among three SGLT2 inhibitors. However, these processes were not dominant over the cellular uptake of the three SGLT2 inhibitors into HEK293-mock cells (i.e., passive diffusion), which is evident from two-fold increases in HEK293-OAT1 or -OAT3 cells compared with mock cells (Figure 5C). Therefore, OAT1- and OAT3-mediated active transport and passive diffusion all contributed to the highly permeable absorptive process of DWP16001 in the kidney, and dapagliflozin and ipragliflozin also showed higher uptake levels into HEK293 cells via passive diffusion.

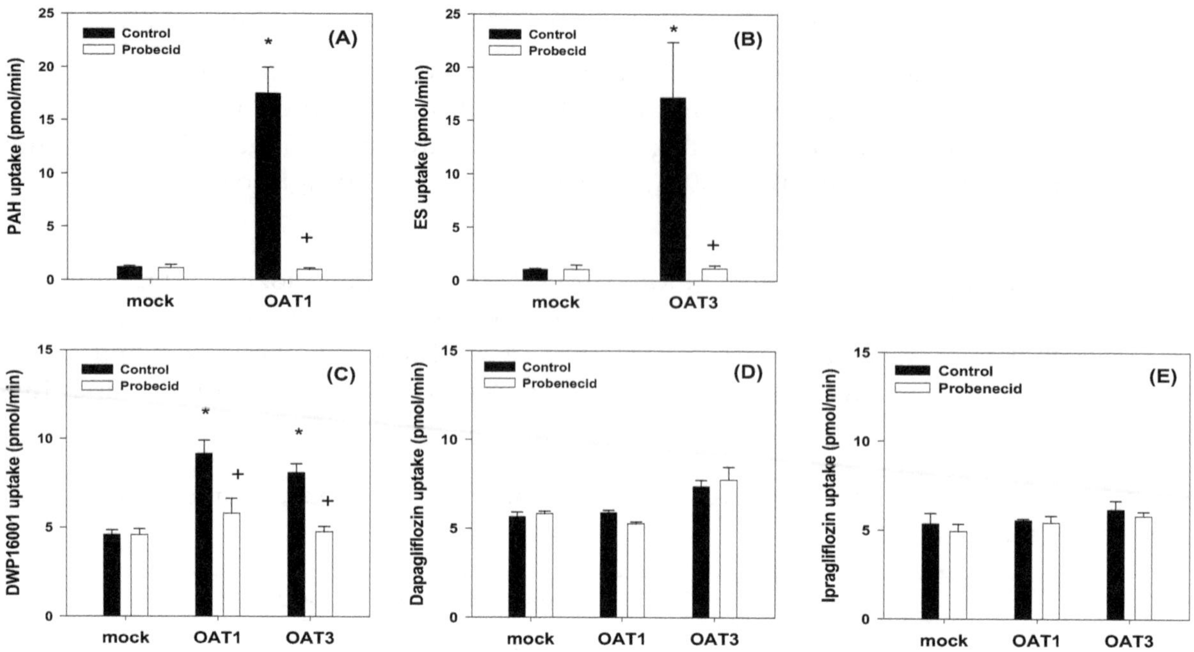

Figure 5. (**A**) Uptake of 0.1 μM [^{3}H]para-aminohippuric acid (PAH) was measured in HEK293-mock and –OAT1 cells in the presence and absence of 20 μM probenecid for 5 min. (**B**) Uptake of 0.1 μM [^{3}H]Estrone-3-sulfate (ES) was measured in HEK293-mock and –OAT3 cells in the presence and absence of 20 μM probenecid. Uptake of (**C**) DWP16001, (**D**) dapagliflozin, and (**E**) ipragliflozin (2 μM each) into HEK293-mock and HEK293 cells expressing OAT1 and OAT3 was measured for 5 min. Each data point represents the mean±standard deviation of triplicate experiments. *: $p < 0.05$, compared with mock cells; +: $p < 0.05$, compared with control group.

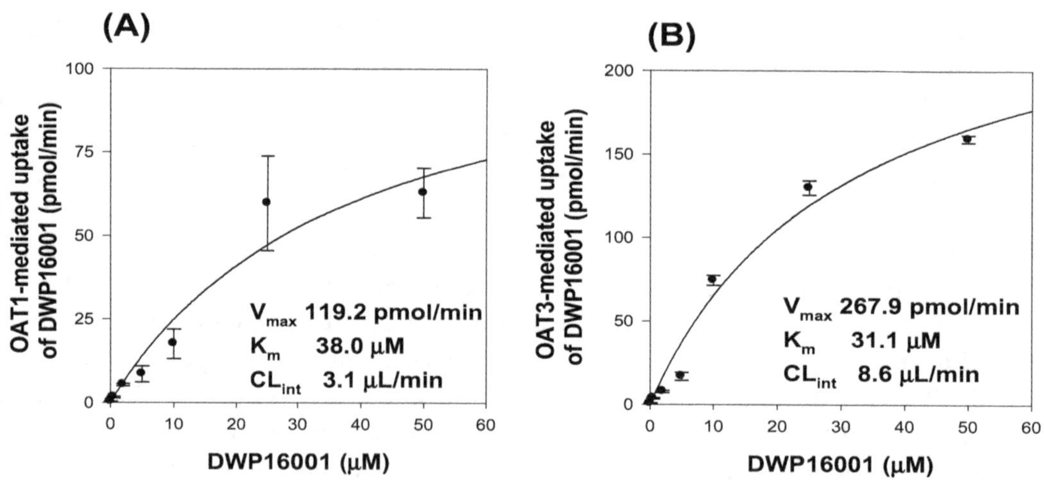

Figure 6. (**A**) OAT1- and (**B**) OAT3-mediated uptake of DWP16001. Concentration dependent uptake of DWP16001 was measured for 5 min into HEK293-mock cells and HEK293 cells expressing OAT1 and OAT3. The transporter-mediated uptake rate was obtained by subtracting the uptake in HEK293-mock cells (passive diffusion) from those in HEK293 cells expressing OAT1 and OAT3 (total uptake). Each data point represents the means ± standard deviation from triplicate experiments.

3.4. Inhibition Potential of DWP16001, Dapagliflozin, Ipragliflozin on SGLT1 and SGLT2 Activities

3.4.1. Comparison of IC_{50} Values of DWP16001, Dapagliflozin, and Ipragliflozin on SGLT1 and SGLT2

To confirm the functionality of CHO-SGLT1 cells, we measured the time-dependent uptake of AMG, a representative substrate for SGLT1 [11,18]. As shown in Figure 7A, AMG uptake was increased with incubation time, and the optimal incubation time was selected as 2 h from the linear phase of the slope. AMG uptake into CHO-SGLT1 cells was 42-fold greater than that into CHO-mock cells and significantly inhibited by the presence of known inhibitors, such as dapagliflozin and ipragliflozin [3,5] (Figure 7B). With the same experimental condition, the inhibitory effect of DWP16001, dapagliflozin, and ipragliflozin on the AMG uptake into CHO-SGLT1 cells was measured in a concentration range of 1–50,000 nM and IC_{50} values were calculated (Figure 7C–E; Table 3).

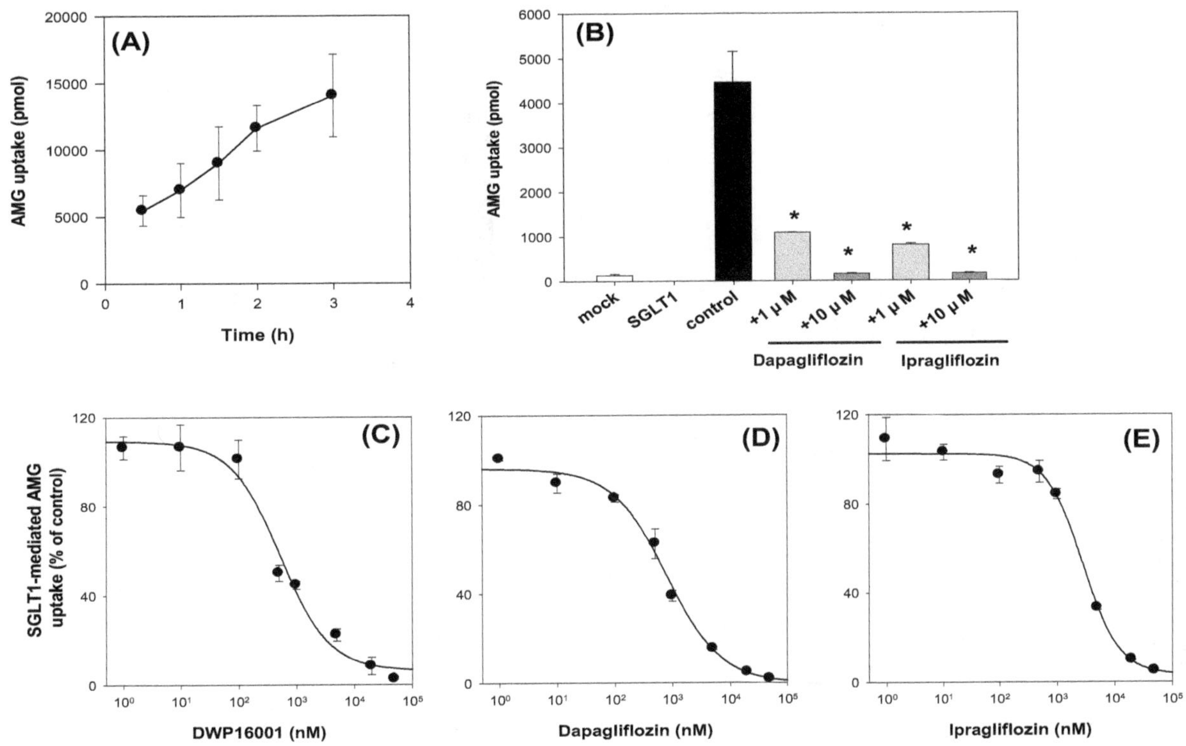

Figure 7. (**A**) Uptake of 10 μM [^{14}C]methyl-a-D-glucopyranoside (AMG) was measured in CHO-sodium-glucose cotransporter 1 (SGLT1) cells with a various incubation time (0.5–3 h). (**B**) Inhibitory effect of dapagliflozin and ipragliflozin (1, 10 μM) on the uptake of 10 μM [^{14}C]AMG in CHO-mock and -SGLT1 cells was measured for 2 h. Concentration dependent inhibition of DWP16001 (**C**), dapagliflozin (**D**), and ipragliflozin (**E**) on the SGLT1-mediated uptake of [^{14}C]AMG. SGLT1-mediated uptake of [^{14}C]AMG was calculated by subtracting the uptake of 10 μM [^{14}C]AMG for 2 h in CHO-mock cells from that in CHO-SGLT1 cells in a concentration range of 1–50,000 nM of DWP16001, dapagliflozin, and ipragliflozin. Each data point represents the mean ± standard deviation of three independent experiments. *: $p < 0.05$, compared with control group.

Table 3. Inhibition potential of DWP16001, dapagliflozin, and ipragliflozin on SGLT1 and SGLT2 activities.

	IC_{50} (nM)		Selectivity
	SGLT1	SGLT2	(IC_{50} Ratio of SGLT1/SGLT2)
DWP16001	549.3 ± 139.6	0.8 ± 0.3	667
Ipragliflozin	2328.7 ± 377.6	8.9 ± 1.7	261
Dapagliflozin	803.0 ± 96.8	1.6 ± 0.3	493

Data were expressed as mean ± SD from triplicate measurement.

Similarly, the functionality of CHO-SGLT2 cells was confirmed from the time-dependent uptake of AMG, a representative substrate for SGLT2 [3,5]. As shown in Figure 8A, AMG uptake was increased with incubation time, and the optimal incubation time was selected as 2 h from the linear phase of the slope. AMG uptake into CHO-SGLT1 cells was 9.8-fold greater than that into CHO-mock cells and significantly inhibited by the presence of known inhibitors, such as dapagliflozin and ipragliflozin [3] (Figure 8B). With the same experimental conditions, the inhibitory effect of DWP16001, dapagliflozin, and ipragliflozin on the AMG uptake into CHO-SGLT2 cells was measured in a concentration range of 0.001–100 nM, and IC_{50} values were calculated (Figure 8C–E; Table 3).

DWP16001 showed greater affinity for SGLT2 compared with dapagliflozin and ipragliflozin. Moreover, the affinity to SGLT1 was also greater with DWP16001 compared with dapagliflozin and ipragliflozin. When compared with selectivity, which was calculated from the SGLT1/SGLT2 IC_{50} ratio, the selectivity of DWP16001 was high relative to that of dapagliflozin and ipragliflozin (Table 3).

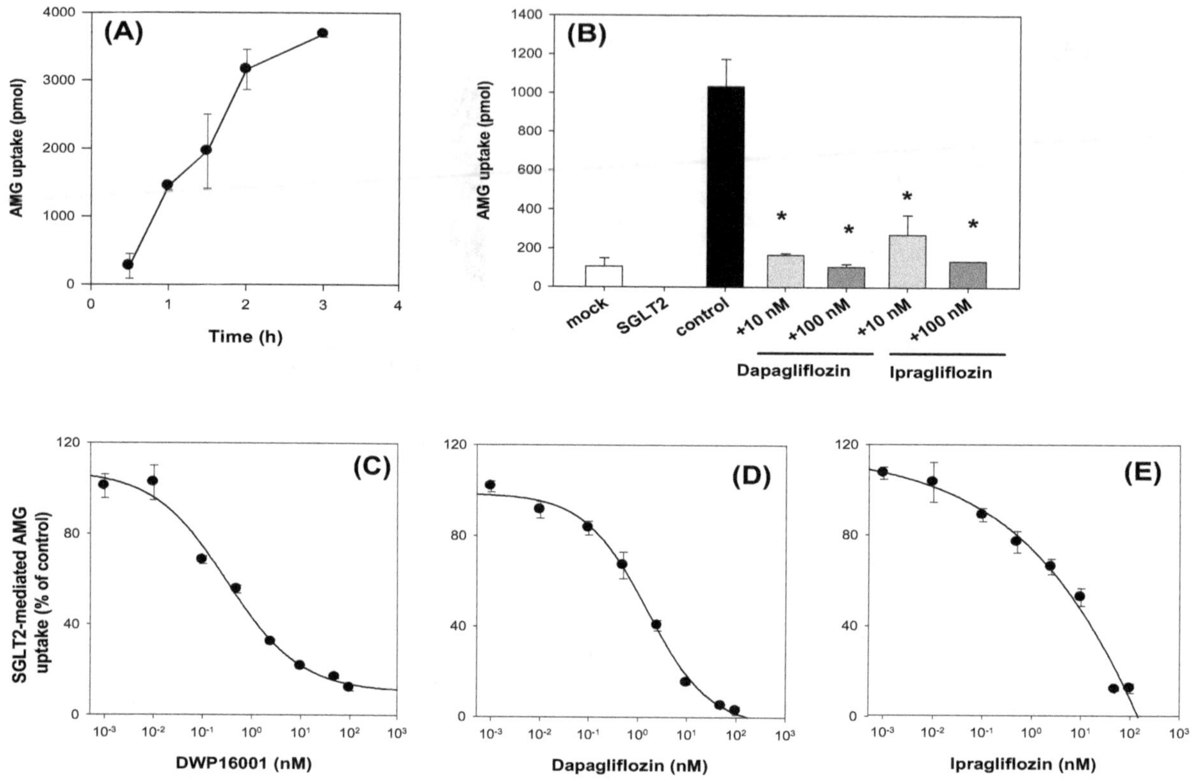

Figure 8. (**A**) The uptake of 10 μM [^{14}C]methyl-a-D-glucopyranoside (AMG) was measured in CHO-SGLT2 cells with a various incubation time (0.5, 1, 1.5, 2, 3 h). (**B**) Inhibitory effect of dapagliflozin and ipragliflozin (10, 100 nM) on the uptake of 10 μM [^{14}C]AMG in CHO-mock and –SGLT2 cells was measured for 2 h. Representative concentration dependent inhibition of DWP16001 (**C**), dapagliflozin (**D**), and ipragliflozin (**E**) on the SGLT2-mediated uptake of [^{14}C]AMG. SGLT2-mediated uptake of [^{14}C]AMG was calculated by subtracting the uptake of 10 μM [^{14}C]AMG for 2 h in CHO-mock cells from that in CHO-SGLT2 cells in a concentration range of 1–100 nM of DWP16001, dapagliflozin, and ipragliflozin. Each data point represents the mean±standard deviation of three independent experiments. *: $p < 0.05$, compared with control group.

3.4.2. Mode of Inhibition

To investigate whether the inhibition of SGLT2 was time-dependent, the inhibitory effects of DWP16001, dapagliflozin, and ipragliflozin on SGLT2-mediated uptake of AMG were measured with or without pretreatment with DWP16001, dapagliflozin, and ipragliflozin, respectively. Figure 9 shows that the inhibitory potential of DWP16001, dapagliflozin, and ipragliflozin on SGLT2 did not change with different pretreatment times, suggesting that all the DWP16001, dapagliflozin, and ipragliflozin inhibited SGLT2 function in a time-independent manner.

To determine the mode of inhibition on SGLT2, the inhibitory effects of DWP16001, dapagliflozin, and ipragliflozin on the AMG uptake into CHO-SGLT2 cells were measured with different substrate concentrations, and the results were expressed as Dixon plots (Figure 10A–C) and a replot of the Dixon slopes (Figure 10D–F) [13,19,20]. Dixon transformation of inhibition profile by DWP16001 (0.001–250 nM) for different concentrations of AMG indicated competitive inhibition of DWP16001 on SGLT2 activity (Figure 10A). A replot of the Dixon slopes vs 1/S produced a straight line converging on the zero (Figure 10D), suggesting competitive and reversible inhibition of DWP16001. Similar results were shown in case of dapagliflozin and ipragliflozin (Figure 10B,C,E,F). The results collectively suggested that the inhibition of SGLT2 by DWP16001, dapagliflozin, and ipragliflozin is reversible and competitive.

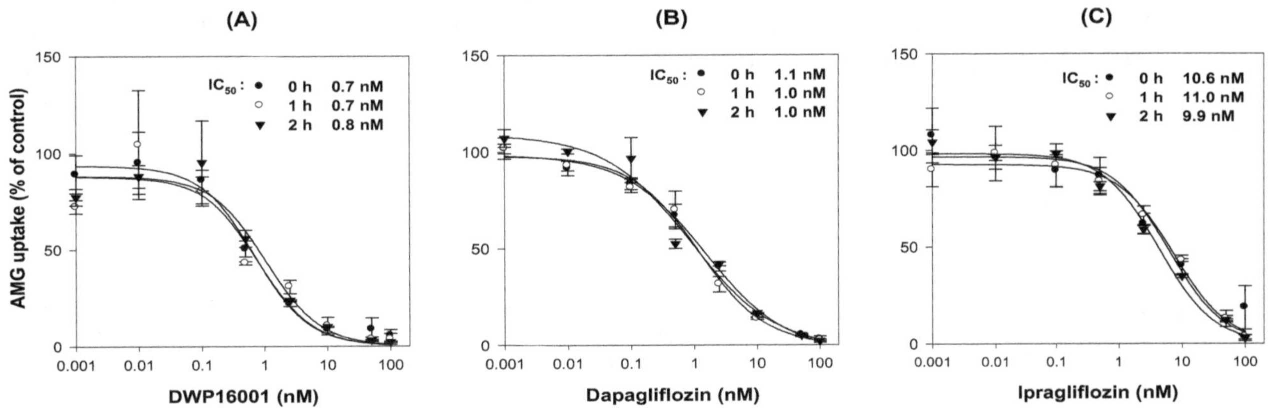

Figure 9. Inhibitory effect of (**A**) DWP16001, (**B**) dapagliflozin, and (**C**) ipragliflozin on the SGLT2-mediated uptake of 10 μM [^{14}C]methyl-a-D-glucopyranoside (AMG) was measured with preincubation time for 1 and 2 h or without preincubation of DWP16001, dapagliflozin, and ipragliflozin, respectively, in a concentration range of 0.001–100 nM. Each data point represents the mean±standard deviation of three independent experiments.

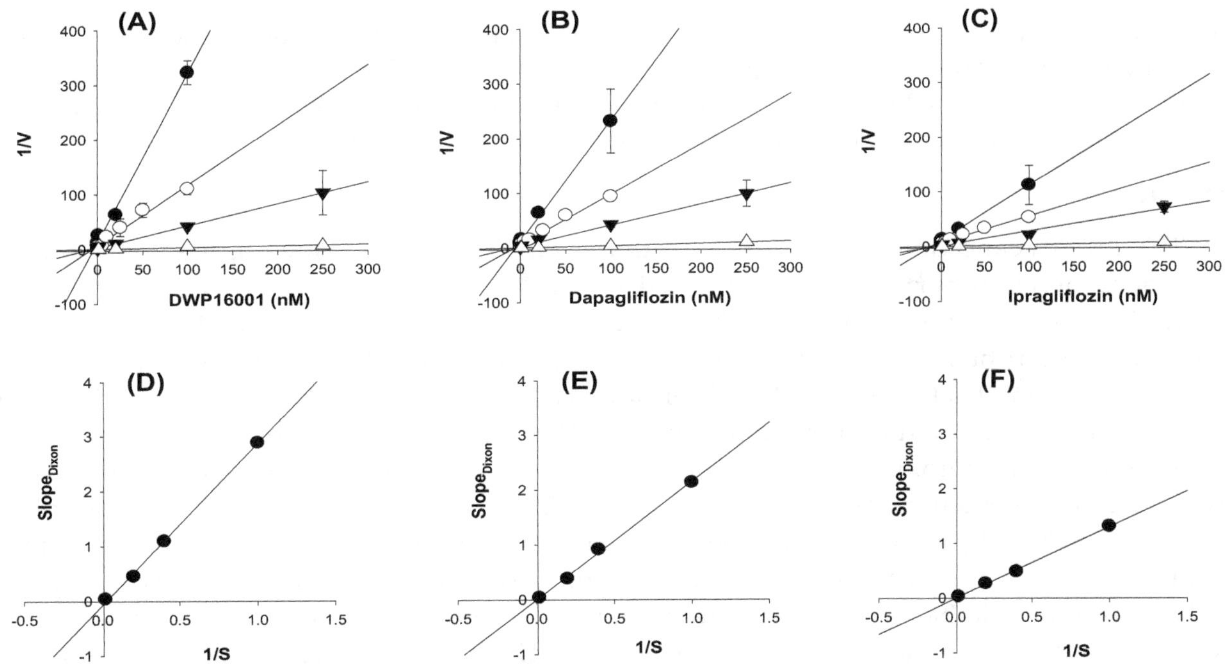

Figure 10. Dixon plot for the inhibitory effect of (**A**) DWP16001, (**B**) dapagliflozin, and (**C**) ipragliflozin on the uptake of [^{14}C]methyl-a-D-glucopyranoside (AMG) in CHO-SGLT2 cells. Each symbol represents the concentration of [^{14}C]AMG: •, 1 μM; ○, 2.5 μM; ▼, 5 μM; △, 50 μM. Replot of the slopes of Dixon plot (slopes vs 1/[S]) was shown for (**D**) DWP16001, (**E**) dapagliflozin, and (**F**) ipragliflozin. V indicates the SGLT2-mediated uptake rate of [^{14}C]AMG and S indicates the concentration of [^{14}C]AMG. The data are the means±standard deviations of triplicate measurements.

3.4.3. Retained Inhibition Potential of DWP16001 Compared to Dapagliflozin and Ipragliflozin

The recovery of SGLT2 activities depending on the washout period after 24 h exposure of DWP16001, ipragliflozin, and dapagliflozin in CHO-SGLT2 cells was investigated. As shown in Figure 11, the activity of reduced SGLT2 by treatment with DWP16001, dapagliflozin, and ipragliflozin for 24 h in CHO-SGLT2 cells revealed differences in the recovery of SGLT2 depending on the time of drug removal from the medium, as well as SGLT2 inhibitors. In the case of DWP16001, the activity tended to gradually recover as the washout time increased. When treated at a high concentration (200 nM), the activity did not recover even 8 h after the drug was removed from the medium (Figure 11A). However, when dapagliflozin and ipragliflozin were used, SGLT2 activity was recovered to the control level 4 h after the removal of dapagliflozin and ipragliflozin (Figure 11B,C). The results indicate that the dissociation of DWP16001 to SGLT2 is slower and more incomplete than that of dapagliflozin and ipragliflozin and that the binding affinity to SGLT2 is stronger than that of dapagliflozin and ipragliflozin.

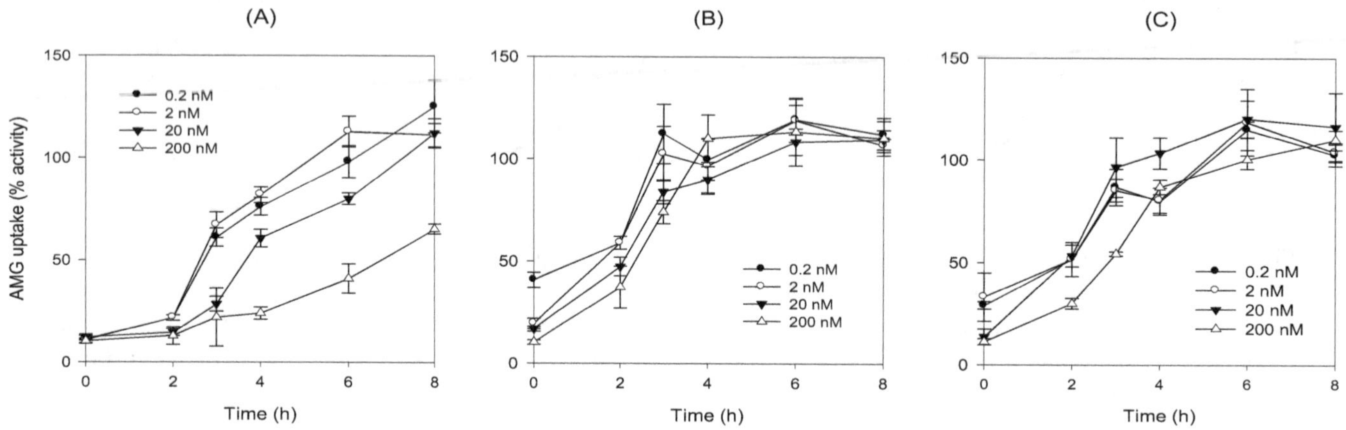

Figure 11. Recovery of SGLT2 transport function with different washout time following 24 h of incubation with (**A**) DWP16001, (**B**) dapagliflozin, and (**C**) ipragliflozin (0.2–200 nM) was measured through the uptake of [^{14}C]methyl-a-D-glucopyranoside (AMG) in CHO-SGLT2 cells. Each data point represents the mean±standard deviation of three independent experiments.

4. Discussion

DWP16001 is a candidate SGLT2 inhibitor that is currently under development. As a first step, the pharmacokinetic properties and in vitro SGLT2 inhibition were compared with currently used SGLT2 inhibitors. Dapagliflozin and ipragliflozin were selected based on their high kidney distributions and long elimination half-lives ($t_{1/2}$) in the kidney [5], which are thought to be important for the efficacy and duration of action of SGLT2 inhibitors. DWP16001 showed higher kidney distributions compared with dapagliflozin and ipragliflozin. DWP16001 also had longer $t_{1/2}$ in the kidney than dapagliflozin and ipragliflozin, as well as a comparable plasma profile with ipragliflozin (Table 1). Moreover, the kidney concentration of DWP16001 was maintained over 72 h following oral administration of 1 mg/kg DWP16001 (Figure 4). Taken together, these pharmacokinetic results show that the duration of action of DWP16001 is greater than that of dapagliflozin and ipragliflozin and that the oral therapeutic dose of DWP16001 could be reduced compared with both dapagliflozin and ipragliflozin.

To investigate the underlying mechanisms of highest kidney distribution and maintained concentration of DWP16001 in the kidney, we measured the kidney tissue binding and involvement of OAT1 and OAT3 transporters of the three SGLT2 inhibitors. All three SGLT2 inhibitors showed high protein binding, but the kidney tissue binding performances of these three SGLT2 inhibitors were not different from their plasma protein binding capabilities (Table 2). However, DWP16001 was a substrate for both OAT1 and OAT3, which are dominantly expressed in the kidney, whereas dapagliflozin and ipragliflozin were not (Figures 5 and 6). Although this could not solely explain the high kidney distribution, OAT1- and OAT3-mediated transport process may contribute to the high kidney distribution.

Next, we compared the in vitro SGLT2 inhibition and selectivity of SGLT2 inhibition over SGLT1. All three SGLT2 inhibitors inhibited SGLT2 and SGLT1 activity in a concentration-dependent manner and IC_{50} values of dapagliflozin and ipragliflozin were in the range of previous reports (1.0–1.3 nM for dapagliflozin; 6.75–8.07 nM for ipragliflozin) [21,22]. IC_{50} values of DWP16001 to SGLT2 and SGLT1 were lower than those of dapagliflozin and ipragliflozin, suggesting a greater affinity to SGLT2 inhibition for DWP16001 with a higher selectivity over SGLT1 than dapagliflozin and ipragliflozin. The mode of inhibition of DWP16001 was not different from the other SGLT2 inhibitors. They all showed reversible and competitive inhibition (Figure 10), which is consistent with other SGLT2 inhibitors [23,24]. However, the affinity to SGLT2 inhibition seemed to be different among the three SGLT2 inhibitors (Table 3). In addition, the recovery of SGLT2 transport activity following the pretreatment of DWP16001, dapagliflozin, and ipragliflozin for 24 h was retained at a higher concentration (200 nM) of DWP16001 compared with dapagliflozin and ipragliflozin. These results suggested that DWP16001 had the highest SGLT2 inhibition potential and that this inhibition potential retained for a longer time compared with dapagliflozin and ipragliflozin. Combined with the higher kidney distribution of DWP16001, retained SGLT2 inhibition with a high concentration of DWP16001 could also potentiate the efficacy of DWP16001 compared with dapagliflozin and ipragliflozin.

The comparative pharmacokinetics and in vitro SGLT2 inhibition findings suggest that DWP16001 might be a superior alternative to dapagliflozin and ipragliflozin; however, we should note that comparisons of the in vivo pharmacologic properties of these agents using therapeutic doses in animals and humans need to be further undertaken.

Author Contributions: Conceptualization, M.-K.C., H.-Y.J and I.-S.S.; Investigation, M.-K.C., S.J.N., H.-Y.J., M.J.P., J.-S.C. and I.-S.S.; Writing-Original Draft Preparation, M.-K.C.; Supervision, I.-S.S.; Writing-Review & Editing, I.-S.S. All authors have read and agreed to the published version of the manuscript.

References

1. Choi, M.-K.; Jin, Q.-R.; Ahn, S.-H.; Bae, M.A.; Song, I.-S. Sitagliptin attenuates metformin-mediated AMPK phosphorylation through inhibition of organic cation transporters. *Xenobiotica* **2010**, *40*, 817–825. [CrossRef]
2. Chao, E.C.; Henry, R.R. SGLT2 inhibition—A novel strategy for diabetes treatment. *Nat. Rev. Drug Discov.* **2010**, *9*, 551–559. [CrossRef]
3. Ferrannini, E.; Solini, A. SGLT2 inhibition in diabetes mellitus: Rationale and clinical prospects. *Nat. Rev. Endocrinol.* **2012**, *8*, 495–502. [CrossRef]
4. Van Baar, M.J.B.; Van Ruiten, C.C.; Muskiet, M.H.A.; Van Bloemendaal, L.; Ijzerman, R.G.; Van Raalte, D.H. SGLT2 inhibitors in combination therapy: From mechanisms to clinical considerations in type 2 diabetes management. *Diabetes Care* **2018**, *41*, 1543–1556. [CrossRef]
5. Tahara, A.; Takasu, T.; Yokono, M.; Imamura, M.; Kurosaki, E. Characterization and comparison of sodium-glucose cotransporter 2 inhibitors: Part 2. Antidiabetic effects in type 2 diabetic mice. *J. Pharmacol. Sci.* **2016**, *131*, 198–208. [CrossRef]
6. Schuhmacher, J.; Buhner, K.; Witt-Laido, A. Determination of the free fraction and relative free fraction of drugs strongly bound to plasma proteins. *J. Pharm. Sci.* **2000**, *89*, 1008–1021. [CrossRef]
7. Jeon, J.H.; Lee, S.; Lee, W.; Jin, S.; Kwon, M.; Shin, C.H.; Choi, M.K.; Song, I.S. Herb-drug interaction of red ginseng extract and ginsenoside Rc with valsartan in rats. *Molecules* **2020**, *25*, 622. [CrossRef] [PubMed]
8. Mathialagan, S.; Piotrowski, M.A.; Tess, D.A.; Feng, B.; Litchfield, J.; Varma, M.V.; Litchfiled, J. Quantitative prediction of human renal clearance and drug-drug interactions of organic anion transporter substrates using in vitro transport data: A relative activity factor approach. *Drug Metab. Dispos.* **2017**, *45*, 409–417. [CrossRef] [PubMed]
9. Song, I.S.; Jeong, H.U.; Choi, M.K.; Kwon, M.; Shin, Y.; Kim, J.H.; Lee, H.S. Interactions between cyazofamid and human drug transporters. *J. Biochem. Mol. Toxic.* **2020**, e22459. [CrossRef]
10. Choi, M.K.; Kwon, M.; Ahn, J.H.; Kim, N.J.; Bae, M.A.; Song, I.S. Transport characteristics and transporter-based drug-drug interactions of TM-25659, a novel TAZ modulator. *Biopharm. Drug Dispos.* **2014**, *35*, 183–194. [CrossRef]
11. Grempler, R.; Thomas, L.; Eckhardt, M.; Himmelsbach, F.; Sauer, A.; Sharp, D.E.; Bakker, R.A.; Mark, M.; Klein, T.; Eickelmann, P. Empagliflozin, a novel selective sodium glucose cotransporter-2 (SGLT-2) inhibitor: Characterisation and comparison with other SGLT-2 inhibitors. *Diabetes Obes. Metab.* **2012**, *14*, 83–90. [CrossRef]
12. Jin, S.; Lee, S.; Jeon, J.H.; Kim, H.; Choi, M.K.; Song, I.S. Enhanced intestinal permeability and plasma concentration of metformin in rats by the repeated administration of red ginseng extract. *Pharmaceutics* **2019**, *11*, e189. [CrossRef] [PubMed]

13. Choi, M.K.; Jin, Q.R.; Choi, Y.L.; Ahn, S.H.; Bae, M.A.; Song, I.S. Inhibitory effects of ketoconazole and rifampin on OAT1 and OATP1B1 transport activities: Considerations on drug-drug interactions. *Biopharm. Drug Dispos.* **2011**, *32*, 175–184. [CrossRef] [PubMed]
14. Kim, S.; Choi, W.G.; Kwon, M.; Lee, S.; Cho, Y.Y.; Lee, J.Y.; Kang, H.C.; Song, I.S.; Lee, H.S. In vitro inhibitory effects of APINACA on human major Cytochrome P450, UDP-Glucuronosyltransferase enzymes, and drug transporters. *Molecules* **2019**, *24*, e3000. [CrossRef] [PubMed]
15. Harvey, A.L.; Edrada-Ebel, R.; Quinn, R.J. The re-emergence of natural products for drug discovery in the genomics era. *Nat. Rev. Drug Discov.* **2015**, *14*, 111–129. [CrossRef] [PubMed]
16. Vallon, V.; Eraly, S.A.; Rao, S.R.; Gerasimova, M.; Rose, M.; Nagle, M.; Anzai, N.; Smith, T.; Sharma, K.; Nigam, S.K.; et al. A role for the organic anion transporter OAT3 in renal creatinine secretion in mice. *Am. J. Physiol. Renal Physiol.* **2012**, *302*, F1293–F1299. [CrossRef] [PubMed]
17. Jeong, H.U.; Kwon, M.; Lee, Y.; Yoo, J.S.; Shin, D.H.; Song, I.S.; Lee, H.S. Organic anion transporter 3-and organic anion transporting polypeptides 1B1-and 1B3-mediated transport of catalposide. *Drug Des. Dev. Ther.* **2015**, *9*, 643–653.
18. Yamamoto, K.; Uchida, S.; Kitano, K.; Fukuhara, N.; Okumura-Kitajima, L.; Gunji, E.; Kozakai, A.; Tomoike, H.; Kojima, N.; Asami, J.; et al. TS-071 is a novel, potent and selective renal sodium-glucose cotransporter 2 (SGLT2) inhibitor with anti-hyperglycaemic activity. *Br. J. Pharmacol.* **2011**, *164*, 181–191. [CrossRef]
19. Meneilly, G.S.; Demuth, H.U.; McIntosh, C.H.S.; Pederson, R.A. Effect of ageing and diabetes on glucose-dependent insulinotropic polypeptide and dipeptidyl peptidase IV responses to oral glucose. *Diabetic Med.* **2000**, *17*, 346–350. [CrossRef]
20. Lorey, S.; Stockel-Maschek, A.; Faust, J.; Brandt, W.; Stiebitz, B.; Gorrell, M.D.; Kahne, T.; Mrestani-Klaus, C.; Wrenger, S.; Reinhold, D.; et al. Different modes of dipeptidyl peptidase IV (CD26) inhibition by oligopeptides derived from the N-terminus of HIV-1 Tat indicate at least two inhibitor binding sites. *Eur. J. Biochem.* **2003**, *270*, 2147–2156. [CrossRef]
21. Ohkura, T. Ipragliflozin: A novel sodium-glucose cotransporter 2 inhibitor developed in Japan. *World J. Diabetes* **2015**, *6*, 136–144. [CrossRef] [PubMed]
22. Obermeier, M.; Yao, M.; Khanna, A.; Koplowitz, B.; Zhu, M.; Li, K.; Komoroski, B.; Kasichayanula, S.; Discenza, L.; Washburn, W.; et al. In vitro characterization and pharmacokinetics of dapagliflozin (BMS-512148), a potent sodium-glucose cotransporter type II Inhibitor, in animals and humans. *Drug Metab. Dispos.* **2010**, *38*, 405–414. [CrossRef] [PubMed]
23. Demaris, K.M.; White, J.R. Dapagliflozin, an SGLT2 inhibitor for the treatment of type 2 diabetes. *Drugs Today* **2013**, *49*, 289–301. [CrossRef] [PubMed]
24. Takasu, T.; Yokono, M.; Tahara, A.; Takakura, S. In vitro pharmacological profile of ipragliflozin, a sodium glucose co-transporter 2 Inhibitor. *Biol. Pharm. Bull.* **2019**, *42*, 507–511. [CrossRef]

12

Pharmacokinetic Drug-Drug Interaction and Responsible Mechanism between Memantine and Cimetidine

Young A. Choi [1], Im-Sook Song [2] and Min-Koo Choi [1,*]

[1] College of Pharmacy, Dankook University, Cheon-an 31116, Korea; ayha06@gmail.com
[2] College of Pharmacy and Research Institute of Pharmaceutical Sciences, Kyungpook National University, Daegu 41566, Korea; isssong@knu.ac.kr
* Correspondence: minkoochoi@dankook.ac.kr

Abstract: A sensitive and simple chromatography-tandem mass spectrometry (LC-MS/MS) method was developed to evaluate memantine in rat plasma. Memantine and propranolol (internal standard) in rat plasma was extracted using a methanol precipitation method. The standard curve value was 0.2–1000 ng/mL and selectivity, linearity, inter-day and intra-day accuracy and precision were within acceptance criteria. Using this validated method, drug-drug interactions between memantine and cimetidine was measured following co-administration of memantine and cimetidine intravenously and orally. Plasma exposure of memantine was increased by 1.6- and 3.0-fold by co-medication with cimetidine intravenously and orally, respectively. It suggested that the drug interaction occurred during the gut absorption process, which was consistent with the results showing that the intestinal permeability of memantine in the presence of cimetidine was 3.2-fold greater than that of memantine alone. Inhibition of cimetidine on hepatic elimination of memantine rather than renal excretion was also attributed to the drug-drug interaction between memantine and cimetidine, which explained the decreased clearance of memantine by co-medication with cimetidine. In conclusion, the newly developed simple and sensitive LC-MS/MS analytical method was applied to investigate the pharmacokinetic drug-drug interactions of memantine. Plasma exposure of memantine by co-administration with cimetidine was increased because of its enhanced intestinal permeability and the decreased metabolic activity of memantine.

Keywords: mematine; drug interaction; liquid chromatography-tandem mass spectrometry; pharmacokinetics

---

1. Introduction

Alzheimer's disease is among the most common dementia and is progressed by memory loss, confusion, impaired judgement and disorientation [1]. Currently drugs that can completely cure Alzheimer's disease are not available [2]. Accessible medications focus on symptomatic treatment and only reduce disease progression [2]. Memantine (Namenda®) is *N*-methyl-D-aspartate antagonist in the brain [3] which has been approved by US Food and Drug Administration (FDA) to treat moderate to severe dementia. Memantine also inhibits the neurodegenerative effects of glutamate [4] and protects neuron cells [5]. Based on this mode of action, memantine showed promising clinical and preclinical effects on several psychiatric disorders such as bipolar disorder, depression, schizophrenia and anxiety disorders as mono or add-on therapy [6]. Therefore, memantine has been prescribed alone or in combination with other cognitive drugs such as donepezil (Aricept®), rivastigmine (Exelon®) and galantamine (Razadyne®) as well as anti-psychotic drugs [6,7]. It has been reported that no drug-drug interaction between memantine and donepezil, rivastigmine and galantamine was observed [8–10]. However, it may interact with other *N*-methyl-D-aspartate receptor ligands such as dextromethorphan, ketamine and phencyclidine and anti-psychotic drugs such as amantadine and dopamine antagonists [6]. Drug-drug interaction may change the pharmacokinetic features and therapeutic response of memantine. In addition, Dizziness and vomiting are common adverse events of memantine, which may be associated with the high plasma concentrations of memantine [5].

Because of its pharmacokinetic-pharmacodynamic relationship, the therapeutic drug monitoring of Alzheimer's disease drugs as well as anti-psychotic drugs is increasingly necessary for studying individual variations, metabolic and kinetic alterations in some patients, responsible mechanisms for decreasing effectiveness and to make a decision to adherence or changing existed therapy [11]. Moreover, to investigate the mechanisms responsible for the possible interaction between memantine and other drugs which may cause the high plasma concentration of memantine, it is necessary to establish an accurate, sensitive and simple bioanalysis method for the detection of memantine in diverse matrices.

Therefore, the aim of this study was to develop and validate a sensitive and simple liquid chromatography tandem mass spectrometry (LC-MS/MS) method for measuring memantine focusing on lowering the required plasma volume and simplifying the overall process. The method was fully validated according to the FDA Guideline for Bioanalytical Method for its linearity, selectivity, accuracy, precision, recovery, stability and matrix effects [12].

To examine application of this analytical method, we investigated pharmacokinetic drug–drug interactions between memantine and cimetidine. To understand the underlying mechanisms of the drug-drug interaction between memantine and cimetidine, we administered memantine with or without cimetidine intravenously as well as orally. Cimetidine was selected because it inhibits cytochrome P 450 (Cyp)-mediated metabolism and the organic cation transporter (Oct)-mediated transport process [13,14]. In addition to Cyp and Oct inhibition, cimetidine, an H2 receptor antagonist, is used to treat peptic ulcers and is the most prescribed over-the-counter drug that is easily accessed by patients [15,16]. Cimetidine is well-absorbed from the gut through the paracellular transport and mainly excreted via the renal route in rats (70% of oral dose was eliminated via the renal route for 72 h) with limited metabolism and low plasma protein binding (approximately 20%) [17,18], suggesting that a high plasma concentration of cimetidine is maintained. Thus, the plausibility of concomitant administration of memantine and cimetidine and drug-drug interaction between memantine and cimetidine seems to be high.

2. Materials and Methods

2.1. Materials

Memantine, cimetidine and propranolol was purchased from Sigma-Aldrich (St. Louis, MO, USA). Methanol and water was of HPLC grade (Burdick & Jackson Korea, Seoul, Korea). All other reagents and solvents were of reagent or analytical grade.

2.2. Animals

Male Sprague-Dawley rats (7–8 weeks, 220−250 g) were purchased from Samtako (Osan, Kyunggi-do, Korea). They were acclimatized to the circumstances for 5 days with water and food ad libitum. Rats were provided a cereal-based maintenance diet, altromin 1320 pellet formula (Altromin, Lage, Germany). Energy density of this diet is about 3227 kcal/kg consisting of 11% of fat, 24% of protein and 65% of carbohydrates. All rats were housed in light (light: 07:00–19:00, dark: 19:00–07:00), temperature (22 ± 2 °C) and humidity (55 ± 5%)-controlled room.

All animal procedures were approved by the Animal Care and Use Committee of Kyungpook National University (2015-0098) and conducted in accordance with the National Institutes of Health guidance for the care and the use of laboratory animals.

2.3. LC-MS/MS Analysis of Memantine

Memantine in each sample was determined by an Agilent 6430 Triple Quadrupole LC-MS/MS system (Agilent, Wilmington, DE, USA). The isocratic mobile phase consisting a mixture of water and methanol (15:85, v/v) containing 0.1% formic acid was used at a flow rate of 0.20 mL/min to elute memantine and propranolol peak from the rat plasma matrix. The separation was performed on a Polar RP column (150 × 4.6 mm, 5 μm particle size; Pheonomenex, Torrance, CA, USA).

Mass transition was monitored using multiple reaction monitoring (MRM) mode at m/z 180.1 → 163.1 for memantine and m/z 260.0 → 116.0 for propranolol (internal standard, IS) in positive ion mode with a collision energy of 10–15 eV. The analytical data were quantified using mass Hunter (version B.06.00, Agilent, Wilmington, DE, USA).

2.4. Method Validation

2.4.1. Selectivity

The representative MRM chromatograms of the standard lower limit of quantification (LLoQ) concentrations of memantine or propranolol (IS) and plasma samples obtained from a rat 10 h after the oral administration of memantine (5 mg/kg) were compared with those of blank plasma [19].

2.4.2. Linearity of Standard Curves

The calibration curve (0.2, 0.5, 2, 10, 50, 200, 1000 ng/mL) was prepared using an internal standard method. Aliquots of standard curve samples (50 μL) were added to 250 μL of methanol containing 20 ng/mL of propranolol (IS). After vortex-mixing and centrifugation for 10 min at 13,200 rpm, an aliquot (2 μL) of the supernatant was injected into the LC-MS/MS system. Linearity of the calibration standard was calculated from the peak response ratio of memantine to IS with the weight adjusted method ($1/x^2$).

2.4.3. Precisions and Accuracy

The precision and accuracy of inter- and intra-day assays were assessed from five measurements of the quality control (QC) samples (0.6, 20, 500 ng/mL) of memantine. Precision was evaluated from the relative standard deviation (RSD) of five measurements. The accuracy of inter-day and intra-day assays was calculated by dividing the measured QC concentration by the spiked QC concentration. Analytical sample preparations were identical during the validation process.

2.4.4. Matrix Effect and Recovery

Matrix effects were monitored by dividing the peak areas of QC samples in water by those in blank plasma [20]. Recovery was calculated by comparing the peak response of QC in the post-extraction spiked samples with those of the pre-extraction spiked samples [20].

2.4.5. Stability

The stability of memantine and IS in the rat plasma was tested from the low and high QC samples exposed to different conditions [19]. Short-term stability was calculated by comparing QC samples that were stored for 12 h at 25 °C with the untreated QC samples. The freeze-thaw stability was analyzed by comparing QC samples that underwent three freeze–thaw cycles (−80 °C to 25 °C as one cycle) with the untreated QC samples. Post-preparative stability was evaluated by analyzing the extracted QC samples maintained in the autosampler at 6 °C for 24 h compared with the untreated QC samples [19].

2.5. Pharmacokinetic (PK) Interaction Study

Before oral administration or rat jejunum resection, the rats were fasted for 12 h but water ad libitum. On the day of study, the femoral arteries and femoral veins of rats were cannulated with PE50 tubing (Jungdo, Seoul, Korea) under anesthesia with isoflurane (30 mmol/kg).

Cimetidine solution (10 mg/kg/mL in water, four rats) or vehicle solution (1 mL/kg of water, four rats) was injected intravenously to rats at 10 Am and, 5 min later, memantine solution (3 mg/kg/mL in water) was injected intravenously to the same rat. Blood samples (250 μL) were collected from the femoral artery at 0, 0, 0.25, 0.5, 0.75, 1, 1.5, 2, 3, 6, 9, 24 h after intravenous bolus injection of memantine and/or cimetidine. Blood samples were centrifuged for 10 min at 13,200 rpm and aliquots of plasma samples (50 μL) were stored at −80 °C until the analysis. Urine samples were collected for 24 h and pooled urine samples were weighed. 50 μL aliquot of urine samples was stored at −80 °C until the analysis.

Similarly, cimetidine solution (50 mg/kg, dissolved in 2 mL water, four rats) or vehicle solution (2 mL/kg of water, four rats) was administered orally to rats at 10 Am and 30 min later, memantine solution (5 mg/kg, dissolved in 2 mL water) was administered orally to the same rat. Blood samples (250 μL) were collected from the femoral artery at 0, 0.083, 0.25, 0.5, 1, 2, 3, 6, 9, 24 h after oral administration of memantine and/or cimetidine. Blood samples were centrifuged for 10 min at 13,200 rpm and aliquots of plasma samples (50 μL) were stored at −80 °C until the analysis.

Memantine concentrations in plasma and urine samples were analyzed using a LC-MS/MS system.

2.6. Intestinal Permeability Test

Apparent permeability (P_{app}) of memantine in the presence or absence of cimetidine was determined with slight modification of a method of Kwon et al. [21]. Briefly, the rat jejunum segments mounted on the inserts of the Ussing chambers were acclimatized with Hank's balanced salt solution (HBSS) for 15 min. Carbogen gas (5% CO_2/ 95% O_2) was bubbled into the Ussing chambers at a rate of 150 drops/min during the experiment for the jejunum segment viability. The experiments started with changing the HBSS with preheated HBSS containing memantine (0.5 mg/mL) with or without cimetidine (5 mg/mL) to the apical (A) side of jejunum. Aliquots (400 μL) of HBSS in the basal side (B) were withdrawn at 0, 30, 60, 90 and 120 min and compensated with an equal volume of fresh, preheated HBSS. Aliquots of 50 μL of samples were analyzed using a LC-MS/MS system applied to the same sample preparation method.

For system feasibility, P_{app} of caffeine, propranolol, ofloxacin and atenolol were monitored as marker compounds for high, moderate and low permeable drugs. P_{app} value of caffeine and propranolol, positive controls of high permeability, was 36.8×10^{-6} and 23.7×10^{-6} cm/s, respectively, which is consistent with the findings of other studies [22]. P_{app} value of ofloxacin and atenolol, a positive control of moderate and poor permeability, respectively, was 4.5×10^{-6} and 0.04×10^{-6} cm/s, respectively, which corroborates with the findings of other studies [23].

2.7. Microsomal Stability

The metabolic stability of memantine (1 μM) in the presence or absence or cimetidine (0, 2 and 20 μM) in the rat liver microsomes was measured as previously described [24]. Briefly, memantine solution (1 μM) in 100 mM potassium phosphate buffer (pH 7.4) containing 0.5 mg of liver microsomes (from Sprague-Dawley rats; Corning, Tewksbury, MA, USA) and an NADPH-generating system incubated at 37 °C for 0, 15, 30, 45 and 60 min in a shaking water bath. The reaction was quenched by adding ice-cold methanol containing 20 ng/mL of propranolol (250 μL). After undergoing the sample preparation procedure, memantine concentration was measured.

We also measured the metabolic stability of 1 μM metformin and 1 μM propranolol by the same procedure to ensure system feasibility [24]. The percent of remaining metformin and propranolol after 60 min incubation in the rat liver microsomes was 63.4% and 12.2%, respectively.

2.8. Data Analysis and Statistics

PK parameters were calculated using the WinNonlin 2.0 (Pharsight Co., Certara, NJ, USA) and the data are expressed as the means ± standard deviation (SD).

A value of $p < 0.05$ was determined to be statistically significant, using a Mann Whitney test between the two means for unpaired data.

3. Results

3.1. Validation of Analytical Method

3.1.1. Selectivity

Representative MS/MS chromatograms memantine and IS (Figure 1) showed that the memantine and IS peaks were well-separated with no interfering peaks at the respective retention times. The selectivity of the analytes was confirmed in six different rat blank plasma and rat plasma samples obtained after memantine administration. The retention times of memantine and IS were 3.62 and 3.14 min, respectively and the total run time was 4.0 min.

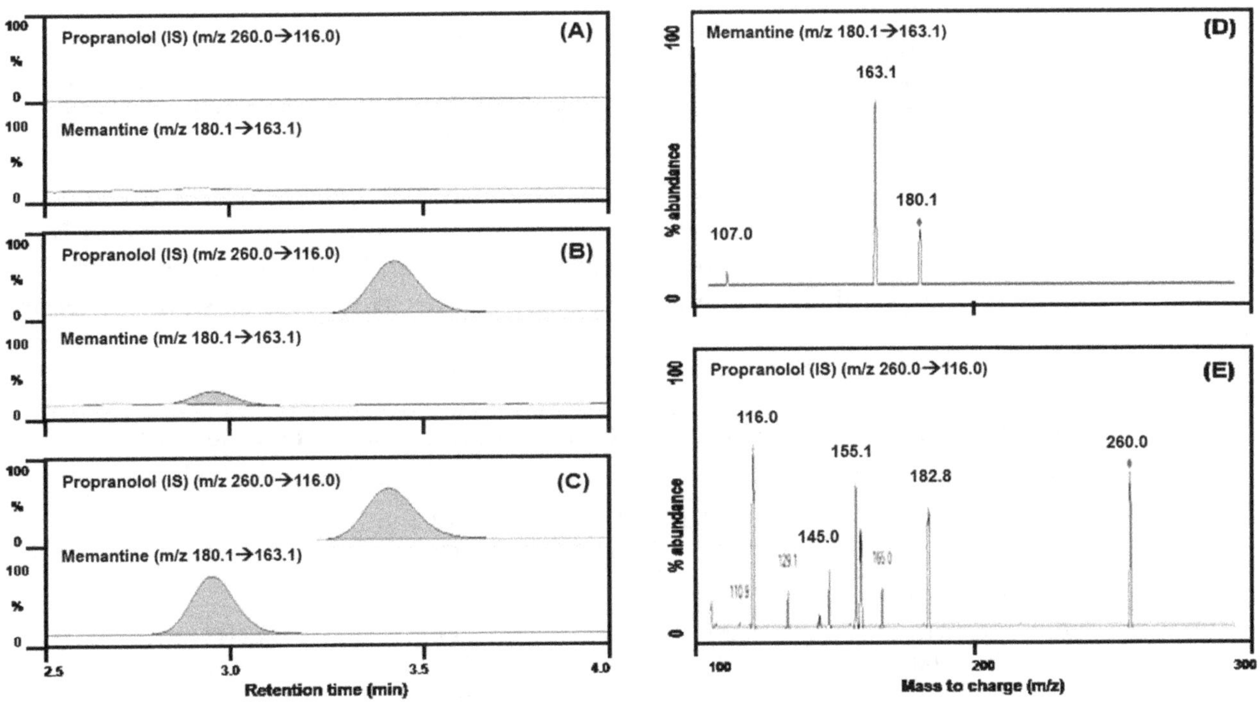

Figure 1. Representative MS/MS chromatograms of memantine and IS in rat (**A**) double blank plasma, (**B**) blank plasma spiked with memantine at lower limit of quantification (LLoQ; 0.2 ng/mL) and propranolol and (**C**) plasma samples following single oral administration of memantine is shown in the left panel. Product ion spectra of memantine (**D**) and propranolol (**E**) are shown in the right panel.

3.1.2. Precision and Accuracy

The precision and accuracy of intra-day and inter-day assays are shown in Table 1. For inter-day validation, the precision was in the range of 8.10 to 11.4%. The accuracy ranged from 101.2 to 108.6%. In intra-day validation, the precision and accuracy ranged from 1.68 to 14.1% and 109.9 to 113.8%, respectively (Table 1).

Table 1. Intra-day and inter-day precision and accuracy of memantine.

Memantine	Spiked (ng/mL)	Inter-day			Intra-day		
		Measured (ng/mL)	Accuracy (%)	Precision (%)	Measured (ng/mL)	Accuracy (%)	Precision (%)
Low QC	0.6	0.62 ± 0.05	101.2	8.10	0.68 ± 0.10	113.8	14.1
Medium QC	20	20.6 ± 2.13	108.6	10.3	21.98 ± 0.37	109.9	1.68
High QC	500	497.6 ± 56.9	104.2	11.4	555.6 ± 23.5	111.2	4.23

Data represent the means ± SD of five measurements.

3.1.3. Matrix Effect and Recovery

The mean recoveries of memantine in the low, medium and high QC samples ranged from 87.5 to 91.2% with an RSD of less than 3.70%. The matrix effects ranged from 91.1 to 108.2% with an RSD of less than 12.6%. These results indicate that no significant interference occurred during the ionization and methanol precipitation process. The matrix effect of the IS at 20 ng/mL was 102.9% and the recovery of IS was 87.7% (Table 2).

Table 2. Matrix effect and recovery of memantine.

Compounds		Spiked (ng/mL)	Recovery (%)	Matrix Effect (%)
Propranolol	IS	20	87.7 ± 1.96 (2.2)	102.9 ± 1.20 (1.2)
Memantine	Low QC	0.6	90.7 ± 3.11 (3.4)	108.2 ± 13.7 (12.6)
	Medium QC	20	91.2 ± 3.38 (3.7)	92.7 ± 5.43 (5.9)
	High QC	500	87.5 ± 3.18 (3.6)	91.1 ± 7.55 (8.3)

Data represent the means ± SD of five measurements.

3.1.4. Stability

The stabilities of memantine and propranolol are summarized in Table 3. Low and high QC samples were stable after being exposed to three freeze-thaw cycles and stable for at least 12 h at 25 °C. Post-preparative samples were stable after storage at 24 h in the autosampler after sample preparation.

Table 3. Stability of memantine.

Spiked (ng/mL)	Measured (ng/mL)	Accuracy (%)	Precision (%)
Bench-top stability for 12 h in plasma			
Low QC (0.6)	0.67 ± 0.10	112.2	14.9
High QC (500)	532.7 ± 27.6	106.6	5.2
Three freeze-thaw cycles			
Low QC (0.6)	0.51 ± 0.05	85.1	10.7
High QC (500)	539.3 ± 16.4	107.9	3.1
Post treatment stability for 24 h			
Low QC (0.6)	0.59 ± 0.04	98.4	7.6
High QC (500)	540.1 ± 13.7	108	2.5

Data represent the means ± SD of five measurements.

3.2. PK Interaction of Memantine and Cimetidine in Rats

The PK profiles of memantine following intravenous injection (3 mg/kg) in the presence or absence of cimetidine (10 mg/kg) are shown in Figure 2A and PK profiles of memantine following oral administration (5 mg/kg) in the presence or absence of cimetidine (50 mg/kg) are shown in Figure 2B. Their related PK parameters are presented in Table 4. The pharmacokinetic parameters of memantine were comparable to those reported previously [3,7,25].

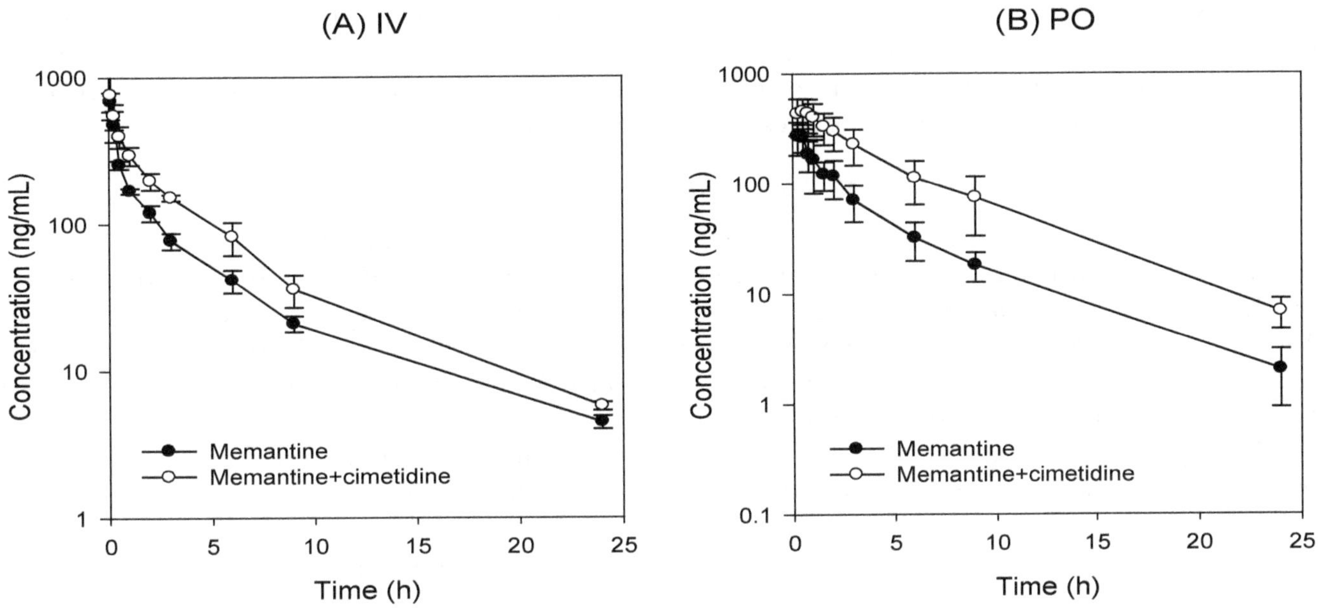

Figure 2. Plasma concentration-time profile of memantine after single intravenous (IV; **A**) and oral (PO; **B**) administration of memantine (3 and 5 mg/kg, respectively) in the presence (○) or absence (●) of cimetidine (10 and 50 mg/kg, respectively) in rats. Data points are the means ± SD of four rats.

Table 4. PK parameters of memantine after single intravenous (IV) and oral (PO) administration of memantine in the presence or absence of cimetidine in rats.

PK Parameters		IV		PO	
		Memantine (3 mg/kg)	Memantine (3 mg/kg) + Cimetidine (10 mg/kg)	Memantine (5 mg/kg)	Memantine (5 mg/kg) + Cimetidine (50 mg/kg)
C_{max}	μg/mL	686.84 ± 100.75	759.04 ± 240.18	293.45 ± 90.90	486.78 ± 140.75 *
T_{max}	h			0.35 ± 0.14	0.50 ± 0.18
AUC_{24h}	μg·h/mL	1089.58 ± 116.55	1724.52 ± 241.36 *	811.38 ± 238.01	2392.69 ± 950.06 *
AUC_{∞}	μg·h/mL	1121.98 ± 116.74	1765.56 ± 237.78 *	825.60 ± 241.92	2439.28 ± 951.72 *
$t_{1/2}$	h	5.06 ± 0.38	4.98 ± 0.59	4.51 ± 0.92	4.70 ± 0.75
$V_{d,ss}$	L/kg	19.70 ± 3.32	12.50 ± 3.16		
CL	mL/min/kg	44.87 ± 4.40	28.67 ± 3.92 *		
CL/F	mL/min/kg			107.63 ± 28.83	39.06 ± 16.00 *
CL_{renal}	mL/min/kg	12.88 ± 3.89	10.64 ± 5.73		

Data were expressed as mean ± SD from four rats per group. *: $p < 0.05$ compared with the memantine group. C_{max}: maximum plasma concentration; T_{max}: time to reach C_{max}. AUC_{24h} or AUC_{∞}: Area under plasma concentration-time curve from zero to 24 h or infinity. $t_{1/2}$: elimination half-life; $V_{d,ss}$: volume of distribution at steady-state CL or CL/F: systemic clearance; CL_{renal}: renal clearance.

There was no significant difference in the C_{max}, $t_{1/2}$ and $V_{d,ss}$ values of memantine between two groups (memantine alone vs. memantine + cimetidine). However, the AUC value of memantine + cimetidine was increased by 1.6-fold compared to that of memantine alone and, consequently, the CL of memantine decreased by co-injection with cimetidine.

Interestingly, the drug–drug interaction between memantine and cimetidine administered orally was greater than that of intravenous injection. For example, the AUC value of memantine + cimetidine was increased by 3.0-fold compared to that of memantine alone without changing the T_{max} and $t_{1/2}$ values. These results suggest that a major drug–drug interaction between memantine and cimetidine occurred during the absorption process. Moreover, systemic clearance (CL and CL/F) of memantine was decreased by co-administration of memantine and cimetidine by both the oral and intravenous routes, suggesting that memantine elimination is affected by the presence of cimetidine.

To investigate the underlying mechanism of the drug interaction in the absorption process, we investigated the effect of cimetidine on the intestinal permeability of memantine.

For the elimination process, we investigated the changes in metabolic stability in the rat liver microsomes because renal elimination (CL_{renal}) was not significantly altered by the presence of cimetidine (Table 4) and, therefore, non-renal clearance of memantine (calculated by subtracting CL_{renal} from CL) was decreased by the presence of cimetidine.

3.3. Effect of Cimetidine on the Intestinal Permeability of Memantine

To mimic the intestinal situation that occurred when memantine and cimetidine were concomitantly administered to rats via oral route, the concentrations of memantine and cimetidine were determined based on the oral dose of these drugs used in pharmacokinetic analysis and fluid volume of the stomach. For example, memantine and cimetidine were administered at doses of 5 and 50 mg/kg (dissolved in 2 mL/kg water), respectively, to rats with stomach fluid volumes of 3.4–4.6 mL [26], which resulted in 8–10-fold dilution.

The apparent permeability of memantine (0.5 mg/mL) in the presence of cimetidine (5 mg/mL) was significantly increased compared to that of memantine alone (Figure 3).

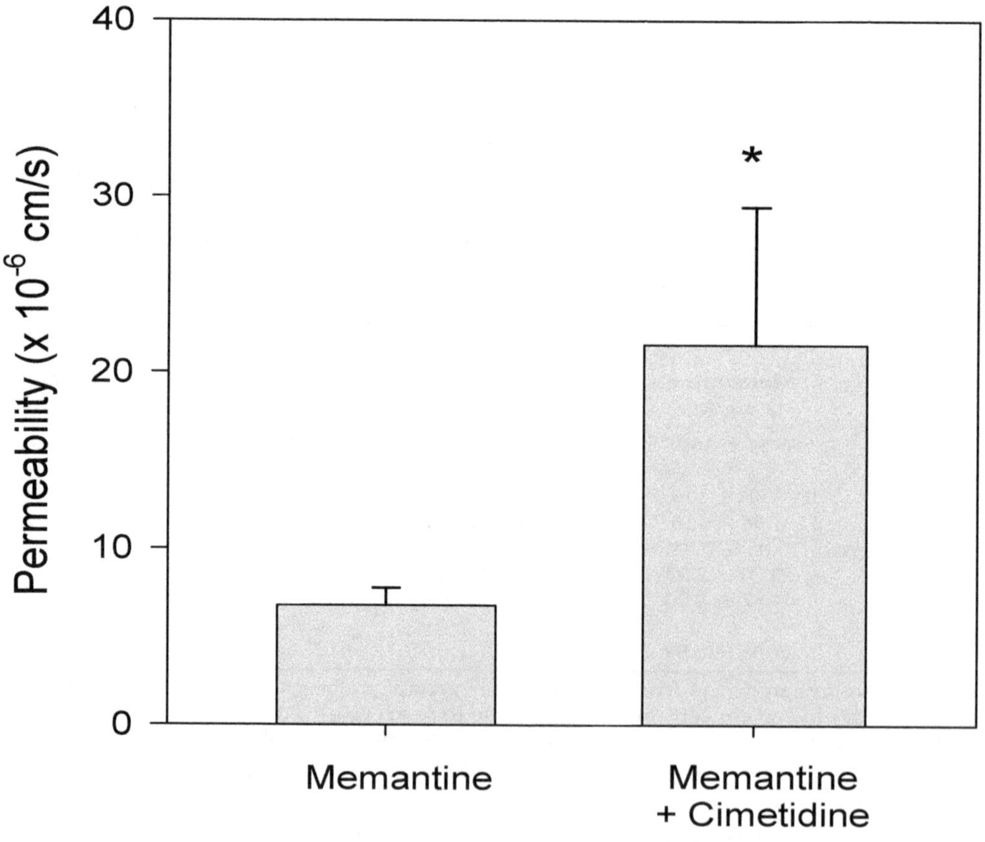

Figure 3. The apparent permeability (P_{app}) of memantine (0.5 mg/mL) in the absence or presence of cimetidine (5 mg/mL) was measured in rat jejunum using the Ussing system. Bar represents the mean ± SD of three independent experiments. * $p < 0.05$ compared with the memantine group.

3.4. Effect of Cimetidine on the Metabolic Stability of Memantine

Approximately 45% of memantine was degraded after 1 h incubation of memantine in the rat liver microsomes (Figure 4), which is consistent with the results of a previous study showing that memantine exhibits rat-specific Cyp-dependent moderate to high intrinsic clearance [3]. Adding 2 and 20 μM cimetidine and 1 μM memantine to the rat liver microsomes showed that the metabolic rate of memantine decreased with increasing concentrations of cimetidine (Figure 4).

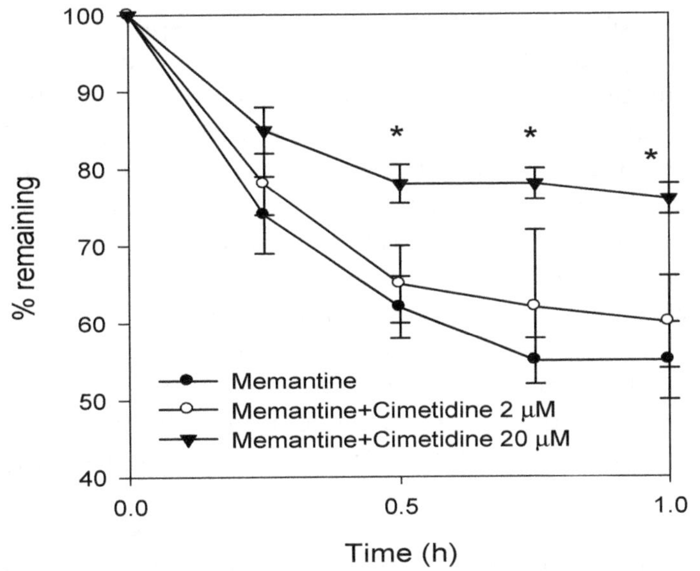

Figure 4. The effect of cimetidine on the metabolic stability of memantine with rat liver microsomes. Memantine (1 μM) in the absence or presence of cimetidine (0, 2 and 20 μM) was incubated with 0.5 mg rat liver microsomes for 60 min at 37 °C. Data represents the mean ± SD of three independent experiments. * $p < 0.05$ compared with the memantine group.

4. Discussion

The newly developed analytical method for memantine using an LC-MS/MS system showed comparable sensitivity (i.e., LLoQ 0.2 ng/mL) as previously published methods (i.e., LLoQ 0.1–1 ng/mL) despite the use of a small volume (50 μL) of plasma samples compared with previous methods [7,27–31]. Additionally, previously established methods used solid-phase extraction or liquid-liquid extraction which requires costly reagents and large volume of plasma samples (100–1000 μL) [27–31]. Noetzli et al. applied the protein-precipitation method and sample preparations were processed by evaporation and reconstitution [29]. However, we used a protein-precipitation method involving methanol containing an internal standard rather than previously described solid-phase extraction or liquid–liquid extraction methods and then directly injected an aliquot of the supernatant after the centrifugation of protein-precipitated plasma samples. Finally, we developed and fully validated a rapid, simple and sensitive analytical method for memantine in biological samples with total run time of 4.0 min. This method can easily be applied in the bioanalysis and pharmacokinetic study of memantine in small experimental animals. Moreover, following appropriate validation, the present method can be extended to determine the routine drug monitoring of memantine in human plasma and thus applied to clinical pharmacokinetic studies.

Memantine showed non-linear pharmacokinetic properties in a single oral dose range of 1–10 mg/kg. Beconi et al. reported that the active process mediated by rat-specific Cyp and active tubular secretion modulated the non-linear pharmacokinetics of memantine [3]. Cimetidine (as a perpetrator) increased the plasma concentration of the victim drug by inhibiting Cyp-mediated metabolism [14] and organic cation-mediated renal tubular secretion [13,14].

Based on these pharmacokinetic properties, the pharmacokinetics drug-drug interaction between memantine and cimetidine could be summarized as follows: (1) the AUC increase of memantine by co-administration with cimetidine was much greater following oral administration of memantine and cimetidine than that following intravenous injection. This suggests that the drug interaction was dominantly induced during the gut absorption process, which was supported by the increased permeability of memantine following addition of cimetidine (Figure 3). Although the intestinal absorption process of memantine has not been fully postulated, memantine absorption increased from 36.3% to 84.9% when oral dose increased from 1 mg/kg to 10 mg/kg, suggesting the presence of active process [3]. The involvement of pH-dependent transport mechanism via Octn1 has been reported in the distribution of memantine [32,33] and cimetidine could efficiently increase the influx of memantine through the inhibition of Octn1 by the inhibition of inwardly directed proton gradient and increase of gut pH [32,33]. (2) The AUC increase of memantine by co-administration of memantine and cimetidine intravenously may be attributed to the decreased clearance of memantine because of the decreased metabolic activity of memantine in the presence of cimetidine (Figure 4). This was also consistent with the previous reports that the intrinsic clearance calculated as moderate to high for rats, in which rat Cyp2c11 is responsible for the memantine metabolism [3] and cimetidine could inhibit hepatic Cyp2C6 and Cyp2C11 enzymes [34]. (3) Inhibition of organic cation-mediated renal tubular secretion of memantine by co-administration with cimetidine was not observed in this study, possibly because the renal clearance of memantine was not significantly decreased by the presence of cimetidine (Table 4). In conclusion, taken together, the pharmacokinetic interaction between memantine and cimetidine in rats was occurred not only at hepatic metabolism but also at intestinal membrane.

The clinical drug-drug between memantine and cimetidine was not investigated yet. However, approximately 48% of memantine was excreted as its unchanged form via renal route in human, in which multidrug and toxin extrusion protein (MATE) 1 was known to be involved [6,35]. The remaining 50% of memantine is metabolized into N-glucuronide conjugate, 6-hydroxy memantine and 1-nitroso deaminated memantine [6]. Since cimetidine acts as inhibitors of MATE1 and CYP enzymes [14,34], possibility of clinical drug-drug interaction between memantine and cimetidine should be carefully considered at high dose administration of cimetidine with memantine.

Author Contributions: Conceptualization, Y.A.C. and M.-K.C.; Methodology, Y.A.C. and I.-S.S.; Investigation, Y.A.C., I.-S.S. and M.-K.C.; Writing-Original Draft Preparation, Y.A.C. and I.-S.S.; Supervision, M.-K.C.; Writing-Review & Editing, M.-K.C.

References

1. Jahn, H. Memory loss in Alzheimer's disease. *Dialogues Clin. Neurosci.* **2013**, *15*, 445–454. [PubMed]
2. Greig, N.H.; Lahiri, D.K. Advances in understanding alzheimer's disease, and the contributions of current alzheimer research: Ten years on and beyond. *Curr. Alzheimer Res.* **2014**, *11*, 107–109. [CrossRef] [PubMed]
3. Beconi, M.G.; Howland, D.; Park, L.; Lyons, K.; Giuliano, J.; Dominguez, C.; Munoz-Sanjuan, I.; Pacifici, R. Pharmacokinetics of memantine in rats and mice. *PLoS Curr.* **2011**, *3*. [CrossRef] [PubMed]
4. Molinuevo, J.L.; Llado, A.; Rami, L. Memantine: Targeting glutamate excitotoxicity in alzheimer's disease and other dementias. *Am. J. Alzheimer's Dis. Other Dement.* **2005**, *20*, 77–85. [CrossRef] [PubMed]
5. McShane, R.; Areosa Sastre, A.; Minakaran, N. Memantine for dementia. *Cochrane Database Syst. Rev.* **2006**. [CrossRef] [PubMed]
6. Sani, G.; Serra, G.; Kotzalidis, G.D.; Romano, S.; Tamorri, S.M.; Manfredi, G.; Caloro, M.; Telesforo, C.L.; Caltagirone, S.S.; Panaccione, I.; et al. The role of memantine in the treatment of psychiatric disorders other than the dementias: A review of current preclinical and clinical evidence. *CNS Drugs* **2012**, *26*, 663–690. [CrossRef] [PubMed]
7. Bhateria, M.; Ramakrishna, R.; Pakala, D.B.; Bhatta, R.S. Development of an lc-ms/ms method for simultaneous determination of memantine and donepezil in rat plasma and its application to pharmacokinetic study. *J. Chromatogr. B Anal. Technol. Biomed. Life Sci.* **2015**, *1001*, 131–139. [CrossRef] [PubMed]
8. Periclou, A.P.; Ventura, D.; Sherman, T.; Rao, N.; Abramowitz, W.T. Lack of pharmacokinetic or pharmacodynamic interaction between memantine and donepezil. *Ann. Pharmacother.* **2004**, *38*, 1389–1394. [CrossRef] [PubMed]
9. Figiel, G.S.; Koumaras, B.; Meng, X.; Strigas, J.; Gunay, I. Long-term safety and tolerability of rivastigmine in patients with alzheimer's disease switched from donepezil: An open-label extension study. *Prim. Care Companion J. Clin. Psychiatry* **2008**, *10*, 363–367. [CrossRef] [PubMed]
10. Yao, C.; Raoufinia, A.; Gold, M.; Nye, J.S.; Ramael, S.; Padmanabhan, M.; Walschap, Y.; Verhaeghe, T.; Zhao, Q. Steady-state pharmacokinetics of galantamine are not affected by addition of memantine in healthy subjects. *J. Clin. Pharmacol.* **2005**, *45*, 519–528. [CrossRef] [PubMed]

11. Lostia, A.M.; Mazzarini, L.; Pacchiarotti, I.; Lionetto, L.; De Rossi, P.; Sanna, L.; Sani, G.; Kotzalidis, G.D.; Girardi, P.; Simmaco, M.; et al. Serum levels of risperidone and its metabolite, 9-hydroxyrisperidone: Correlation between drug concentration and clinical response. *Ther. Drug Monit.* **2009**, *31*, 475–481. [CrossRef] [PubMed]
12. Zimmer, D. New us fda draft guidance on bioanalytical method validation versus current fda and ema guidelines: Chromatographic methods and isr. *Bioanalysis* **2014**, *6*, 13–19. [CrossRef] [PubMed]
13. Ito, S.; Kusuhara, H.; Yokochi, M.; Toyoshima, J.; Inoue, K.; Yuasa, H.; Sugiyama, Y. Competitive inhibition of the luminal efflux by multidrug and toxin extrusions, but not basolateral uptake by organic cation transporter 2, is the likely mechanism underlying the pharmacokinetic drug-drug interactions caused by cimetidine in the kidney. *J. Pharmacol. Exp. Ther.* **2012**, *340*, 393–403. [CrossRef] [PubMed]
14. Matsushima, S.; Maeda, K.; Inoue, K.; Ohta, K.Y.; Yuasa, H.; Kondo, T.; Nakayama, H.; Horita, S.; Kusuhara, H.; Sugiyama, Y. The inhibition of human multidrug and toxin extrusion 1 is involved in the drug-drug interaction caused by cimetidine. *Drug Metab. Dispos. Boil. Fate Chem.* **2009**, *37*, 555–559. [CrossRef] [PubMed]
15. Hoffman, A.; Perlstein, I.; Habib, G.; Pinto, E.; Gilhar, D. The effect of cimetidine on the pharmacodynamics of theophylline-induced seizures and ethanol hypnotic activity. *Pharmacol. Toxicol.* **1999**, *85*, 130–132. [CrossRef] [PubMed]
16. Rafi, J.A.; Frazier, L.M.; Driscoll-Bannister, S.M.; O'Hara, K.A.; Garnett, W.R.; Pugh, C.B. Effect of over-the-counter cimetidine on phenytoin concentrations in patients with seizures. *Ann. Pharmacother.* **1999**, *33*, 769–774. [CrossRef] [PubMed]
17. Kurata, T.; Muraki, Y.; Mizutani, H.; Iwamoto, T.; Okuda, M. Elevated systemic elimination of cimetidine in rats with acute biliary obstruction: The role of renal organic cation transporter OCT2. *Drug Metab. Pharmacokinet.* **2010**, *25*, 328–334. [CrossRef] [PubMed]
18. Piyapolrungroj, N.; Zhou, Y.S.; Li, C.; Liu, G.; Zimmermann, E.; Fleisher, D. Cimetidine absorption and elimination in rat small intestine. *Drug Metab. Dispos. Boil. Fate Chem.* **2000**, *28*, 65–72.
19. Guo, P.; Dong, L.; Yan, W.; Wei, J.; Wang, C.; Zhang, Z. Simultaneous determination of linarin, naringenin and formononetin in rat plasma by lc-ms/ms and its application to a pharmacokinetic study after oral administration of bushen guchi pill. *Biomed. Chromatogr.* **2015**, *29*, 246–253. [CrossRef] [PubMed]
20. Huang, P.; Zhang, L.; Chai, C.; Qian, X.C.; Li, W.; Li, J.S.; Di, L.Q.; Cai, B.C. Effects of food and gender on the pharmacokinetics of ginkgolides a, b, c and bilobalide in rats after oral dosing with ginkgo terpene lactones extract. *J. Pharm. Biomed. Anal.* **2014**, *100*, 138–144. [CrossRef] [PubMed]
21. Kwon, M.; Ji, H.K.; Goo, S.H.; Nam, S.J.; Kang, Y.J.; Lee, E.; Liu, K.H.; Choi, M.K.; Song, I.S. Involvement of intestinal efflux and metabolic instability in the pharmacokinetics of platycodin d in rats. *Drug Metab. Pharmacokinet.* **2017**, *32*, 248–254. [CrossRef] [PubMed]
22. Levin, V.A. Relationship of octanol/water partition coefficient and molecular weight to rat brain capillary permeability. *J. Med. Chem.* **1980**, *23*, 682–684. [CrossRef] [PubMed]
23. Stewart, B.H.; Chan, O.H.; Lu, R.H.; Reyner, E.L.; Schmid, H.L.; Hamilton, H.W.; Steinbaugh, B.A.; Taylor, M.D. Comparison of intestinal permeabilities determined in multiple in vitro and in situ models: Relationship to absorption in humans. *Pharm. Res.* **1995**, *12*, 693–699. [CrossRef] [PubMed]
24. Choi, M.K.; Lee, J.; Nam, S.J.; Kang, Y.J.; Han, Y.; Choi, K.; Choi, Y.A.; Kwon, M.; Lee, D.; Song, I.S. Pharmacokinetics of jaspine b and enhancement of intestinal absorption of jaspine b in the presence of bile acid in rats. *Mar. Drugs* **2017**, *15*, 279. [CrossRef] [PubMed]
25. Lee, S.H.; Kim, S.H.; Noh, Y.H.; Choi, B.M.; Noh, G.J.; Park, W.D.; Kim, E.J.; Cho, I.H.; Bae, C.S. Pharmacokinetics of memantine after a single and multiple dose of oral and patch administration in rats. *Basic Clin. Pharmacol. Toxicol.* **2016**, *118*, 122–127. [CrossRef] [PubMed]
26. McConnell, E.L.; Basit, A.W.; Murdan, S. Measurements of rat and mouse gastrointestinal ph, fluid and lymphoid tissue, and implications for in-vivo experiments. *J. Pharm. Pharmacol.* **2008**, *60*, 63–70. [CrossRef] [PubMed]
27. Qiu, H.W.; Xia, L.; Gong, L.M.; Ruan, L.M.; Zhao, Y.G. Rapid determination of memantine in human plasma by using nanoring carboxyl-functionalized paramagnetic molecularly imprinted polymer d-mu-spe and uflc-ms/ms. *Drug Test. Anal.* **2015**, *7*, 535–543. [CrossRef] [PubMed]

28. Suresh, P.S.; Mullangi, R.; Sukumaran, S.K. Highly sensitive lc-ms/ms method for determination of galantamine in rat plasma: Application to pharmacokinetic studies in rats. *Biomed. Chromatogr.* **2014**, *28*, 1633–1640. [CrossRef] [PubMed]
29. Noetzli, M.; Ansermot, N.; Dobrinas, M.; Eap, C.B. Simultaneous determination of antidementia drugs in human plasma: Procedure transfer from hplc-ms to uplc-ms/ms. *J. Pharm. Biomed. Anal.* **2012**, *64–65*, 16–25. [CrossRef] [PubMed]
30. Konda, R.K.; Challa, B.R.; Chandu, B.R.; Chandrasekhar, K.B. Bioanalytical method development and validation of memantine in human plasma by high performance liquid chromatography with tandem mass spectrometry: Application to bioequivalence study. *J. Anal. Methods Chem.* **2012**, *2012*. [CrossRef] [PubMed]
31. Almeida, A.A.; Campos, D.R.; Bernasconi, G.; Calafatti, S.; Barros, F.A.; Eberlin, M.N.; Meurer, E.C.; Paris, E.G.; Pedrazzoli, J. Determination of memantine in human plasma by liquid chromatography-electrospray tandem mass spectrometry: Application to a bioequivalence study. *J. Chromatogr. B Anal. Technol. Biomed. Life Sci.* **2007**, *848*, 311–316. [CrossRef] [PubMed]
32. Mehta, D.C.; Short, J.L.; Nicolazzo, J.A. Memantine transport across the mouse blood-brain barrier is mediated by a cationic influx h+ antiporter. *Mol. Pharm.* **2013**, *10*, 4491–4498. [CrossRef] [PubMed]
33. Yabuuchi, H.; Tamai, I.; Nezu, J.; Sakamoto, K.; Oku, A.; Shimane, M.; Sai, Y.; Tsuji, A. Novel membrane transporter octn1 mediates multispecific, bidirectional, and ph-dependent transport of organic cations. *J. Pharmacol. Exp. Ther.* **1999**, *289*, 768–773. [PubMed]
34. Levine, M.; Law, E.Y.; Bandiera, S.M.; Chang, T.K.; Bellward, G.D. In vivo cimetidine inhibits hepatic CYP2C6 and CYP2C11 but not cyp1a1 in adult male rats. *J. Pharmacol. Exp. Ther.* **1998**, *284*, 493–499. [PubMed]
35. Muller, F.; Weitz, D.; Derdau, V.; Sandvoss, M.; Mertsch, K.; Konig, J.; Fromm, M.F. Contribution of mate1 to renal secretion of the nmda receptor antagonist memantine. *Mol. Pharm.* **2017**, *14*, 2991–2998. [CrossRef] [PubMed]

13

Revisiting the Latency of Uridine Diphosphate-Glucuronosyltransferases (UGTs)—How Does the Endoplasmic Reticulum Membrane Influence their Function?

Yuejian Liu and Michael W. H. Coughtrie *

Faculty of Pharmaceutical Sciences, The University of British Columbia, Vancouver, BC V6T 1Z3, Canada; yuejian.liu@alumni.ubc.ca

* Correspondence: michael.coughtrie@ubc.ca

Abstract: Uridine diphosphate-glucuronosyltransferases (UGTs) are phase 2 conjugation enzymes mainly located in the endoplasmic reticulum (ER) of the liver and many other tissues, and can be recovered in artificial ER membrane preparations (microsomes). They catalyze glucuronidation reactions in various aglycone substrates, contributing significantly to the body's chemical defense mechanism. There has been controversy over the last 50 years in the UGT field with respect to the explanation for the phenomenon of latency: full UGT activity revealed by chemical or physical disruption of the microsomal membrane. Because latency can lead to inaccurate measurements of UGT activity in vitro, and subsequent underprediction of drug clearance in vivo, it is important to understand the mechanisms behind this phenomenon. Three major hypotheses have been advanced to explain UGT latency: compartmentation, conformation, and adenine nucleotide inhibition. In this review, we discuss the evidence behind each hypothesis in depth, and suggest some additional studies that may reveal more information on this intriguing phenomenon.

Keywords: UDP-glucuronosyltransferase; latency; microsomes; glucuronidation; regulation

1. Introduction

Uridine diphosphate-glucuronosyltransferases (UGTs) comprise a superfamily of phase 2 conjugation enzymes that catalyze the glucuronidation of numerous substrates at functional groups such as –OH, –COOH, $–NH_2$, –SH, and C–C [1]. They are arguably the most important conjugation enzymes facilitating the excretion of various endobiotics such as bilirubin, steroid and thyroid hormones, bile acids, and retinoids, as well as xenobiotics including environmental chemicals, pollutants, and drugs [2]. These substrates are mostly hydrophobic and are conjugated by the UGTs with the glucuronic acid moiety derived from the co-substrate, uridine diphosphate-glucuronic acid (UDPGA). The resulting glucuronide conjugates that are generally more polar and water-soluble are substrates for numerous membrane transporters and thus they can eventually be excreted out of the body in bile and urine (Figure 1).

UGTs are type-I transmembrane glycoproteins mainly located within the smooth endoplasmic reticulum (ER), although some isoforms can be found in the nuclear envelope [3,4]. UGTs demonstrate protein–protein interactions within the superfamily (homo- and hetero-dimers and possibly higher order structures) or with other enzymes such as the cytochromes P450 [5–12], as demonstrated by studies using co-immunoprecipitation, fluorescence microscopy, and Förster resonance energy transfer (FRET), among many other approaches (as summarized in [6]). The interactions have been shown to alter kinetic properties of UGTs [7,9,10].

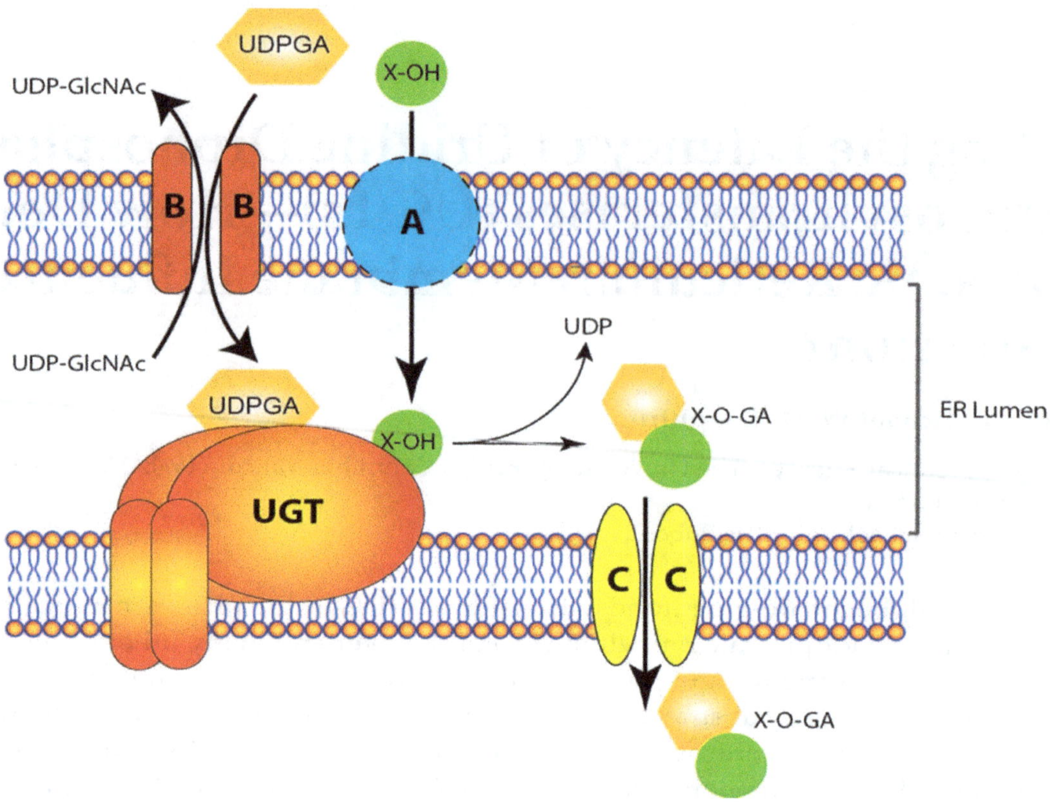

Figure 1. The glucuronidation system in the endoplasmic reticulum. Substrates (X-OH) enter the lumen by diffusion (A), and UDPGA is transported via the UDPGA/UDP-GlcNAc antiporter (UGTrel7, B). Following the conjugation reaction, the glucuronide products (X-O-GA) are removed from the lumen by glucuronide transporter(s) (C). UDPGA: Uridine diphosphate-glucuronic acid; UDP-GLcNAc: UDP-*N*-acetylglucosamine.

Detoxification is divided into two phases [13]. The basic principle is that oxidative metabolism by phase 1 enzymes (such as cytochromes P450, CYP) results in the addition or revealing of a functional group (e.g., –OH, –COOH or $–NH_2$) such that the compounds can be conjugated by phase 2 enzymes such as the UGTs. This necessitates the phase 1 metabolites crossing the ER membrane in order to access the UGT active site. Evidence suggests a functional interaction between the UGT and CYP proteins to facilitate the multistep detoxification process [5,12,14,15].

Besides detoxification, glucuronidation can activate substrates such as certain procarcinogens, as well as morphine that can be converted to morphine 3- and 6-glucuronides, where the latter is a more potent analgesic than the parent drug [16]. Glucuronidation also produces toxic metabolites such as steroid D-ring glucuronides that may be responsible for intrahepatic cholestasis of pregnancy [17]. The human UGT superfamily is divided into five subfamilies: UGT1A, 2A, 2B, 3A, and 8. They are mainly expressed in liver, but are also prevalent in extrahepatic tissues including gastrointestinal tract, kidney, lung, brain, and reproductive tissues [1,18]. The human UGT1A isoforms are generated from a single gene located at chromosome 2q37.1 through alternative splicing. Specifically, there are 13 first exons, including 4 pseudogenes, each of which is controlled by an individual promoter (1A1, 1A2p, 1A3, 1A4, 1A5, 1A6, 1A7, 1A9, 1A13p, 1A10, 1A8, 1A11p, and 1A12p). These 13 exon/promoter pairs are upstream of a second region that consists of 5 common exons under the regulation of a single promoter (exons 2, 3, 4, 5a, and 5b). The mRNA for each UGT1A isoform is generated by splicing one of the first exons with the group of common exons. This mechanism of alternative splicing is conserved in human, mouse, and rat UGTs [19].

2. UGTs and Latency

The majority of the UGT enzyme protein, including its catalytic site, is believed to reside inside the ER lumen (and partially associate with the ER membrane); thus there are physical and physiological barriers to substrates accessing the active site of the enzymes within the ER lumen, as well as to the egress of reaction products from the ER and, subsequently, from the cell. This leads to the phenomenon of latency of UGT activity in preparations of ER (i.e., microsomes). The phenomenon of latency derives from experimental observations that in isolated microsomal preparations, UGTs generally show increased activities after the membranes are physically or chemically disrupted [20–28]. Other enzymes present in the lumen of the ER, such as glucose-6-phosphatase, also display latency [29]. Although the latency of UGTs has been known for more than half a century, the exact mechanism(s) underlying it remain incompletely understood, and this has generated several hypotheses and much heated debate during this time. The phenomenon of latency is an important factor in the consistent underprediction of drug clearance in vivo based on in vitro measurement of UGT activity [30], since it is of particular importance to be able to accurately measure UGT activity in microsomal preparations. Examples of treatments that disrupt microsomal membranes and reveal UGT latency (to different extents) include grinding in sand, sonication, high hydrostatic pressure, detergents, phospholipase A or C, staphylococcal α-toxin, or the pore-forming antibiotic alamethicin [22,23,28,31–39]. It has been postulated that these agents, or physical stressors, act in different ways, for example by allowing unlimited access of substrate and co-substrate to the enzyme's catalytic site; by inducing an alteration in the conformation of the enzyme; by releasing UGT inhibitors from the microsomal lumen; or a combination of these mechanisms which of course are all dependent to some extent on the ER membrane.

Three major hypotheses have been developed over the years to explain latency: compartmentation, conformation, and adenine-nucleotide inhibition. The first two hypotheses mainly address whether the ER membrane limits UGT activity by acting as a barrier blocking access of UDPGA (and potentially aglycone substrate) to the luminal space and thus the UGT active site, or by regulating the conformation of the UGT protein through lipid–protein (or potentially protein–protein) interactions. The last hypothesis was the most recently proposed, based on the inhibitory effects of adenine-containing nucleotides on the UGTs. Under this hypothesis, the membranes might limit UGT activity by sequestering these natural inhibitors in the lumen.

The latency phenomenon makes accurate measurement of UGT activity in microsomal preparations challenging, however it is one of the most important factors to take into consideration in the design of UGT enzyme assays. Different methods of preparation of the microsomal fraction can have major impact on measurable latency, since the level of intactness of the membrane preparation clearly influences the enzyme activity. For example, it has been shown that preparation of microsomal fractions from freshly isolated liver is significantly preferable over frozen tissue, which tends to produce microsomal fractions with much lower levels of intactness [40]. Similarly, microsomes prepared from rat lung tissue exhibited far lower latency levels than those from rat liver, although this may derive from the harsher treatment required to homogenize rat lung tissue [41]. The nature of the disrupting agent also has an impact on the latency—for example some detergents appear to be much harsher than others, resulting in inhibition of UGT activity. In our experience, Lubrol PX has been the most effective detergent for the disruption of the microsomal membrane, and for the solubilization of the UGT protein from the microsomal membrane for purification (e.g., [41,42]). It is generally accepted that the pore-forming antibiotic alamethicin is the membrane disruptor of choice for UGT assays since the UGT enzymes seem less sensitive to variations in its concentration than they are to various detergents [34]. Where liver microsomal preparations are used to generate glucuronide metabolites at a semi-preparative scale, for example for metabolite identification, the issue of latency is also important. For instance, long incubations in the presence of detergents could result in inhibition of the UGT activity, so careful choice of membrane perturbation method would be of particular importance.

Here we review the major hypotheses that have been proposed to explain the phenomenon of latency as it applies to UGTs, and discuss future studies that might be needed to gain a greater understanding of its origins and implications.

3. Compartmentation Hypothesis

This hypothesis is based on the assumption that the highly hydrophilic co-substrate for the glucuronidation reaction, UDPGA, (and possibly certain aglycone substrates) is not able to diffuse across the ER membrane, and therefore that disruption of the membrane integrity is required to reveal the full extent of in vitro UGT activity in microsomal preparations. The discovery of transporters for nucleotide sugars, including UDPGA, has provided very strong evidence in support of this hypothesis.

The barrier function of microsomal membranes was proposed by Winsnes in 1972 [38] and was later elaborated by Berry and Hallinan, who firstly proposed the compartmentation model to explain latency based on previous experimental results [43]. In this model, UGT located on the luminal side of the ER is partially embedded in the membrane, together with a transmembrane UDPGA permease and a lumenal nucleoside diphosphatase (NDPase). This model predicts that UDPGA needs to be transported by the permease into the microsomal lumen where UGT catalyzes glucuronidation reactions, then the NDPase hydrolyzes UDP, a co-product besides the glucuronide conjugate, to facilitate the forward reaction since UDP is an inhibitor of UGTs. Later evidence strongly supports this model, including the prediction of UGT topology and the discovery of UDPGA transporters.

The identification of complete cDNA sequences improved the understanding of many aspects of UGTs such as the ER targeting process and topology [1]. Initial reports on the sequences came from Jackson et al. and Mackenzie et al. for rat liver UGTs [44,45], and allowed researchers to synthesize UGT proteins for studies on post-translational modifications [1,46,47]. In general, UGTs are synthesized as precursors of approximately 530 amino acid residues, and are targeted to the ER by an N-terminal signal sequence. A C-terminal di-lysine motif has been found in several human UGT sequences, and could act as an ER retention signal [48]. Following membrane integration, the N-terminal signal peptide is cleaved and the enzyme is *N*-glycosylated in the ER lumen. Notably, other internal topological elements within the UGTs might be required to regulate the integration process, as demonstrated for UGT1A6 [49,50]. In this way, the UGTs become mature ER enzymes of just over 500 residues [1]. Although significant portions of the protein may associate with the membrane, approximately 95% of the polypeptide chain is predicted to be luminal, and is connected to the cytosolic C-terminal tail through a 17-residue alpha helix that spans the lipid bilayer.

Although the intimate association between UGT protein and the ER membrane has so far prevented the generation of a complete crystal structure, the predicted topology of UGTs has been well developed. Vanstapel and Blanckaert predicted the catalytic site of bilirubin UGT faces ER lumen [51], which was followed by the development of a more complete topology model by Shepherd et al. [52]. This model was proposed based on the evidence from the authors' own results indicating that the majority of bilirubin UGT (UGT1A1) was not exposed to the cytosol, hydropathy plot analysis [53], and complete cDNA sequences of androsterone UGT [54,55], and rat phenol UGT (UGT1A6) [56]. Site-directed mutagenesis experiments have also confirmed that the UGT proteins are comprised of two domains, one binding the UDPGA (in the conserved C-terminal part of the protein) and one that presumably confers substrate preference located in the less-well conserved N-terminal region [57]. The determination of an X-ray crystal structure (1.8-Å resolution) for the C-terminal domain of human UGT2B7 is another strong piece of evidence confirming the presence of a nucleotide-binding site in the C-terminal half of the UGT proteins [58]. Above all, the sequence information together with recombinant DNA technology have allowed the development of a topology model that is generally accepted today (Figure 1). Compared to the topology proposed by Shepherd et al. [52], the most significant advances include the more specific locations of substrate and co-substrate binding sites, and the presence of transporters for UDPGA and glucuronides. If the binding sites are luminal as predicted, then the rate of glucuronidation might be constrained by the membrane barrier limiting the access of UDPGA, a highly charged molecule synthesized in the cytoplasmic space [59], to the reaction center. Although the complete crystal structure of a UGT protein is unsolved, homology modeling has been used to predict the three-dimensional structure [57]. For example, human UGT1A1 and UGT1A10 were homology-modeled using plant UGT71G1 and UDP-galactose 4-epimerase from *Escherichia coli*, respectively [60,61].

In addition, a transporter (or transporters) might be needed to facilitate the efflux of polar glucuronides out of the ER; this transporting activity has been biochemically demonstrated with a rate comparable to the rate of glucuronide synthesis [62]. Interestingly, the authors suggested that glucuronide efflux could be another rate-limiting step besides UDPGA import, because the rate of glucuronidation is highly variable among intact microsomes and it is unlikely that transport of UDPGA, the universal co-substrate for all glucuronidation reactions, is responsible for all of the variation observed. The identity of glucuronide efflux transporter(s) is still unknown and in contrast to this, UDPGA transporters have been intensively studied and identified, as described below. The role of UDP-*N*-acetylglucosamine (UDP-GlcNAc) has been key to advancing the compartmentation hypothesis.

It is well known that UDP-GlcNAc can activate UGT activity in microsomal preparations in the presence of UDPGA, having been first demonstrated by Pogell and Leloir, who suggested the effect was partly due to inhibition of the breakdown of UDPGA [24]. Later work suggested that UDP-GlcNAc acted as an allosteric effector of UGT [63]. However, it was Berry and Hallinan who proposed the existence of a "UDPGA permease" [43], following on from the suggestion made by Winsnes that UDP-GlcNAc might increase the permeability of the microsomal membrane to UDPGA, thus activating the enzyme [38]. UDP-GlcNAc stimulated UGT activities only when UDPGA was added to preparations of intact microsomes, but not when it was generated in situ by trans-glucuronidation or reverse glucuronidation reactions [64,65], which indicates the stimulation effect of UDP-GlcNAc occurs at the step of UDPGA transport into microsomes. The integrity of microsomal membranes needs to be maintained for UDP-GlcNAc stimulation of UGT activity, because UDP-GlcNAc no longer activated UGTs when microsomal membranes were disrupted by Triton X-100 treatment, sonication, or Lubrol PX treatment [28,31,41]. Interestingly, UGT activity in rat lung microsomes (with 1-naphthol as substrate) was insensitive to UDP-GlcNAc stimulation, unlike in rat liver microsomes [41], although this may be due to excessive mechanical disruption of the membranes during homogenization resulting from the nature of the lung tissue. Taken together, this evidence suggested that UDP-GlcNAc activates UGTs through an indirect mechanism that requires an intact microsomal membrane, presumably by enhancing the transport and access of UDPGA to the catalytic site. Evidence supporting this presumption includes the observation that glucuronidation rate was increased by UDP-GlcNAc when the concentration of UDPGA was high or saturating [24]. Additionally, Berry and Hallinan demonstrated that UDP, UTP, and UDP-glucose showed inhibitory effects on UGT activities only after microsomal membranes were disrupted [43], whereas native UGTs were resistant to the inhibitors, suggesting that these compounds are not transported by the presumptive UDPGA permease [63,66]. Therefore, it was concluded that the presumptive permease has a regulatory role in UGT activities by selectively transporting UDPGA.

Further evidence came from the observations that addition of *N*-ethylmaleimide (NEM) blocked the activation effect of UDP-GlcNAc on native UGT activity within intact microsomes, without a direct inhibition on the enzyme's catalytic site [67]. This piece of evidence suggested the presence of membrane permease-containing thiol groups that are required for the action of UDP-GlcNAc. Indeed, later studies showed that NEM inhibited UDPGA transport into the ER of permeabilized rat hepatocytes, which in turn inhibited glucuronidation of 4-methylumbelliferone (4-MU), a non-selective substrate metabolized by many UGT isoforms [68,69]. However, when microsomal and ER membranes were permeabilized, glucuronidation was not affected by NEM treatment [69].

The discovery of UDPGA transporters was preceded by studies recognizing a carrier-mediated, UDPGA transport activity at the rat liver ER membrane [68–71]. The common question raised by these studies was as to how important UDPGA transport could be to glucuronidation reactions. Bossuyt and Blanckaert carried out a series of studies characterizing the transport activities of UDPGA and UDP-GlcNAc across microsomal membranes [68,72], and were able to connect the two transport systems when UDPGA uptake into the microsomes preloaded with UDP-GlcNAc showed an overshoot effect [69]. Hence, UDP-GlcNAc might be exported by a bidirectional carrier to trans-stimulate the import of UDPGA for UGT catalysis. It turned out that UDPGA transport was both required and necessary for glucuronidation, because the inhibition or stimulation of UDPGA transport by NEM or UDP-GlcNAc, as partly mentioned above, inhibited or stimulated glucuronidation respectively towards 4-MU in microsomes and permeabilized hepatocytes [73]. Indeed, UDPGA transport seemed to be the rate-limiting step of glucuronidation reactions, which formed the basis of the compartmentation hypothesis in that the release of the transport constraint would significantly increase the glucuronidation rate.

A number of nucleotide sugar transporters (NSTs) have now been cloned, expressed and functionally characterized. UDP-galactose transporter-related protein 7 (UGTrel7), a human NST, was shown to transport both UDPGA and UDP-*N*-acetylgalactosamine (UDP-GalNAc) into microsomal vesicles when expressed in *Saccharomyces cerevisiae* [74]. Kobayashi et al. molecularly and functionally characterized four human NSTs, namely UGTrel1, UGTrel7, huYEA4, and huYEA4S, the last two being newly identified human NSTs that are splice variants of each other [75]. These transporters all mediated UDP-GlcNAc-dependent UDPGA uptake into the microsomes isolated from recombinant V79 cells expressing the NST cDNAs, although UGTrel7 was by far the most efficient. These authors also demonstrated that UGTs themselves, at least UGT1 family members, were not significantly involved in the transport of UDPGA. Muraoka et al. subsequently confirmed that UGTrel7 (expressed in *S. cerevisiae*) transported UDPGA in a manner that was much enhanced by UDP-GlcNAc and showed that UGTrel7 was a UDPGA/UDP-GlcNAc antiporter [76]. Therefore, after more than 50 years since the discovery that UDPGA was the co-substrate and glucuronic acid donor for UGTs [77,78], these two papers provided the most direct evidence of how the highly charged co-substrate is delivered to the UGTs in the microsomal lumen, and how UDP-GlcNAc enhances this process. The rapid advance in gene editing technology, such as the CRISPR/Cas9 system, provides an alternate approach to investigating the role of UDPGA transporters in the latency of UGTs. It should be possible, for example, to delete a UDPGA transporter such as UGTrel7 in a cell line (or embryonically in an animal model) to determine the contribution of individual NSTs to UGT latency.

UDPGA transport is a complex process, and probably involves other transport molecules, as described by Rowland et al. who demonstrated that UDPGA uptake into human liver microsomes involves more than one transporter [79]. Other NSTs capable of transporting UDPGA at ER membrane have been identified. For instance, Selva et al. and Goto et al. identified the gene fringe connection (*frc*) that encodes an NST transporting UDPGA, UDP-GlcNAc, and UDP-xylose from the cytoplasm to the lumen of ER/Golgi in *Drosophila* [80,81]. Interestingly, this transporter is important in growth-factor signaling pathways including Wnt/Wingless-, Hedgehog-, fibroblast growth factor-, and Notch-dependent pathways, by transporting UDP-sugars into the Golgi to facilitate the synthesis of heparan sulfate proteoglycan and the glycosylation and maturation of Notch receptor. Lastly, Suda et al. identified the gene *hfrc 1* homologous to *frc* (*Drosophila melanogaster*), *sqv-7* (*Caenorhabditis elegans*), and *UGTrel7* (human) [82]. It encodes an NST that is located at the Golgi and transports UDP-GlcNAc, UDP-glucose, and UDP-mannose.

4. Conformation Hypothesis

The concept that the conformation of the UGT enzyme protein is subject to influence by the hydrophobic lipid environment in the ER membrane, and it is this that controls the activity of enzymes, is the underlying basis of the conformation hypothesis. In contrast to the compartmentation hypothesis, the conformation hypothesis explains latency by assuming that the catalytic site of UGTs is accessible by substrates and UDPGA and the membrane disruption induces the formation of different kinetic forms of the enzyme with increased activity [39].

According to Vessey and Zakim, treatments altering the lipid portion of bovine liver microsomes increased UGT activity at V_{max} towards *p*-nitrophenol, including the addition of phospholipase A or Triton X-100, and sonication [37]. These treatments can alter the lipid composition as well as the integrity of the microsomal membrane. For instance, phospholipase A produces lysophospholipids that can act as detergents when present at high concentrations within the membrane. Therefore, the increase in V_{max} of UGTs could be due to a change in the protein–lipid interaction or greater access of substrates to the catalytic site after the membrane integrity had been lost, or a combination of both. Because Triton treatment only sped up the forward reaction which is the glucuronidation reaction catalyzed by UGTs [37], the activation effect was restricted to the UGTs (not other microsomal components) when the luminal space was fully accessible. Besides, phospholipase A treatment has been shown to alter the binding specificity for UDPGA, allowing for the competitive binding from other UDP-sugars to the UGTs [63,83]. Hence, phospholipase A seems to induce a change in the conformation of the co-substrate binding site that can fit the structures of other UDP-sugars. Overall, these experiments suggested that the effect of membrane perturbants is mainly the alteration of lipid composition which directly affects the enzyme itself, as Zakim and Dannenberg argued [39]. They concluded that the enzyme might exist in different functional states demonstrating different kinetic properties, and the lipid environment controls the enzyme activity by intimately regulating its conformation.

The interaction between substrate and co-substrate binding sites within a single UGT protein was another piece of evidence used to support the existence of multiple conformational forms [84,85]. Vessey and Zakim proposed that *p*-nitrophenol UGTs follow a random order kinetic mechanism after they carried out product inhibition and isotope exchange studies, and so the enzymes can firstly bind substrate or co-substrate and form rapid equilibrium [85]. Interestingly, under high concentrations of *p*-nitrophenol, UGTs showed increased values of V_{max} and $K_{m\ UDPGA}$, which suggested that occupation of the substrate binding site decreased the binding affinity for the co-substrate. The interaction between substrate and co-substrate binding sites was further investigated by Hochman and Zakim who used an enzyme reconstitution system where a delipidated form of purified UGT, called GT_{2p}, was reconstituted into different species of phospholipids to study their influence on the enzyme properties [84]. GT_{2p} represented the second peak of eluted UGT after a hydroxylapatite column purification from pig liver microsomes, and showed a single band of protein following sodium dodecyl sulfate—polyacrylamide (7.5%) gel electrophoresis (SDS-PAGE) [86]. It was shown that the nature of phospholipids used to reconstitute GT_{2p} activity affected the extent to which substrate binding decreased the binding affinity of the co-substrate. In parallel with this result, the α-glucuronidase activity of GT_{2p} was differentially affected by the binding of structural variants of aromatic ethers that only occupy the substrate binding site without being conjugated. Therefore, the binding of a substrate seems to induce a conformational change in the enzyme that possesses an altered co-substrate binding affinity, which is dependent on the surrounding lipid environment.

Further experiments suggested that the physical properties, rather than the chemical structures, of phospholipids surrounding UGTs seemed to play a role in the interaction with the enzymes and regulation of their kinetic patterns. For example, when GT_{2p} was reconstituted into bilayers of 1,2-dimyristoylphosphatidylcholine or 1,2-dipalmitoylphosphatidylcholine lipids in the gel phase, the enzyme displayed non-Michaelis–Menten kinetics, however when the lipids were heated to liquid–crystal phase, the enzyme(s) displayed Michaelis–Menten kinetics [87,88]. The change in enzyme kinetics was solely due to the phase transition of phospholipids independent from a direct effect of increasing temperature. Furthermore, the GT_{2p} demonstrating non-Michaelis–Menten kinetics had two different binding sites for UDPGA per molecule of enzyme, and the appearance of Michaelis–Menten kinetics after phase transition occurred was in parallel with the disappearance of one binding site [87]. These results could be explained by the conformational hypothesis in that the physical state of the phospholipids seems to determine the number of functional binding sites for UDPGA by changing enzyme conformation, although it is possible that the change in membrane fluidity promotes the association/disassembly of UGT monomers by modulating protein–protein interactions. The length and degree of saturation of phospholipid acyl chains are important for regulating membrane fluidity, and have been shown to affect the activity of UGTs [89]. For instance, for the purified pig liver GT_{1p}, the first eluted fraction from a hydroxylapatite column as described by Hochman and Zakim [90], the lysophosphatidylcholine species that had longer acyl chains with more unsaturated bonds led to greater activation at V_{max}. This result further suggested that the interaction between UGTs and phospholipids does not depend on the specific chemical structures of phospholipids. Rather, as Rotenberg and Zakim suggested, the interaction occurs through a non-specific mechanism depending on the physical state of phospholipids [91].

The experiments described above repeatedly emphasize the role of the lipid environment in the regulation of UGT conformation. The change in conformation can in turn alter the rate of glucuronidation presumably by changing the catalytic mechanism, as demonstrated for GT_{2p} reconstituted into different species of lysophosphatidylcholine [86,92]. Specifically, changing the lipids used to reconstitute GT_{2p} from oleoyl lysophosphatidylcholine to stearoyl lysophosphatidylcholine led to changes in the rate of glucuronidation depending on the specific aglycone substrates: a 20-fold decline for *p*-nitrophenol, no change for 1-naphthol and phenol, and a 3-fold decline for *p*-bromophenol. Hence, the specific lipid environment has a selective effect on the glucuronidation rate towards different aglycones. Two mechanisms have been proposed as to how the lipid–protein interaction affects the catalytic rate of UGT (in this case, purified GT_{2p}). Firstly, phospholipids may regulate enzyme–substrate interactions and determine how much inherent binding energy to UDPGA can be shared for catalysis to enhance the reaction rate [92]. Only certain species of lysophosphatidylcholine could influence the enzyme in a way that more inherent binding energy is used for catalysis. Alternatively, phospholipids like oleoyl lysophosphatidylcholine speed up glucuronidation by facilitating the bond breaking between the C1 of glucuronic acid and UDP [86].

Besides kinetic properties and avidity for substrate binding, the lipid environment also regulates the thermal stability of UGTs [91]. Rotenberg and Zakim's data suggest that the GT_{2p} fraction of UGTs existed in three forms through conformational changes: the active form (E), inactive form (E′), and denatured form. The change between E and E′ is controlled by temperature and is reversible, whereas the denatured form is obtained by heating E′ to a certain extent. The specific temperatures required for the occurrence of these conformational changes are dependent on a specific lipid environment. In general, the reconstitution of pure, delipidated GT_{2p} into different species of phosphatidylcholine, such as distearoylphosphatidylcholine, dioleoylphosphatidylcholine, or 1-stearoyl-2-oleoylphosphatidylcholine, stabilized the E form with a greater change in the entropy of the whole system rather than the enthalpy, and slowed down denaturation rate of the E′ form. However, each of these phospholipids affected the thermal stability of GT_{2p} to a different extent depending on the nature of the acyl chains, so the increase in temperature might alter enzyme conformation through modulating the physical state of phospholipids. Using the reconstitution method, Hochman and Zakim showed that only gel-phase phospholipids could reconstitute the sensitivity of the purified GT_{2p} fraction to stimulation by UDP-GlcNAc, a physiological activator of UGTs [90]. Also, GT_{2p} seems to have a favorable interaction with viscous lipids [87]. These data suggest UGTs are restricted by certain forces within a subregion of the ER membrane where the lipids are gel-like, hence it is less likely that the enzymes randomly interact with the bulk phase of lipids within the ER membrane [87,90]. The forces could come from the interactions between UGTs and specific acyl chains in the lipid bilayer, or between different UGT isoforms that preferentially aggregate in the gel-like regions.

Alternatively, the gel-like regions might be formed by lipid rafts, membrane microdomains that are enriched in cholesterol, sphingolipids, and specific proteins such as glycosylphosphatidylinositol (GPI)-anchored proteins and Src-family kinases [93]. These microdomains could be formed by the phase segregation of membrane lipids [93], and/or by anchoring of the lipids to actin filaments [94].

More importantly, the rafts have various functions including endo-, exo-, and transcytosis, polarized intracellular trafficking of specific membrane proteins, and signal transduction [93,95,96]. They can transiently recruit membrane and intracellular proteins to initiate a cellular signaling event [97]. Since the intracellular transport of UGTs to the ER membrane is not fully understood, it is likely that UGTs functionally interact with lipid rafts for the purposes of intracellular transport, ER localization, and/or regulation of the enzyme stability and activity. In vitro and in vivo experiments have demonstrated the effect of cholesterol, a major component of lipid rafts, on the activity of UGTs [98,99]. Specifically, the addition of cholesterol to guinea pig liver microsomes increased UGT activity at V_{max}; diet supplementation that increased the membrane content of cholesterol in guinea pig liver ER showed similar results to that of the in vitro data. In both cases, the activity of UGTs was studied under the native membrane environment. Rotenberg and Zakim reconstituted delipidated GT_{2p} into different phospholipids to study the influence of the lipid environment on the observed cholesterol effect [100]. They showed that the modulation of UGT activity and stability by cholesterol was dependent on specific types of phospholipids surrounding the enzyme. For example, the addition of cholesterol to the bilayers of distearoylphosphatidylcholine decreased enzyme activity but increased stability of the enzyme against thermal denaturation, whereas cholesterol in the bilayers of dioleoylphosphatidylcholine showed little effect on the properties of the enzyme. In order to address the effects of lipid rafts on the activity and stability of UGTs, it is worthwhile to compare the effects of cholesterol in the contexts of raft associated lipids and phospholipids.

Because lipid rafts have been extensively studied with much evidence supporting their existence in living cells, technologies have been developed to monitor raft dynamics such as single molecule tracking together with advanced microscopic analyses [94,97]. These technologies allow researchers to precisely follow the dynamic interactions between raft lipids and raft-associated proteins despite the crowding environment within a cell, and so could be extended to UGTs to follow their interactions with microsomal lipids in real time. A possible experiment would be to use a recombinant system, such as human embryonic kidney 293 (HEK293) cells, where a UGT enzyme and a raft lipid can each be tagged with a Fab-conjugated fluorescent molecule. This would be followed by fluorescence microscopy that records the trajectories of the labeled molecules. The measurement on the time length of co-localization between the enzyme and raft lipid could indicate whether there is a significant interaction between them.

The challenges of using purified membrane protein preparations on the outcome of these experiments has been mentioned several times by Zakim's group [86,87,90]. Integral membrane proteins tend to associate with detergents and other membrane components after they have been isolated, and form mixed micelles with the detergents and phospholipids used to reconstitute the enzymes. Therefore, the properties displayed by the reconstituted GT_{2p} may be artificially affected by other components more than the phosphatidylcholine variants, and may not faithfully reveal UGT–phospholipid interactions. Also, the native structure and function of membrane proteins might be altered during purification before the enzymes are reconstituted into a new lipid environment. Lastly, if UGTs truly have a significant interaction with surrounding phospholipids in the ER membrane, then it is essential that the enzymes are reconstituted into a native lipid environment for functional studies [87]. The studies reported by Zakim and colleagues on the conformational change of UGTs, especially GT_{2p} reconstituted in phosphatidylcholine variants, were mainly carried out on pig liver microsomes, since the activity of *p*-nitrophenol UGTs was greater than that from cow liver microsomes and so was easier to measure [85]. It would be interesting to carry out these studies using liver from other species, particularly humans, to investigate if lipid–protein interaction is a universal mechanism in the regulation of UGT activity, and how much variation among different species that the influence of the lipid environment could have on the enzymes. Nevertheless, Vessey and Zakim observed latency among all the species examined: guinea pigs, mice, rats, cows, rabbits, and humans, using phospholipase A and the detergent *p*-chloromercuribenzoate as the membrane perturbants [101]. The extent of activation by the addition of either reagent varied among the species.

Additionally, most of the kinetic assays were carried out using the substrate *p*-nitrophenol which can be glucuronidated by more than one isoform such as UGT1A6 and 1A1 [102]. This means that the kinetic properties revealed by UGTs could reflect the action of one or multiple isomers. Since protein–protein interactions exist among UGT isoforms, then after altering the lipid phase by changing temperature, the measured kinetic data may not solely represent the regulation from lipid-protein interactions. Above all, the superfamily of UGTs contains many isoforms with overlapping substrate specificity, and these enzymes are widely distributed in the nature from coral and insects to mammals [1]. It is especially important to take these properties into consideration when measuring UGT activity.

It is true that the compartmentation hypothesis is more widely accepted in the field, however the studies by Zakim and colleagues, and others, provide a rich reservoir of data that do indicate that the regulation of UGT activity within the ER membrane environment is complex and may well involve multiple mechanisms.

5. Adenine Nucleotide Inhibition Effect

Recently, the inhibitory effects of adenine and adenine-containing nucleotides on UGT activities have been proposed as another explanation of latency [103–105]. The first report came from Hallinan et al. who demonstrated that activities of UGTs toward *p*-nitrophenol, estradiol, and estrone were suppressed by 4 mM ATP (adenosine triphosphate) in guinea pig liver microsomes [104,106]. Then, Nishimura et al. found that adenine, ATP, NAD^+ (nicotinamide adenine dinucleotide, oxidized), and $NADP^+$ (nicotinamide adenine dinucleotide phosphate, oxidized) inhibited the glucuronidation of 4-MU and estradiol by allosteric binding to UGTs at a site independent from the substrate and co-substrate binding sites, and proposed that membrane perturbations could lead to the release of these inhibitors and hence an increase in glucuronidation activities [105]. AMP (adenosine monophosphate) by itself barely inhibited UGTs, but decreased the potency of inhibitory nucleotides. It is likely that AMP antagonizes the inhibitory nucleotides by competing for the allosteric binding site, as suggested in a later publication [103]. When Nishimura et al. tested 4-MU UGT activity in rat liver microsomes, latency and inhibitory effects of ATP and $NADP^+$ were observed on the UGTs after Brij58 solubilization of the membranes, which suggests the allosteric binding site is luminal [105]. This evidence indirectly supports the compartmentation model since adenine nucleotides must pass the membrane barrier if the UGTs exhibit the native topology, except that the compartmentation model was originally rationalized upon the limited supply of UDPGA for glucuronidation reactions. Lastly, human UGT is also regulated by adenine nucleotides [105]. In microsomes isolated from human embryonic kidney 293 (HEK293) cells that express human UGT1A1, the glucuronidation activity towards estradiol was gradually inhibited by increasing concentrations of ATP, NAD^+, or $NADP^+$.

In 2012, Ishii et al. compared alamethicin- and Brij58-treated microsomes from rat and human livers, and showed the inhibitory potency of adenine nucleotides was lower in the alamethicin-disrupted microsomes [103]. The luminal concentration of ATP in rat liver ER can be as high as 30 μM which is similar to the IC_{50} value measured from Brij58-treated human liver microsomes (33.8 μM), but much lower than that from rat liver microsomes (66.8 μM). Therefore, under physiological conditions, the level of ATP in the ER lumen might be sufficient to suppress UGT activity. These authors also showed that Brij58 and alamethicin treatments could lead to the release of ATP from rat liver microsomes in vitro. Two structural components have been thought to be important for inhibitory nucleotides to bind the allosteric effector site of UGTs [104,105]. The first one is the adenine skeleton. This is because AMP decreased the inhibitory effects of ATP, adenine, NAD^+, and $NADP^+$, and so was thought to compete with the other adenine nucleotides for the common allosteric binding site. The second structural component is a di- or triphosphate moiety attached to the 5′-position of ribose, because neither AMP nor adenosine showed an inhibitory effect on the UGT activity. However, because adenine was able to inhibit UGT and lacks a phosphate group, the significance of the number of phosphates attached to ribose on the inhibitory effect of adenine nucleotides is called into question. Besides adenine-containing nucleotides, GTP and CTP are the only guanine- and cytidine nucleotides that inhibited UGTs, respectively, using 4-MU as the aglycone substrate [104,105]. CTP and ATP had similar IC_{50} values, and so comparable inhibitory effects. GTP, however, was much less potent than ATP.

UDP is a well-known inhibitor of UGTs. However, unlike adenine nucleotides, UDP is believed to compete with the co-substrate UDPGA for binding to UGTs, hence exerting the inhibitory effect on glucuronidation [104,107,108]. The inhibition of UGT by UDP can be prevented by the inclusion of a divalent metal ion in the incubation mixture, for example 10 mM Mg^{2+}.

Despite being a possible explanation of latency, the adenine nucleotides, particularly $NADP^+$, could play a role in the regulation of glucocorticoid levels [105,109]. Specifically, 11 β-hydroxysteroid dehydrogenase reduces $NADP^+$ to produce cortisone from cortisol in hepatic ER lumen. As the level of $NADP^+$ decreases, the inhibitory effect on the UGTs is also decreased, which enables UGTs to glucuronidate excess cortisol. Above all, information on the ER concentrations of adenine nucleotides relative to their cytosolic concentrations and IC_{50} values is needed to further investigate the physiological effects of the nucleotides on glucuronidation and metabolism.

6. Conclusions and Future Direction

The controversy over the underlying mechanisms that explain the latency of UGT activity that is observed in vitro in microsomal preparations has continued for more than half a century. It is clear that disruption of the microsomal membrane by physical and chemical treatments is necessary to reveal full UGT enzyme activity in vitro. Based on the available evidence, it is likely that much of the effect is due to the disruption of the membrane allowing increased access of UDPGA (and potentially also aglycone substrates) to the active site of the enzymes. Critical evidence for this comes from the existence of transporter(s) for UDPGA that presumably regulate access of the co-substrate to the enzyme in vivo. However, it is equally clear that UGT enzyme activity can be regulated by membrane components including phospholipids, cholesterol and indeed other proteins, including other UGTs and CYPs. Some of the effects of membrane disrupting agents such as detergents may well be mediated through their impact on the membrane environment as well as on the UGT proteins themselves.

Readers may ask "why does this matter?", particularly in a time when we know much about the biology, genetics and regulation of UGTs and glucuronidation. One of the main reasons it remains important is that we are still unable to accurately extrapolate in vitro measurements of UGT activity to estimates of in vivo clearance of drugs that are metabolized by glucuronidation. This in vitro–in vivo extrapolation (IVIVE) consistently underpredicts clearance in vivo for such drugs despite significant advances in physiologically-based pharmacokinetic (PBBK) analysis and a far more sophisticated understanding of the physiological factors that influence UGT activity [110,111]. We believe that increasing our understanding of the underlying mechanisms of UGT latency will help to further refine IVIVE for many drugs that are glucuronidated in humans. Advances in analytical tools such as Förster resonance energy transfer, mass spectrometry, etc. provide the technological basis for advancing our knowledge of this important feature of one of the body's key chemical defense mechanisms.

Acknowledgments: Yuejian Liu is supported by the James E. Axelson Outstanding Graduate Scholar Award.

Author Contributions: Yuejian Liu and Michael W. H. Coughtrie reviewed the literature and wrote the paper.

References

1. Radominska-Pandya, A.; Czernik, P.J.; Little, J.M.; Battaglia, E.; Mackenzie, P.I. Structural and functional studies of UDP-glucuronosyltransferases. *Drug Metab. Rev.* **1999**, *31*, 817–899. [CrossRef] [PubMed]
2. Dutton, G.J. *Glucuronidation of drugs and other compounds*; CRC Press: Boca Raton, FL, USA, 1980; ISBN 9780849352959.
3. Fry, D.J.; Wishart, G.J. Apparent induction by phenobarbital of uridine diphosphate glucuronyltransferase activity in nuclear envelopes of embryonic-chick liver. *Biochem. Soc. Trans.* **1976**, *4*, 265–266. [CrossRef] [PubMed]

4. Wishart, G.J.; Fry, D.J. Uridine diphosphate glucuronyltransferase activity in nuclei and nuclear envelopes of rat liver and its apparent induction by phenobarbital. *Biochem. Soc. Trans.* **1977**, *5*, 705–706. [CrossRef]
5. Fremont, J.J.; Wang, R.W.; King, C.D. Coimmunoprecipitation of UDP-glucuronosyltransferase isoforms and cytochrome P450 3A4. *Mol. Pharmacol.* **2005**, *67*, 260–262. [CrossRef] [PubMed]
6. Fujiwara, R.; Nakajima, M.; Oda, S.; Yamanaka, H.; Ikushiro, S.; Sakaki, T.; Yokoi, T. Interactions between human UDP-glucuronosyltransferase (UGT) 2B7 and UGT1A enzymes. *J. Pharm. Sci.* **2010**, *99*, 442–454. [CrossRef] [PubMed]
7. Fujiwara, R.; Nakajima, M.; Yamanaka, H.; Katoh, M.; Yokoi, T. Interactions between human UGT1A1, UGT1A4, and UGT1A6 affect their enzymatic activities. *Drug Metab. Dispos.* **2007**, *35*, 1781–1787. [CrossRef] [PubMed]
8. Ghosh, S.S.; Sappal, B.S.; Kalpana, G.V.; Lee, S.W.; Chowdhury, J.R.; Chowdhury, N.R. Homodimerization of human bilirubin-uridine-diphosphoglucuronate glucuronosyltransferase-1 (UGT1A1) and its functional implications. *J. Biol. Chem.* **2001**, *276*, 42108–42115. [CrossRef] [PubMed]
9. Ikushiro, S.; Emi, Y.; Iyanagi, T. Protein-protein interactions between UDP-glucuronosyltransferase isozymes in rat hepatic microsomes. *Biochemistry* **1997**, *36*, 7154–7161. [CrossRef] [PubMed]
10. Lewis, B.C.; Mackenzie, P.I.; Miners, J.O. Homodimerization of UDP-glucuronosyltransferase 2B7 (UGT2B7) and identification of a putative dimerization domain by protein homology modeling. *Biochem. Pharmacol.* **2011**, *82*, 2016–2023. [CrossRef] [PubMed]
11. Operana, T.N.; Tukey, R.H. Oligomerization of the UDP-glucuronosyltransferase 1A proteins: Homo- and heterodimerization analysis by fluorescence resonance energy transfer and co-immunoprecipitation. *J. Biol. Chem.* **2007**, *282*, 4821–4829. [CrossRef] [PubMed]
12. Taura, K.I.; Yamada, H.; Hagino, Y.; Ishii, Y.; Mori, M.A.; Oguri, K. Interaction between cytochrome P450 and other drug-metabolizing enzymes: Evidence for an association of CYP1A1 with microsomal epoxide hydrolase and UDP-glucuronosyltransferase. *Biochem. Biophys. Res. Commun.* **2000**, *273*, 1048–1052. [CrossRef] [PubMed]
13. Williams, R.T. *Detoxication Mechanisms*, 2nd ed.; Chapman & Hall: London, UK, 1959.
14. Ishii, Y.; Iwanaga, M.; Nishimura, Y.; Takeda, S.; Ikushiro, S.; Nagata, K.; Yamazoe, Y.; Mackenzie, P.I.; Yamada, H. Protein-protein interactions between rat hepatic cytochromes P450 (P450s) and UDP-glucuronosyltransferases (UGTs): Evidence for the functionally active UGT in P450-UGT complex. *Drug Metab. Pharmacokinet.* **2007**, *22*, 367–376. [CrossRef] [PubMed]
15. Takeda, S.; Ishii, Y.; Iwanaga, M.; Mackenzie, P.I.; Nagata, K.; Yamazoe, Y.; Oguri, K.; Yamada, H. Modulation of UDP-glucuronosyltransferase function by cytochrome P450: Evidence for the alteration of UGT2B7-catalyzed glucuronidation of morphine by CYP3A4. *Mol. Pharmacol.* **2005**, *67*, 665–672. [CrossRef] [PubMed]
16. Abbott, F.V.; Palmour, R.M. Morphine-6-glucuronide: Analgesic effects and receptor binding profile in rats. *Life Sci.* **1988**, *43*, 1685–1695. [CrossRef]
17. Vore, M.; Slikker, W. Steroid D-ring glucuronides: A new class of cholestatic agents. *Trends Pharmac. Sci.* **1985**, *6*, 256–259. [CrossRef]
18. Riches, Z.; Collier, A.C. Posttranscriptional regulation of uridine diphosphate glucuronosyltransferases. *Expert. Opin. Drug Metab. Toxicol.* **2015**, *11*, 949–965. [CrossRef] [PubMed]
19. Caspersen, C.S.; Reznik, B.; Weldy, P.L.; Abildskov, K.M.; Stark, R.I.; Garland, M. Molecular cloning of the baboon UDP-glucuronosyltransferase 1A gene family: Evolution of the primate UGT1 locus and relevance for models of human drug metabolism. *Pharmacogenet. Genomics* **2007**, *17*, 11–24. [CrossRef] [PubMed]
20. Halac, E.; Bonevard, E. Solubilization and activation of liver UDP glucuronyltransferase by EDTA. *Biochim. Biophys. Acta* **1963**, *67*, 498–500. [CrossRef]
21. Heirwegh, K.P.; Meuwissen, J.A. Activation in vitro and solubilization of glucuronyltransferase (assayed with bilirubin as acceptor) with digitonin. *Biochem. J.* **1968**, *110*, 31P–32P. [CrossRef] [PubMed]
22. Isselbacher, K.J.; Chrabas, M.F.; Quinn, R.C. The solubilization and partial purification of a glucuronyl transferase from rabbit liver microsomes. *J. Biol. Chem.* **1962**, *237*, 3033–3036. [PubMed]
23. Lueders, K.K.; Kuff, E.L. Spontaneous and detergent activation of a glucuronyltransferase in vitro. *Arch. Biochem. Biophys.* **1967**, *120*, 198–203. [CrossRef]
24. Pogell, B.M.; Leloir, L.F. Nucleotide activation of liver microsomal glucuronidation. *J. Biol. Chem.* **1961**, *236*, 293–298. [PubMed]

25. Stevenson, I.; Greenwood, D.; McEwen, J. Hepatic UDP-glucuronyltransferase in Wistar and Gunn rats - in vitro activation by diethylnitrosamine. *Biochem. Biophys. Res. Commun.* **1968**, *32*, 866–872. [CrossRef]
26. Tomlinson, G.A.; Yaffe, S.J. The formation of bilirubin and p-nitrophenyl glucuronides by rabbit liver. *Biochem. J.* **1966**, *99*, 507–512. [CrossRef] [PubMed]
27. Van Roy, F.P.; Heirwegh, K.P. Determination of bilirubin glucuronide and assay of glucuronyltransferase with bilirubin as acceptor. *Biochem. J.* **1968**, *107*, 507–518. [CrossRef] [PubMed]
28. Winsnes, A. Studies on the activation in vitro of glucuronyltransferase. *Biochim. Biophys. Acta* **1969**, *191*, 279–291. [CrossRef]
29. Burchell, A.; Waddell, I.D. The molecular basis of the hepatic microsomal glucose-6-phosphatase system. *Biochim. Biophys. Acta* **1991**, *1092*, 129–137. [CrossRef]
30. Lin, J.H.; Wong, B.K. Complexities of glucuronidation affecting in vitro in vivo extrapolation. *Curr. Drug Metab.* **2002**, *3*, 623–646. [CrossRef] [PubMed]
31. Berry, C.; Stellon, A.; Hallinan, T. Guinea pig liver microsomal UDP-glucuronyltransferase: Compartmented or phospholipid-constrained? *Biochim. Biophys. Acta* **1975**, *403*, 335–344. [CrossRef]
32. Dannenberg, A.; Wong, T.; Zakim, D. Effect of brief treatment at alkaline pH on the properties of UDP-glucuronosyltransferase. *Arch. Biochem. Biophys.* **1990**, *277*, 312–317. [CrossRef]
33. Dannenberg, A.J.; Kavecansky, J.; Scarlata, S.; Zakim, D. Organization of microsomal UDP-glucuronosyltransferase. Activation by treatment at high pressure. *Biochemistry* **1990**, *29*, 5961–5967. [CrossRef] [PubMed]
34. Fisher, M.B.; Campanale, K.; Ackermann, B.L.; VandenBranden, M.; Wrighton, S.A. In vitro glucuronidation using human liver microsomes and the pore-forming peptide alamethicin. *Drug Metab. Dispos.* **2000**, *28*, 560–566. [PubMed]
35. Graham, A.B.; Wood, G.C. The phospholipid-dependence of UDP-glucuronyltransferase. *Biochem. Biophys. Res. Commun.* **1969**, *37*, 567–575. [CrossRef]
36. Mulder, G.J. The effect of phenobarbital on the submicrosomal distribution of uridine diphosphate glucuronyltransferase from rat liver. *Biochem. J.* **1970**, *117*, 319–324. [CrossRef] [PubMed]
37. Vessey, D.A.; Zakim, D. Regulation of microsomal enzymes by phospholipids. II. Acitvation of hepatic uridine diphosphate-glucuronyltransferase. *J. Biol. Chem.* **1971**, *246*, 4649–4656. [PubMed]
38. Winsnes, A. Kinetic properties of different forms of hepatic UDP glucuronyltransferase. *Biochim. Biophys. Acta* **1972**, *284*, 394–405. [CrossRef]
39. Zakim, D.; Dannenberg, A.J. How does the microsomal membrane regulate UDP-glucuronosyltransferases? *Biochem. Pharmacol.* **1992**, *43*, 1385–1393. [CrossRef]
40. Coughtrie, M.W.H.; Blair, J.N.R.; Hume, R.; Burchell, A. Improved procedure for the preparation of hepatic microsomes to be used in the in vitro diagnosis of inherited disorders of the glucose-6-phosphatase system. *Clin. Chem.* **1991**, *37*, 739–742. [PubMed]
41. Coughtrie, M.W.H. A Molecular Analysis of Biological Variations in UDP-Glucuronosyltransferase Activities. Ph.D. Thesis, University of Dundee, Dundee, UK, 1986.
42. Coughtrie, M.W.H.; Burchell, B.; Bend, J.R. Purification and properties of rat kidney UDP-glucuronosyltransferase. *Biochem. Pharmacol.* **1987**, *36*, 245–251. [CrossRef]
43. Berry, C.; Hallinan, T. Summary of a novel, three-component regulatory model for uridine diphosphate glucuronyltransferase. *Biochem. Soc. Trans.* **1976**, *4*, 650–652. [CrossRef] [PubMed]
44. Jackson, M.R.; McCarthy, L.R.; Corser, R.B.; Barr, G.C.; Burchell, B. Cloning of cDNAs coding for rat hepatic microsomal UDP-glucuronyltransferases. *Gene* **1984**, *34*, 147–153. [CrossRef]
45. Mackenzie, P.I.; Gonzalez, F.J.; Owens, I.S. Cloning and characterization of DNA complementary to rat liver UDP-glucuronosyltransferase mRNA. *J. Biol. Chem.* **1984**, *259*, 12153–12160.
46. Mackenzie, P.I.; Owens, I.S. Cleavage of nascent UDP glucuronosyltransferase from rat liver by dog pancreatic microsomes. *Biochem. Biophys. Res. Commun.* **1984**, *122*, 1441–1449. [CrossRef]
47. Rowland, A.; Miners, J.O.; Mackenzie, P.I. The UDP-glucuronosyltransferases: Their role in drug metabolism and detoxification. *Int. J. Biochem. Cell Biol.* **2013**, *45*, 1121–1132. [CrossRef] [PubMed]
48. Jackson, M.R.; Nilsson, T.; Peterson, P.A. Identification of a consensus motif for retention of transmembrane proteins in the endoplasmic reticulum. *EMBO J.* **1990**, *9*, 3153–3162. [PubMed]
49. Ouzzine, M.; Magdalou, J.; Burchell, B.; Fournel-Gigleux, S. Expression of a functionally active human hepatic UDP-glucuronosyltransferase (UGT1A6) lacking the N-terminal signal sequence in the endoplasmic reticulum. *FEBS Lett.* **1999**, *454*, 187–191. [PubMed]

50. Ouzzine, M.; Magdalou, J.; Burchell, B.; Fournel-Gigleux, S. An internal signal sequence mediates the targeting and retention of the human UDP-glucuronosyltransferase 1A6 to the endoplasmic reticulum. *J. Biol. Chem.* **1999**, *274*, 31401–31409. [CrossRef] [PubMed]
51. Vanstapel, F.; Blanckaert, N. Topology and regulation of bilirubin UDP-glucuronyltransferase in sealed native microsomes from rat liver. *Arch. Biochem. Biophys.* **1988**, *263*, 216–225. [CrossRef]
52. Shepherd, S.R.; Baird, S.J.; Hallinan, T.; Burchell, B. An investigation of the transverse topology of bilirubin UDP-glucuronosyltransferase in rat hepatic endoplasmic reticulum. *Biochem. J.* **1989**, *259*, 617–620. [CrossRef] [PubMed]
53. Kyte, J.; Doolittle, R.F. A simple method for displaying the hydropathic character of a protein. *J. Mol. Biol.* **1982**, *157*, 105–132. [CrossRef]
54. Jackson, M.R.; Burchell, B. The full length coding sequence of rat liver androsterone UDP-glucuronyltransferase cDNA and comparison with other members of this gene family. *Nucleic Acids Res.* **1986**, *14*, 779–795. [CrossRef] [PubMed]
55. Mackenzie, P.I. Rat liver UDP-glucuronosyltransferase. cDNA sequence and expression of a form glucuronidating 3-hydroxyandrogens. *J. Biol. Chem.* **1986**, *261*, 14112–14117. [PubMed]
56. Iyanagi, T.; Haniu, M.; Sogawa, K.; Fujii-Kuriyama, Y.; Watanabe, S.; Shively, J.E.; Anan, K.F. Cloning and characterization of cDNA encoding 3-methylcholanthrene inducible rat mRNA for UDP-glucuronosyltransferase. *J. Biol. Chem.* **1986**, *261*, 15607–15614. [PubMed]
57. Fujiwara, R.; Yokoi, T.; Nakajima, M. Structure and protein-protein interactions of human UDP-glucuronosyltransferases. *Front. Pharmacol.* **2016**, *7*, 388. [CrossRef] [PubMed]
58. Miley, M.J.; Zielinska, A.K.; Keenan, J.E.; Bratton, S.M.; Radominska-Pandya, A.; Redinbo, M.R. Crystal structure of the cofactor-binding domain of the human phase II drug-metabolism enzyme UDP-glucuronosyltransferase 2B7. *J. Mol. Biol.* **2007**, *369*, 498–511. [CrossRef] [PubMed]
59. Axelrod, J.; Kalckar, H.M.; Maxwell, E.S.; Strominger, J.L. Enzymatic formation of uridine diphosphoglucuronic acid. *J. Biol. Chem.* **1957**, *224*, 79–90. [PubMed]
60. Banerjee, R.P.; Pennington, M.W.; Garza, A.; Owens, I.S. Mapping the UDP-glucuronic acid binding site in UDP-glucuronosyltransferase 1A10 by homology-based modeling: Confirmation with biochemical evidence. *Biochemistry* **2008**, *47*, 7385–7392. [CrossRef] [PubMed]
61. Locuson, C.W.; Tracy, T.S. Comparative modelling of the human UDP-glucuronosyltransferases: Insights into structure and mechanism. *Xenobiotica* **2007**, *37*, 155–168. [CrossRef] [PubMed]
62. Revesz, K.; Toth, B.; Staines, A.G.; Coughtrie, M.W.; Mandl, J.; Csala, M. Luminal accumulation of newly synthesized morphine-3-glucuronide in rat liver microsomal vesicles. *Biofactors* **2013**, *39*, 271–278. [CrossRef] [PubMed]
63. Zakim, D.; Vessey, D.A. Membrane dependence of uridine diphosphate glucuronyltransferase: Effect of the membrane on kinetic properties. *Biochem. Soc. Trans.* **1974**, *2*, 1165–1167. [CrossRef]
64. Berry, C.; Hallinan, T. 'Coupled transglucuronidation': A new tool for studying the latency of UDP-glucuronyl transferase. *FEBS Lett.* **1974**, *42*, 73–76. [CrossRef]
65. Vessey, D.A.; Zakim, D. Stimulation of microsomal uridine diphosphate glucuronyltransferase by glucuronic acid derivatives. *Biochem. J.* **1974**, *139*, 243–249. [CrossRef] [PubMed]
66. Winsnes, A. Inhibition of hepatic UDP glucuronyltransferase by nucleotides. *Biochim. Biophys. Acta* **1972**, *289*, 88–96. [CrossRef]
67. Winsnes, A. The effects of sulfhydryl reacting agents on hepatic UDP-glucuronyltransferase in vitro. *Biochim. Biophys. Acta* **1971**, *242*, 549–559. [CrossRef]
68. Bossuyt, X.; Blanckaert, N. Carrier-mediated transport of intact UDP-glucuronic acid into the lumen of endoplasmic-reticulum-derived vesicles from rat liver. *Biochem. J.* **1994**, *302*, 261–269. [CrossRef] [PubMed]
69. Bossuyt, X.; Blanckaert, N. Mechanism of stimulation of microsomal UDP-glucuronosyltransferase by UDP-N-acetylglucosamine. *Biochem J.* **1995**, *305*, 321–328. [CrossRef] [PubMed]
70. Hauser, S.C.; Ziurys, J.C.; Gollan, J.L. A membrane transporter mediates access of uridine 5'-diphosphoglucuronic acid from the cytosol into the endoplasmic reticulum of rat hepatocytes: Implications for glucuronidation reactions. *Biochim. Biophys. Acta* **1988**, *967*, 149–157. [CrossRef]
71. Nuwayhid, N.; Glaser, J.H.; Johnson, J.C.; Conrad, H.E.; Hauser, S.C.; Hirschberg, C.B. Xylosylation and glucuronosylation reactions in rat liver golgi apparatus and endoplasmic reticulum. *J. Biol. Chem.* **1986**, *261*, 12936–12941. [PubMed]

72. Bossuyt, X.; Blanckaert, N. Functional characterization of carrier-mediated transport of uridine diphosphate N-acetylglucosamine across the endoplasmic reticulum membrane. *Eur. J. Biochem.* **1994**, *223*, 981–988. [CrossRef]
73. Bossuyt, X.; Blanckaert, N. Carrier-mediated transport of uridine diphosphoglucuronic acid across the endoplasmic reticulum membrane is a prerequisite for UDP-glucuronosyltransferase activity in rat liver. *Biochem. J.* **1997**, *323*, 645–648. [CrossRef] [PubMed]
74. Muraoka, M.; Kawakita, M.; Ishida, N. Molecular characterization of human UDP-glucuronic acid/UDP-N-acetylgalactosamine transporter, a novel nucleotide sugar transporter with dual substrate specificity. *FEBS Lett.* **2001**, *495*, 87–93. [CrossRef]
75. Kobayashi, T.; Sleeman, J.E.; Coughtrie, M.W.; Burchell, B. Molecular and functional characterization of microsomal UDP-glucuronic acid uptake by members of the nucleotide sugar transporter (NST) family. *Biochem. J.* **2006**, *400*, 281–289. [CrossRef] [PubMed]
76. Muraoka, M.; Miki, T.; Ishida, N.; Hara, T.; Kawakita, M. Variety of nucleotide sugar transporters with respect to the interaction with nucleoside mono- and diphosphates. *J. Biol. Chem.* **2007**, *282*, 24615–24622. [CrossRef] [PubMed]
77. Dutton, G.J.; Storey, I.D.E. The isolation of a compound of uridine diphosphate and glucuronic acid from liver. *Biochem. J.* **1953**, *53*, xxxvii–xxxviii. [PubMed]
78. Storey, I.D.E.; Dutton, G.J. Uridine compounds in glucuronic acid metabolism. 2. The isolation and structure of 'uridine-diphosphate-glucuronic acid'. *Biochem. J.* **1955**, *59*, 279–288. [CrossRef] [PubMed]
79. Rowland, A.; Mackenzie, P.I.; Miners, J.O. Transporter-mediated uptake of UDP-glucuronic acid by human liver microsomes: Assay conditions, kinetics, and inhibition. *Drug Metab. Dispos.* **2015**, *43*, 147–153. [CrossRef] [PubMed]
80. Goto, S.; Taniguchi, M.; Muraoka, M.; Toyoda, H.; Sado, Y.; Kawakita, M.; Hayashi, S. UDP-sugar transporter implicated in glycosylation and processing of notch. *Nat. Cell Biol.* **2001**, *3*, 816–822. [CrossRef] [PubMed]
81. Selva, E.M.; Hong, K.; Baeg, G.H.; Beverley, S.M.; Turco, S.J.; Perrimon, N.; Hacker, U. Dual role of the fringe connection gene in both heparan sulphate and fringe-dependent signalling events. *Nat. Cell Biol.* **2001**, *3*, 809–815. [CrossRef] [PubMed]
82. Suda, T.; Kamiyama, S.; Suzuki, M.; Kikuchi, N.; Nakayama, K.; Narimatsu, H.; Jigami, Y.; Aoki, T.; Nishihara, S. Molecular cloning and characterization of a human multisubstrate specific nucleotide-sugar transporter homologous to drosophila fringe connection. *J. Biol. Chem.* **2004**, *279*, 26469–26474. [CrossRef] [PubMed]
83. Dutton, G.J. Commentary: Control of UDP-glucuronyltransferase activity. *Biochem. Pharmacol.* **1975**, *24*, 1835–1841. [CrossRef]
84. Hochman, Y.; Zakim, D. Studies of the catalytic mechanism of microsomal UDP-glucuronyltransferase. Alpha-glucuronidase activity and its stimulation by phospholipids. *J. Biol. Chem.* **1984**, *259*, 5521–5525. [PubMed]
85. Vessey, D.A.; Zakim, D. Regulation of microsomal enzymes by phospholipids. V. Kinetic studies of hepatic uridine diphosphate-glucuronyltransferase. *J. Biol. Chem.* **1972**, *247*, 3023–3028. [PubMed]
86. Magdalou, J.; Hochman, Y.; Zakim, D. Factors modulating the catalytic specificity of a pure form of UDP-glucuronyltransferase. *J. Biol. Chem.* **1982**, *257*, 13624–13629. [PubMed]
87. Dannenberg, A.; Rotenberg, M.; Zakim, D. Regulation of UDP-glucuronosyltransferase by lipid-protein interactions. Comparison of the thermotropic properties of pure reconstituted enzyme with microsomal enzyme. *J. Biol. Chem.* **1989**, *264*, 238–242. [PubMed]
88. Hochman, Y.; Kelley, M.; Zakim, D. Modulation of the number of ligand binding sites of UDP-glucuronyltransferase by the gel to liquid-crystal phase transition of phosphatidylcholines. *J. Biol. Chem.* **1983**, *258*, 6509–6516. [PubMed]
89. Erickson, R.H.; Zakim, D.; Vessey, D.A. Preparation and properties of a phospholipid-free form of microsomal UDP-glucuronyltransferase. *Biochemistry* **1978**, *17*, 3706–3711. [CrossRef] [PubMed]
90. Hochman, Y.; Zakim, D.A. Comparison of the kinetic properties of two different forms of microsomal UDP-glucuronyltransferase. *J. Biol. Chem.* **1983**, *258*, 4143–4146. [PubMed]
91. Rotenberg, M.; Zakim, D. Effect of phospholipids on the thermal stability of microsomal UDP-glucuronosyltransferase. *Biochemistry* **1989**, *28*, 8577–8582. [CrossRef] [PubMed]

92. Hochman, Y.; Zakim, D.; Vessey, D.A. A kinetic mechanism for modulation of the activity of microsomal UDP-glucuronyltransferase by phospholipids. Effects of lysophosphatidylcholines. *J. Biol. Chem.* **1981**, *256*, 4783–4788. [PubMed]
93. Simons, K.; Ikonen, E. Functional rafts in cell membranes. *Nature* **1997**, *387*, 569–572. [CrossRef] [PubMed]
94. Fujiwara, T.; Ritchie, K.; Murakoshi, H.; Jacobson, K.; Kusumi, A. Phospholipids undergo hop diffusion in compartmentalized cell membrane. *J. Cell Biol.* **2002**, *157*, 1071–1081. [CrossRef] [PubMed]
95. Brown, D.A.; London, E. Functions of lipid rafts in biological membranes. *Annu. Rev. Cell Dev. Biol.* **1998**, *14*, 111–136. [CrossRef] [PubMed]
96. Simons, K.; Toomre, D. Lipid rafts and signal transduction. *Nat. Rev. Mol. Cell Biol.* **2000**, *1*, 31–39. [CrossRef] [PubMed]
97. Suzuki, K.G.; Fujiwara, T.K.; Sanematsu, F.; Iino, R.; Edidin, M.; Kusumi, A. GPI-anchored receptor clusters transiently recruit Lyn and G alpha for temporary cluster immobilization and Lyn activation: Single-molecule tracking study 1. *J. Cell Biol.* **2007**, *177*, 717–730. [CrossRef] [PubMed]
98. Castuma, C.E.; Brenner, R.R. Cholesterol-dependent modification of microsomal dynamics and UDP-glucuronyltransferase kinetics. *Biochemistry* **1986**, *25*, 4733–4738. [CrossRef] [PubMed]
99. Castuma, C.E.; Brenner, R.R. Effect of dietary cholesterol on microsomal membrane composition, dynamics and kinetic properties of UDP-glucuronyltransferase. *Biochim. Biophys. Acta* **1986**, *855*, 231–242. [CrossRef]
100. Rotenberg, M.; Zakim, D. Effects of cholesterol on the function and thermotropic properties of pure UDP-glucuronosyltransferase. *J. Biol. Chem.* **1991**, *266*, 4159–4161. [PubMed]
101. Vessey, D.A.; Zakim, D. Regulation of microsomal enzymes by phospholipids. IV. Species differences in the properties of microsomal UDP-glucuronyltransferase. *Biochim. Biophys. Acta* **1972**, *268*, 61–69. [CrossRef]
102. Peters, W.H.; te Morsche, R.H.; Roelofs, H.M. Combined polymorphisms in UDP-glucuronosyltransferases 1A1 and 1A6: Implications for patients with Gilbert's syndrome. *J. Hepatol.* **2003**, *38*, 3–8. [CrossRef]
103. Ishii, Y.; An, K.; Nishimura, Y.; Yamada, H. ATP serves as an endogenous inhibitor of UDP-glucuronosyltransferase (UGT): A new insight into the latency of UGT. *Drug Metab. Dispos.* **2012**, *40*, 2081–2089. [CrossRef] [PubMed]
104. Ishii, Y.; Nurrochmad, A.; Yamada, H. Modulation of UDP-glucuronosyltransferase activity by endogenous compounds. *Drug Metab. Pharmacokinet* **2010**, *25*, 134–148. [CrossRef] [PubMed]
105. Nishimura, Y.; Maeda, S.; Ikushiro, S.; Mackenzie, P.I.; Ishii, Y.; Yamada, H. Inhibitory effects of adenine nucleotides and related substances on UDP-glucuronosyltransferase: Structure-effect relationships and evidence for an allosteric mechanism. *Biochim. Biophys. Acta* **2007**, *1770*, 1557–1566. [CrossRef] [PubMed]
106. Hallinan, T.; Pohl, K.R.; de Brito, R. Studies on the inhibition of hepatic microsomal glucuronidation by uridine nucleotides or adenosine triphosphate. *Med. Biol.* **1979**, *57*, 269–273. [PubMed]
107. Fujiwara, R.; Nakajima, M.; Yamanaka, H.; Katoh, M.; Yokoi, T. Product inhibition of UDP-glucuronosyltransferase (UGT) enzymes by UDP obfuscates the inhibitory effects of UGT substrates. *Drug Metab. Dispos.* **2008**, *36*, 361–367. [CrossRef] [PubMed]
108. Yokota, H.; Ando, F.; Iwano, H.; Yuasa, A. Inhibitory effects of uridine diphosphate on UDP-glucuronosyltransferase. *Life Sci.* **1998**, *63*, 1693–1699. [CrossRef]
109. Agarwal, A.K.; Monder, C.; Eckstein, B.; White, P.C. Cloning and expression of rat cDNA encoding corticosteroid 11 beta-dehydrogenase. *J. Biol. Chem.* **1989**, *264*, 18939–18943. [PubMed]
110. Rostami-Hodjegan, A. Physiologically based pharmacokinetics joined with in vitro-in vivo extrapolation of ADME: A marriage under the arch of systems pharmacology. *Clin. Pharmacol. Ther.* **2012**, *92*, 50–61. [CrossRef] [PubMed]
111. Gill, K.L.; Houston, J.B.; Galetin, A. Characterization of in vitro glucuronidation clearance of a range of drugs in human kidney microsomes: Comparison with liver and intestinal glucuronidation and impact of albumin. *Drug Metab. Dispos.* **2012**, *40*, 825–835. [CrossRef] [PubMed]

14

Revolutionizing Therapeutic Drug Monitoring with the Use of Interstitial Fluid and Microneedles Technology

Tony K.L. Kiang [1], Sahan A. Ranamukhaarachchi [2] and Mary H.H. Ensom [3,*]

1 Faculty of Pharmacy and Pharmaceutical Sciences, University of Alberta, Edmonton, AB T6G 2E1, Canada; tkiang@ualberta.ca

2 Department of Electrical and Computer Engineering, University of British Columbia, Vancouver, BC V6T 1Z4, Canada; sahan@microdermics.com

3 Faculty of Pharmaceutical Sciences, University of British Columbia, Vancouver, BC V6T 1Z3, Canada

* Correspondence: ensom@mail.ubc.ca

Abstract: While therapeutic drug monitoring (TDM) that uses blood as the biological matrix is the traditional gold standard, this practice may be impossible, impractical, or unethical for some patient populations (e.g., elderly, pediatric, anemic) and those with fragile veins. In the context of finding an alternative biological matrix for TDM, this manuscript will provide a qualitative review on: (1) the principles of TDM; (2) alternative matrices for TDM; (3) current evidence supporting the use of interstitial fluid (ISF) for TDM in clinical models; (4) the use of microneedle technologies, which is potentially minimally invasive and pain-free, for the collection of ISF; and (5) future directions. The current state of knowledge on the use of ISF for TDM in humans is still limited. A thorough literature review indicates that only a few drug classes have been investigated (i.e., anti-infectives, anticonvulsants, and miscellaneous other agents). Studies have successfully demonstrated techniques for ISF extraction from the skin but have failed to demonstrate commercial feasibility of ISF extraction followed by analysis of its content outside the ISF-collecting microneedle device. In contrast, microneedle-integrated biosensors built to extract ISF and perform the biomolecule analysis on-device, with a key feature of not needing to transfer ISF to a separate instrument, have yielded promising results that need to be validated in pre-clinical and clinical studies. The most promising applications for microneedle-integrated biosensors is continuous monitoring of biomolecules from the skin's ISF. Conducting TDM using ISF is at the stage where its clinical utility should be investigated. Based on the advancements described in the current review, the immediate future direction for this area of research is to establish the suitability of using ISF for TDM in human models for drugs that have been found suitable in pre-clinical experiments.

Keywords: clinical pharmacokinetics; therapeutic drug monitoring; interstitial fluid; microneedles

1. Introduction

Therapeutic drug monitoring (TDM) is broadly defined as the science or practice of optimizing drug therapy by targeting drug concentrations in biological matrices to the defined therapeutic range in order to increase and decrease the probabilities of efficacy and adverse effects, respectively. Fundamentally, the science of pharmacokinetics (PK) is the underpinning for the practice of TDM; that is, how the absorption, distribution, metabolism, and elimination processes of a drug dictate how TDM is implemented. Not all drugs are subjected to TDM and considerable research is continuing to be conducted on all aspects of TDM today.

From the practical stand point, the traditional gold-standard approach to TDM is to collect blood (hereafter, the term "blood" will be used in this manuscript to infer any biological matrices related to blood, plasma, or serum), because it is relatively easier to obtain compared to other matrices (e.g., organ tissues). Due to the fact that blood remains the gold standard for TDM, the majority of the target range is still being developed in this matrix. However, the primary assumption for using blood for TDM is that drug concentration in the blood compartment is reflective of that attained in the target site, which is not always the case (e.g., concentrations of antibiotics can differ in blood compared to muscle or fat tissues [1]). Moreover, the act of obtaining blood is a relatively invasive procedure which can potentially lead to untoward adverse effects such as iatrogenic infection and psychological unpleasantness [2]. In many patient populations (e.g., elderly, pediatric, anemic) and those with fragile veins, it might be impossible, impractical, or even unethical to obtain this biological fluid for any therapeutic purpose. With the substantial costs associated with collecting and analyzing blood (e.g., salary for nurses, phlebotomists, and lab technicians), it is of great interest for researchers and clinicians to find alternative biological matrices that can be as effective as blood for TDM but without the aforementioned untoward effects.

While many non-blood biological matrices have been investigated in the context of TDM [3], many have limitations that preclude their routine usage in the clinic. One of the few exceptions is interstitial fluid (ISF), which has gained a significant interest and recently fueled the research activities of many laboratories, including ours [1,4–6]. In the context of finding an alternative biological matrix for TDM, this manuscript will provide a qualitative review on: (1) the principles of TDM; (2) alternative matrices for TDM; (3) current evidence supporting the use of ISF for TDM in clinical models; (4) the use of microneedle technologies, which is potentially minimally invasive and pain-free, for the collection of ISF; and (5) future directions.

2. Principles of Therapeutic Drug Monitoring

The term therapeutic drug monitoring is often used interchangeably with clinical pharmacokinetic monitoring. TDM emerged as a clinical discipline in the late 1960s and early 1970s and involves the measurement and interpretation of drug concentrations in order to provide safe and efficacious dosing of drugs. In the past, we applied 4 basic principles to ascertain whether or not to perform routine TDM. These fundamental tenets were: (1) Is there a good relationship between drug concentration and pharmacological response? (2) Does wide interpatient variation exist in drug absorption, distribution, metabolism or excretion? (3) Does the drug have a narrow therapeutic range? and (4) Is the drug's pharmacological response not readily assessable [7,8]?

Given more recent focus on patient-centered care and individualization of dosage regimens as well as judicious use of limited resources, we added to these 4 basic principles and developed a 9-step decision-making algorithm to ascertain whether or not to perform selective TDM for a given patient in a specific scenario. The 9 steps include: (1) Is the patient on the best drug for his/her specific disease state and specific indication? (2) Can the drug be readily measured in the desired biological matrix? (3) Has a good relationship between drug concentration and pharmacologic response been reported in pharmacokinetic studies conducted in humans? (4) Does this relationship still apply to the patient's specific disease state and specific indication? (5) Is the drug's pharmacologic response not readily assessable? (6) Does the drug have a narrow therapeutic range for the specific disease state and indication? (7) Are the pharmacokinetic parameters unpredictable, due to either intrinsic variability or the presence of other confounding factors? (8) Is the duration of drug therapy of a sufficient length for the patient to benefit from clinical pharmacokinetic monitoring? and (9) Will the results of the drug assay make a significant difference in the clinical decision-making process? (i.e., provide more information than sound clinical judgement alone) [7]? If one can answer "yes" to the last question (i.e., quintessential step 9) and "yes" to most of the other questions, then selective TDM is warranted for that particular patient scenario.

From the practical stand point, TDM is usually conducted at steady-state conditions using one or more concentrations. A trough concentration is often used as a surrogate to the area-under-the concentration time curve (AUC), the best marker for drug exposure. Limited sampling strategies (i.e., using 2–4 concentration samples to predict AUC) have become more widely utilized in various disease states as well (e.g., solid organ transplant [9]). Theoretically, once the basic PK characteristics about a drug are known, TDM can be tailored to already-established fundamental PK models (e.g., one, two, three-compartments; oral vs. parenteral; intermittent vs. continuous infusion; linear vs. non-linear (Michaelis-Menten) disposition; well-stirred vs. parallel-tube, etc.). Moreover, a universally accepted idea is that only the free drug is pharmacologically active and subjected to further PK processes (e.g., metabolism or elimination). Because free drug concentrations are not easily accessible, another branch of TDM is the development of static models to "predict" free from total drug concentrations in specific patient populations (e.g., phenytoin [10,11]). Recent advances in physiologically-based PK modeling and population PK modeling [12,13] with Bayesian applications (e.g., so-called "dynamic models" [9]) have further revolutionized the prediction/simulation of drug concentrations for TDM as well.

Since the publication of the decision-making algorithm in 1998, many clinician researchers have used it to critically assess currently available literature and determine the utility of TDM for specific drugs in specific patient scenarios [7]. Examples of papers in various therapeutic classes and special populations are available: central nervous system disorders (e.g., [14,15]), infectious disease (e.g., [16,17]), organ transplant (e.g., [18,19]), pediatric patients (e.g., [20,21]), cancer (e.g., [22]), psychiatric disorders (e.g., [23,24]). This paper will focus on step 2—can the drug be readily measured in the desired biological matrix?

3. Alternative Matrices for Therapeutic Drug Monitoring

Many alternative, less-invasive biological matrices (e.g., ISF, oral fluids, hair, sweat, tears, semen, breast milk, urine) have been investigated for the purpose of TDM [3,25]. In our opinion, with exceptions of a few specific applications where a certain matrix (e.g., tears) is preferred in unique situations (e.g., drug concentrations in eye disorders) [25], only saliva and ISF show the potential to replace blood primarily because drug concentrations can be quantified reliably and consistently in these matrices.

The science and practice of saliva TDM is still undergoing significant evolution [26–29]. Although saliva can be used for the monitoring of illicit drug use (i.e., "doping") [30], the discussion here will focus only on TDM. Saliva is composed of aqueous fluids secreted by three salivary glands [28]. The composition of saliva, with respect to electrolytes and macromolecules, can differ based on intrinsic (e.g., healthy vs. diseased) and extrinsic (e.g., concurrent drugs that modulate the sympathetic or parasympathetic systems; method of saliva simulation) factors [27,28]. A common observation, however, is that protein content is significantly lower in saliva compared to blood [27,28]. There are many advantages and disadvantages of using saliva for diagnostics, which have been extensively reviewed [26–29]. For the purpose of TDM, the primary advantages for using saliva are the non-invasive nature for obtaining this biological fluid and the fact that saliva drug concentration reflects the free (i.e., pharmacologically active) concentration. Because of the latter characteristic, saliva has the distinct benefit over other matrices (e.g., whole tissue, blood) which are protein-rich and require additional analytical techniques to determine free drug concentrations. The primary disadvantages for using saliva for TDM are potential contaminants, drug instability, and lack of phase II metabolites [3,29]. In order for saliva to replace blood for the purpose of TDM, correlations between saliva-blood concentrations also need to be established.

The biochemical properties of xenobiotics (i.e., ionizability, molecular weight, lipophilicity, protein binding) are known to affect the distribution/excretion of drug into saliva [31]. Of these, the ionizability of the drug molecule in saliva appears to play a primary role in the penetration ratio because only unionized drugs can partition into this matrix [29]. Based on these principles, not all drugs are detectable in saliva. The first documented salivary TDM dates back to the 1970s when theophylline [32], digoxin [33], lithium [34], and various anticonvulsant drugs [35] were initially investigated. Since then, the suitability of conducting TDM in saliva for drugs in various therapeutic classes has been reported. While not the primary objective of this paper, the most recent review articles—based on therapeutic classes—on salivary TDM are cited here for the reader's reference: antibiotics [36], anticonvulsants [37], antiretroviral agents [38], and psychotropics [39].

Similar to saliva, ISF has very similar composition as plasma but lower protein content [40]; therefore, drugs are mostly present in ISF in the free (active) form and the matrix is relatively easier to assay compared to blood. Because ISF serves as the connection between vasculature and cells, it acts as a conduit or medium for various signaling molecules and cellular wastes [41], although the exact composition of ISF can differ between organs or locations [40]. In addition to TDM, ISF has been used for other purposes such as diagnostics (e.g., for monitoring the degree of traumatic brain injury) [40] or treatment (e.g., being the primary site for many bacterial infections) [1]. The use of ISF for TDM can have several advantages: potentially pain-free (to be discussed below in the section on sampling techniques, including the use of microneedles), less cumbersome analytical assays (because the matrix is relatively clean and devoid of large macromolecules or cellular debris), and potentially less costly because the collection does not require specially trained personnel. Similar to saliva, however, in order for ISF to replace blood for the purpose of TDM, correlations between ISF-blood concentrations need to be established. On the other hand, unlike saliva, factors influencing the partitioning of drugs between blood and ISF are relatively poorly understood. Although biochemical properties (e.g., ionizability, molecular weight, lipophilicity, protein binding) can theoretically affect drug distribution into ISF, no good correlations have been observed with most of these variables in the currently available literature [1]. Although data are available on drug distribution kinetics (including model-based predictions) into whole tissues (e.g., [42–45]), the ISF compartment would exhibit different physiological properties and warrant an investigation itself. The currently available evidence supporting the use of ISF for TDM in humans is presented in the next section.

4. Current Evidence Supporting the Use of Interstitial Fluid for Therapeutic Drug Monitoring in Clinical Models

For the purpose of this manuscript, data pertaining to cerebral spinal fluid, brain extracellular fluid, tumor ISF, or any internal organ tissue fluid which is not routinely sampled and cannot be characterized non-invasively for the purpose of TDM will be excluded. This approach is similar to exclusion criteria we published previously [1]. Likewise, only studies incorporating microdialysis have been included, because other models (skin blisters, whole tissue) do not adequately reflect the ISF space [1]. Based on our comprehensive investigation in an animal model using an extensive panel of drugs commonly subjected to TDM today [4], a novel scoring algorithm was developed to characterize the suitability of conducting TDM in ISF: directly suitable ("comparable exposure and similar concentration-time profile versus blood"); likely suitable ("different exposure, but similar concentration-time profile versus blood"); unlikely suitable ("detectable in ISF, but different concentration-time profile versus blood"); and not suitable ("not detected in ISF") [4]. We have already used this algorithm to analyze the suitability of using ISF or saliva for TDM in humans for anti-infective drugs [1,36]. The same principles will be employed in this paper to discuss the evidence supporting the use of ISF for TDM of other drug classes. In short, the current state of knowledge on the use of ISF for TDM in humans is still limited. A thorough literature review indicates that only a few drug classes have been investigated (i.e., anti-infectives, anticonvulsants, and miscellaneous other agents). A body of literature is also available on the measurement of drug concentrations in solid tumors [46–52] which is excluded from this paper (i.e., not used routinely for the purpose of TDM) and has been reviewed elsewhere [53,54].

4.1. Anti-Infectives

The majority of the ISF data collected in humans to date is related to anti-infectives because ISF is the primary target compartment of interests for various types of infections [1]. The evidence supporting the use of ISF for TDM for antibiotics has been systematically reviewed by Kiang et al. up to February 2014 [1], which will be summarized briefly. Additional novel data published since this paper will be presented in more detail.

Kiang et al. [1] provided a comprehensive review detailing 87 individual PK comparisons between tissue ISF and blood on various antibiotic classes: penicillins, cephalosporins, fluoroquinolones, carbapenems, oxazolidiones, macrolides, glycopeptides/glycylcycline/lipopeptide and other agents. Overall, different antibiotics exhibited different degrees of penetration into ISF of muscle or adipose tissue [1]. With respect to penicillins, the majority of data were collected on piperacillin, which showed reduced concentration in ISF compared to blood, especially in critically ill (i.e., intensive care) patients. The ability of a specific cephalosporin (i.e., cefaclor, cefixime, cefodizime, cefpirome, cefpodoxime, ceftobiprole, cefuroxime) to penetrate into ISF also appears to be dependent on the type of tissue (i.e., muscle vs. adipose) and the degree of protein binding. In the case of cefpirome, a significant reduction in ISF penetration was observed in critically ill patients, indicating that a potentially more aggressive dosing regimen might be warranted in this patient population [1]. More recently, Roberts et al. [55] compared the pharmacokinetics of cefazolin in subcutaneous ISF and blood in post-trauma critically ill patients ($N = 30$) and found similar exposure (median % penetration ratio of 74%) between the two matrices. Despite the fact that specific pharmacokinetic values were not reported, the concentration-time profiles between the two matrices appear approximately "equivalent", indicating that it is suitable to monitor cefazolin in ISF in this population (albeit cefazolin concentrations are not typically measured in clinical practice). Overall, most of the penicillins and cephalosporins can be categorized as likely suitable drugs for TDM in ISF, due to comparable elimination characteristics but different exposure values in both blood and ISF.

Different degrees of tissue ISF penetration were observed for carbapenems in humans [1]. While doripenem and ertapenem show consistent distribution ratios between different tissues, inconsistent findings were reported for imipenem between muscle and adipose and between studies. The inconsistencies found with imipenem may have been attributed to experimental artifacts, pointing to the potential limitations of comparing findings from multiple sources utilizing different microdialysis calibration techniques. Moreover, imipenem's distribution into ISF in critically ill patients might be dependent on renal function, as evident by contrasting findings shown by Tegeder et al. [56] and Dahyot et al. [57]. More recently, Varghese et al. [58] determined the penetration ratio of meropenem in critically ill patients receiving continuous hemodialysis and noted reduced exposure in subcutaneous ISF (60–74%) compared to blood. Although it was not clear whether the free blood concentration was determined in this study, the concentration-time profiles of meropenem in both matrices exhibited similar characteristics. Overall, the carbapenems can be categorized as likely suitable for TDM in ISF, due to comparable elimination characteristics but different exposure values in both blood and ISF [1].

With respect to the glycopeptides/glycylcycline/lipopeptides, both daptomycin and tigecycline distribute into tissue ISF completely in a manner independent of tissue inflammation or the diagnosis of diabetes [1]. These data suggest that daptomycin and tigecycline could be likely suitable for TDM in ISF (although they are not subjected to routine TDM today). Although vancomycin distributes well into tissues (penetration ratio of 0.8 from comparable exposure in two matrices based on free concentrations) in otherwise healthy subjects with limb infections [59], evidence suggests a reduced penetration in diabetic patients [60,61]. Population modeling also suggests potential suboptimal vancomycin tissue exposure in diabetics which may result in treatment failure [60], but these simulations require further testing in real clinical subjects. The findings for vancomycin in humans of comparable pharmacokinetic characteristics between ISF and blood is consistent with that observed in various animal models, including that published in our own lab [1,62]. Because vancomycin is one of the most frequently monitored drugs in the clinic today, these data suggest that vancomycin could be a potential drug candidate to test the paradigm of using ISF for the purpose of TDM. However, more studies are needed to characterize the effects of intrinsic and extrinsic factors that may affect the disposition characteristics of vancomycin. Further pharmacokinetic modeling is also needed to determine the relationship between ISF and blood concentrations, tailored for the purpose of TDM.

In contrast to the heterogeneity of tissue ISF penetration characteristics observed within many antibiotic classes presented in this manuscript, some consistent class effects of robust tissue distribution could be observed for fluoroquinolones (ciprofloxacin, levofloxacin, moxifloxacin, except for gemifloxacin) and oxazolidinones (linezolid and torezolid) [1], because the distribution ratios appear complete and independent of tissue type (muscle vs. adipose) or disease state (healthy vs. sepsis or diabetes). On the other hand, many macrolide antibiotics (except for telithromycin) penetrate into tissue ISF relatively poorly, resulting in potentially suboptimal drug concentrations at the target site [1]. Based on these characteristics and the available limited data, fluoroquinolones and oxazolidinones in general might be suitable for TDM in ISF whereas the macrolides would not be suitable. While the clinical utility of fluoroquinolone or oxazolidinone TDM still remains to be established, further research is needed to elucidate how drugs in certain classes penetrate into ISF space better than others and careful consideration is needed when selecting and avoiding antibiotic classes for the treatment of tissue infections.

4.2. *Anticonvulsants*

There is a significant interest regarding TDM for anticonvulsants using alternative body fluids [37,63] and ISF is no exception. The majority of the experiments pertaining to ISF have been conducted with valproic acid [64–67] although preliminary data on other agents (topiramate, carbamazepine, phenytoin, and phenobarbital) are also available [68,69]. Given that patients taking these agents are often monitored on an outpatient basis, having a TDM matrix that is more convenient than blood could potentially improve patient care and quality of life. Although these authors indicated collecting extracellular fluid, their approach (i.e., in vivo microdialysis on subcutaneous tissue) is reflective of free drug concentrations in ISF. The data for valproic acid look promising in that there is a good qualitative correlation between free tissue and blood concentrations in epileptic [64] and healthy subjects [65]. Moreover, the concentration-time profiles of free valproic acid in epileptic patients ($N = 3$) receiving a single dose of valproic acid or in one subject under steady-state conditions were virtually superimposable between ISF and blood [66]. However, a subsequent study using a larger sample size indicated a higher free fraction in plasma under steady-state conditions compared to single-dose conditions [67]. Although specific pharmacokinetic parameters were lacking in these studies to allow a systematic categorization of suitability, these data are suggestive of the general appropriateness of using ISF for TDM for valproic acid. Given that valproic acid is a frequently monitored anticonvulsant drug today, further systematic studies are needed to establish the quantitative relationships between ISF and blood (i.e., using compartmental, population modeling) under various conditions (e.g., single-dose vs. steady-state, healthy vs. various diseased populations requiring valproic acid, mono-therapy vs. polypharmacy, etc.) in order to determine the role of ISF for TDM.

In a single epileptic patient receiving doses of topiramate (not under steady-state conditions) co-administered with phenytoin and dextropropoxifen, the concentration-time profiles of free topiramate in subcutaneous ISF and blood were comparable with a high correlation coefficient (0.99) [69]. Likewise, in single case studies of patients undergoing tapering regimens, carbamazepine and phenobarbital [68] also exhibited similar pharmacokinetic characteristics in subcutaneous ISF and blood up to 70 h post-dose. In Lindberger et al. [68], phenytoin was not detectable in tissue ISF due to extensive binding to the microdialysis tubing. The observation of likely suitable nature with phenobarbital is consistent with our observation in rabbits [4]. Although we noticed the same effects (lack of detection in ISF) with phenytoin in our rabbit experiments, it was not due to recovery, indicating other factors that may prevent phenytoin's distribution into ISF should also be considered. Unfortunately, neither study provided quantitative pharmacokinetic data to allow a systematic determination of suitability of conducting TDM in ISF for these anticonvulsants. Given that topiramate drug concentrations can be used occasionally to guide dosing in refractory, resistant seizure cases, and that phenobarbital and carbamazepine are routinely monitored, more studies in larger patient samples are warranted.

4.3. *Miscellaneous Agents*

The concentrations of various other drugs have been determined in ISF and compared to blood. Boschmann et al. [70] compared the concentrations of aliskiren in obese hypertensive subjects ($N = 10$)

in adipose ISF, skeletal muscle ISF, and blood under steady-state conditions. Aliskiren appeared to distribute to skeletal muscle ISF (concentration comparable to blood) to a greater extent compared to adipose ISF. Because pharmacokinetic parameters were not characterized in this study, it was not possible to determine the suitability of conducting TDM in ISF for aliskiren. The concentration-time profile of a single healthy subject administered caffeine was illustrated by Stahle et al. [71]. Caffeine presented in the ISF at higher concentrations than blood (i.e., increased exposure), suggesting that additional mechanisms other than simple diffusion might be responsible for its distribution into the tissue compartment. Based on the five individual ISF concentration-time profiles presented in the study, it appeared that the pharmacokinetics of caffeine exhibit large variability in ISF; however, similar information was not provided in blood to draw any correlations. Pharmacokinetic parameters needed for the assessment for suitability of TDM in ISF were not presented for caffeine by Stahle et al. [71]. Stetina et al. [72] characterized the concentration-time profiles of scopolamine (after a single intravenous dose) in adipose tissue ISF and blood in healthy male subjects ($N = 6$) and found similar pharmacokinetic characteristics between the two matrices. Despite reduced maximum concentration and delayed time-to-reach maximum concentration, the overall exposure of scopolamine between the two matrices was essentially the same, as evident by a distribution ratio approaching unity. These characteristics suggest that scopolamine can potentially be a suitable agent to be monitored in ISF, although TDM for scopolamine is not currently clinically indicated.

5. Microneedle Technologies for Interstitial Fluid Collection for Therapeutic Drug Monitoring

Microneedle technologies have been used in non-clinical and clinical settings for their TDM, diagnostics, and physiological health monitoring using ISF rather than blood, as described here. ISF is trapped in its extracellular matrices of skin [73] leading to difficulties in extracting in biosensing applications. Considering limited availability of ISF in the skin (~20 nL mm^{-2} in the epidermis and ~800 nL mm^{-2} in the dermis [73]), extracting large volumes of ISF for bioanalysis is a major hurdle in developing sensors that rely on ISF extraction. Development of microneedle-integrated biosensors can potentially provide commercially feasible solutions to TDM and diagnostics [74]. A summary of microneedle strategies used for ISF collection and TDM is presented in Table 1.

Table 1. Summary of microneedle strategies used for interstitial fluid (ISF) collection and therapeutic drug monitoring.

Microneedle Device Strategy	Description	Indication	Testing Model	ISF Volume Collected/Required
ISF extraction and off-device analysis	Glass hollow microneedle (0.7–1.5 mm long) and vacuum-assisted ISF collection [75]	Glucose	Tail vein of rats, finger tips of humans	1–10 μL
	Dissolving microneedle "poke" followed by vacuum suction [62]	Vancomycin	Male Wistar rats	2 μL
	Solid microneedle arrays "poked" the skin, and hydrogel "patch" collected ISF [76]	Glucose and sodium ion concentration	Human subjects	<10 μL
	Hydrogel forming microneedle array [77–79]	Theophylline, caffeine, glucose	Pigs, rats, and human subjects	-
ISF extraction and on-device analysis	Hollow microneedles with integrated ISF collection reservoir [80]	Glucose	Human subject	-
	Hollow microneedle array integrated with screen-printed enzyme sensor [81]	Glucose	In vitro bench testing	10 μL
	Hollow microneedle integrated with optofluidic sensor [6]	Vancomycin	In vitro bench testing	0.6 nL
Continuous ISF monitoring	Hollow microneedle integrated with buffer-filled glucose sensor [82]	Glucose	Human subjects	-

5.1. Interstitial Fluid Extraction Devices for Off-Device Analysis

Several studies have successfully demonstrated techniques for ISF extraction from the skin, followed by analysis of its content outside the ISF-collecting microneedle device (hereafter termed "off-device analysis"). For example, Wang et al. [75] used a glass microneedle device to penetrate 0.7–1.5 mm into the skin in hairless rats and healthy adults, and collect 1–10 μL of ISF using a 200–500 mm Hg vacuum for 2 to 10 min for glucose measurement. Sakaguchi et al. [76] overcame vacuum-assisted extraction by applying a solid microneedle array to create micropores on the skin surface followed by a hydrogel patch to collect ISF by swelling action for glucose and sodium ion concentration measurement. Donnelly et al. [77] developed a hydrogel-forming microneedle array, using blends of hydrolyzed poly(methyl-vinylether-*co*-maleic anhydride) and polyethylene glycol crosslinked by esterification, which increased its mass when applied to skin, due to ISF uptake by the hydrogel. Caffarrel-Salvador et al. [78], Romanyuk et al. [79], and Chang et al. [83] showed that extremely small volumes of ISF (<20 μL) can be extracted by similar hydrogel-forming swellable microneedle-arrays over 1 to 2 h in porcine, human (Figure 1) [78], rat [79], and mice [83] skins.

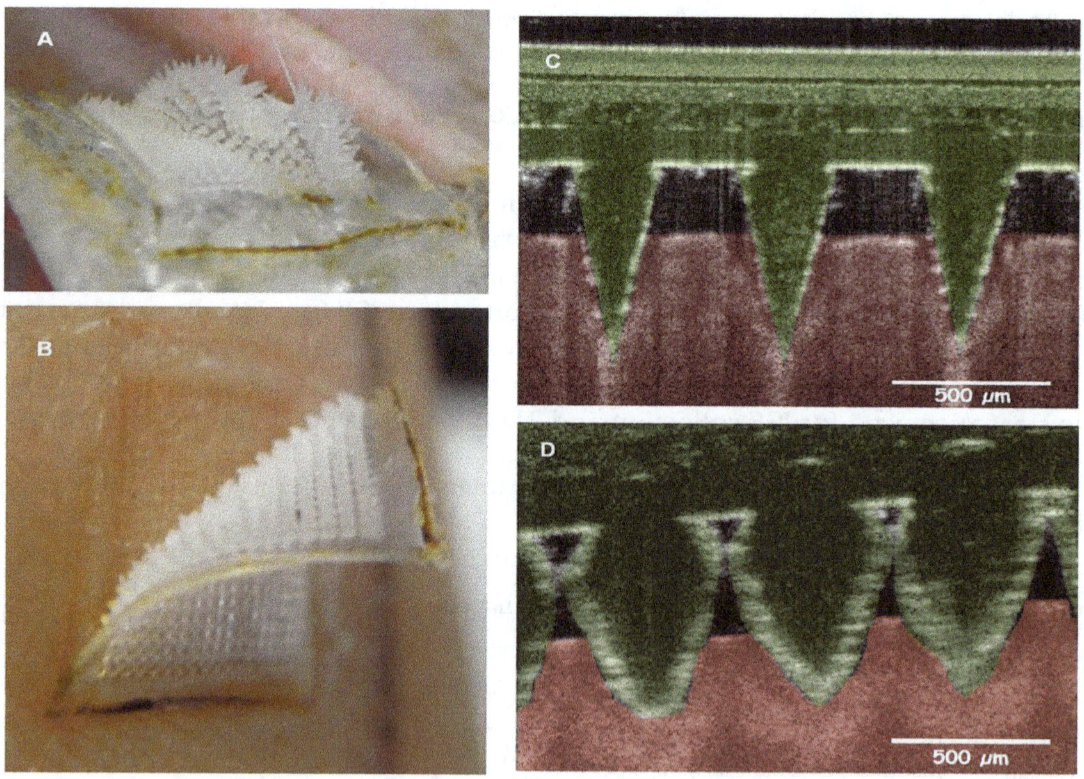

Figure 1. Hydrogel-forming microneedles for extraction of analytes from ISF. Figure obtained from Caffarel-Salvador et al. with permission [78]. A hydrogel forming microneedle array (**A**) before application into the skin and (**B**) after application where microneedles are swollen. Optical coherent tomography images show the microneedle arrays after skin insertion (**C**) before swelling, and (**D**) after swelling.

Research conducted to date have failed to demonstrate commercial feasibility of ISF extraction followed by off-device analysis for various reasons. These include prolonged ISF extraction time, need for multiple steps between sample extraction and bioanalysis, need to further extract and/or transfer the fluid from the collection apparatus to a separate site for analysis, extremely low volume of ISF collected, and evaporation of ISF leading to measurement variability and error [74].

5.2. Interstitial Fluid Extraction for On-Device Analysis

Microneedle-integrated biosensors were built to extract ISF and perform the biomolecule analysis on-device, with a key feature of not needing to transfer ISF to a separate instrument. Mukerjee et al. [80] devised a hollow silicone microneedle-integrated system to collect water, glycerol, ISF, and whole blood. ISF was extracted in vivo from human earlobe skin over a 15 to 20-min period, and analyzed qualitatively for glucose [80]. Zimmerman et al. [84] developed a hollow silicon microneedle array integrated into an enzymatic glucose sensor with a porous dialysis membrane, and showed a significant sensor response after exposure to ISF ex vivo. Strambini et al. [81] developed a similar glucose sensor with hollow silicon-dioxide microneedle arrays (1×10^6 needles cm^{-2}) connected to chip consisting screen-printed enzymatic glucose sensor integrated to the backside of the microneedle array for ISF collection and bioanalysis. Ex vivo evaluation showed rapid detection of glucose [81]. Although more commercially feasible than ISF collection devices for off-device analysis, devices with integrated on-device analytical capabilities consist of some challenges, including the need for microliter-level volumes of ISF for analysis, prolonged time to collect ISF, and transfer of ISF to the backside of the microneedle for bioanalysis.

Ranamukhaarachchi et al. [6] developed a point-of-care TDM device by integrating a gold-coated hollow microneedle with an optofluidic sensing system to detect vancomycin in sub-nanoliter volumes of fluid in vitro. Vancomycin receptors were immobilized inside the microneedle lumen (Figure 2), which collected 0.6 nL of sample (i.e., ISF) within seconds, and caused vancomycin to bind to the microneedle lumen for quantification.

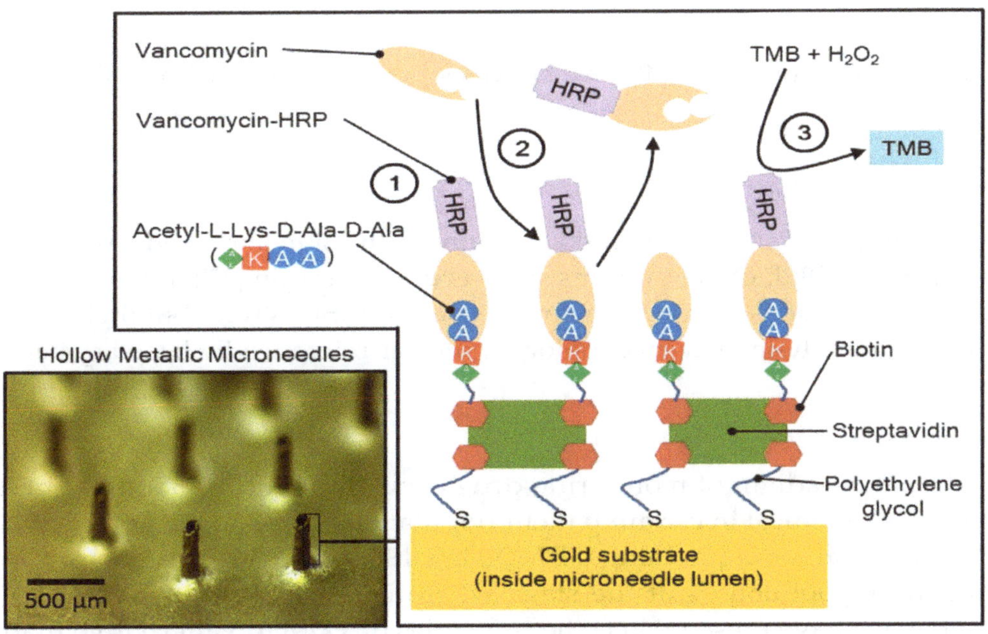

Figure 2. Functionalization of gold-coated hollow microneedle lumens for fluid collection, drug binding, and detection. Figure obtained from Ranamukhaarachchi et al. with permission [6].

The extremely small sample volume, capability to detect low concentration TDM drugs, rapid operation from collection to analysis (altogether less than 5 min TDM time), and lack of need for sample transfer from the collection site to analytical site were key advantages of this system. However, this system needs to be validated in pre-clinical and clinical studies [74].

5.3. Continuous Monitoring Microneedle Devices

The most promising applications for microneedle-integrated biosensors is continuous monitoring of biomolecules from the skin's ISF. Jina et al. [82] developed a hollow microneedle-integrated continuous glucose monitoring (CGM) biosensor, and demonstrated accurate and continuous glucose measurements in humans using ISF up to 72 h. The sensing chamber (Figure 3), located behind the microneedle array, was filled with a buffer solution to transfer glucose passively from ISF to sensor, eliminating the need for removal of ISF from the skin [82]. The main advantages of this system are lack of volume requirement for ISF extraction, real-time bioanalysis, and limited number of steps to obtain bioanalytical results [74].

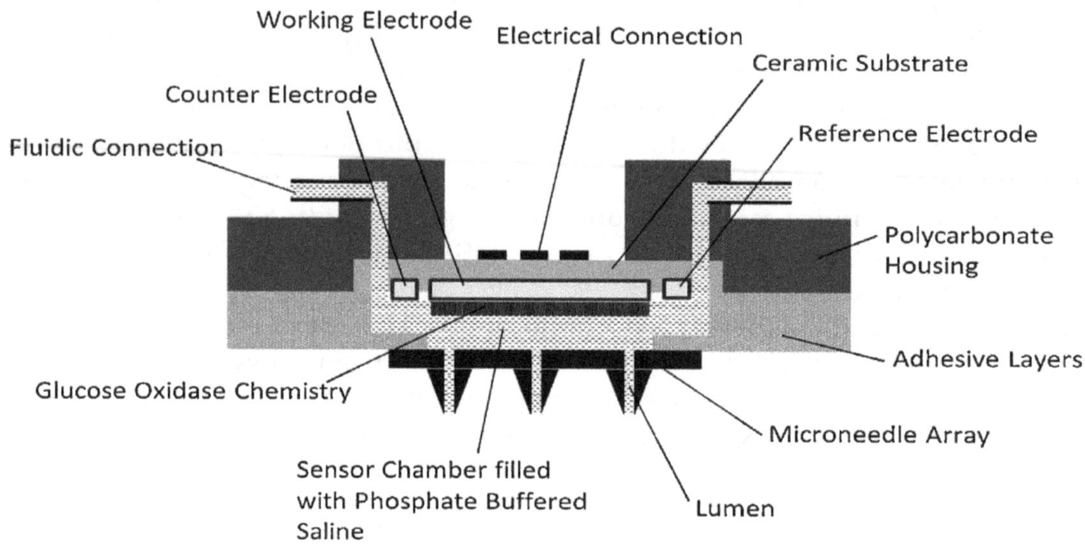

Figure 3. Continuous glucose monitoring biosensor. Figure obtained from Chua et al. with permission [85].

5.4. Other Methods for ISF Extraction

Microdialysis catheters can be implanted in or under the skin and used to extract biomolecules, such as glucose, from ISF [86]. Other systems such as ultrafiltration [87], reverse iontophoresis [88], and sonophoresis [89] have all been used previously to extract ISF as well, but their potential is limited compared to more minimally-invasive technologies such as microneedle-based systems.

6. Future Directions

The conventional paradigm of monitoring drug concentrations in blood might be impractical, costly, and sometimes unethical in certain patient populations (e.g., pediatric, elderly, or those with "bad" veins). A new way of conducting TDM using ISF is gaining momentum in the research community and, in our opinion, is at the stage where its clinical utility should be investigated. In this review paper, we have presented (1) the principles of TDM; (2) alternative matrices for TDM; (3) current evidence supporting the use of ISF for TDM in clinical models; and (4) the use of microneedle technologies, which is potentially minimally invasive and pain-free, for the collection of ISF. Based on these advancements, the immediate future direction for this area of research is to establish the suitability of using ISF for TDM in human models for drugs that have been found "suitable" in pre-clinical experiments. In order to do this, a systematic approach involving compartmental modeling, physiologically-based modeling, and population pharmacokinetic modeling would have to be utilized. The effects of intrinsic and extrinsic factors that can potentially affect the pharmacokinetics of particular drugs in ISF should be incorporated into these clinical studies to fully capture the covariates and variabilities associated with this approach. In the more distant future, microneedle devices, such as those described in this review, that are minimally invasive and potentially pain-free should be tested on humans to determine their utility in the collection of ISF. Ultimately, we envision point-of-care devices where pain-free ISF collection (via a microneedle-like device), drug concentration assessment, and dosing can be done in real time, at the bedside.

Acknowledgments: No sources of funding were received for the preparation of this manuscript. The authors would like to acknowledge Urs O. Häfeli, for his invaluable input and guidance.

References

1. Kiang, T.K.; Hafeli, U.O.; Ensom, M.H. A Comprehensive Review on the Pharmacokinetics of Antibiotics in Interstitial Fluid Spaces in Humans: Implications on Dosing and Clinical Pharmacokinetic Monitoring. *Clin. Pharmacokinet.* **2014**, *53*, 695–730. [CrossRef] [PubMed]
2. Koka, S.; Beebe, T.J.; Merry, S.P.; DeJesus, R.S.; Berlanga, L.D.; Weaver, A.L.; Montori, V.M.; Wong, D.T. The Preferences of Adult Outpatients in Medical or Dental Care Settings for Giving Saliva, Urine or Blood for Clinical Testing. *J. Am. Dent. Assoc.* **2008**, *139*, 735–740. [CrossRef] [PubMed]
3. Pichini, S.; Altieri, I.; Zuccaro, P.; Pacifici, R. Drug Monitoring in Nonconventional Biological Fluids and Matrices. *Clin. Pharmacokinet.* **1996**, *30*, 211–228. [CrossRef] [PubMed]
4. Kiang, T.K.; Schmitt, V.; Ensom, M.H.; Chua, B.; Hafeli, U.O. Therapeutic Drug Monitoring in Interstitial Fluid: A Feasibility Study using a Comprehensive Panel of Drugs. *J. Pharm. Sci.* **2012**, *101*, 4642–4652. [CrossRef] [PubMed]
5. Hafeli, U.O.; Ensom, M.H.; Kiang, T.K.; Stoeber, B.; Chua, B.A.; Pudek, M.; Schmitt, V. Comparison of Vancomycin Concentrations in Blood and Interstitial Fluid: A Possible Model for Less Invasive Therapeutic Drug Monitoring. *Clin. Chem. Lab. Med.* **2011**, *49*, 2123–2125. [CrossRef] [PubMed]
6. Ranamukhaarachchi, S.A.; Padeste, C.; Dubner, M.; Hafeli, U.O.; Stoeber, B.; Cadarso, V.J. Integrated Hollow Microneedle-Optofluidic Biosensor for Therapeutic Drug Monitoring in Sub-Nanoliter Volumes. *Sci. Rep.* **2016**, *6*, 29075. [CrossRef] [PubMed]
7. Ensom, M.H.; Davis, G.A.; Cropp, C.D.; Ensom, R.J. Clinical Pharmacokinetics in the 21st Century. Does the Evidence Support Definitive Outcomes? *Clin. Pharmacokinet.* **1998**, *34*, 265–279. [CrossRef] [PubMed]
8. DiPiro, J.; Blouin, R.; Pruemer, J.; Spruill, W. *Concepts in Clinical Pharmacokinetics: A Self-Instructional Course*, 2nd ed.; American Society of Health-System Pharmacists Inc.: Bethesda, MD, USA, 1996; p. 200.
9. Kiang, T.K.; Ensom, M.H. Therapeutic Drug Monitoring of Mycophenolate in Adult Solid Organ Transplant Patients: An Update. *Expert Opin. Drug Metab. Toxicol.* **2016**, *12*, 545–553. [CrossRef] [PubMed]
10. Kiang, T.K.; Ensom, M.H. A Comprehensive Review on the Predictive Performance of the Sheiner-Tozer and Derivative Equations for the Correction of Phenytoin Concentrations. *Ann. Pharmacother.* **2016**, *50*, 311–325. [CrossRef] [PubMed]
11. Cheng, W.; Kiang, T.K.; Bring, P.; Ensom, M.H. Predictive Performance of the Winter-Tozer and Derivative Equations for Estimating Free Phenytoin Concentration. *Can. J. Hosp. Pharm.* **2016**, *69*, 269–279. [CrossRef] [PubMed]
12. Kiang, T.K.; Sherwin, C.M.; Spigarelli, M.G.; Ensom, M.H. Fundamentals of Population Pharmacokinetic Modelling: Modelling and Software. *Clin. Pharmacokinet.* **2012**, *51*, 515–525. [CrossRef] [PubMed]
13. Sherwin, C.M.; Kiang, T.K.; Spigarelli, M.G.; Ensom, M.H. Fundamentals of Population Pharmacokinetic Modelling: Validation Methods. *Clin. Pharmacokinet.* **2012**, *51*, 573–590. [CrossRef] [PubMed]
14. Bring, P.; Ensom, M.H. Does Oxcarbazepine Warrant Therapeutic Drug Monitoring? A Critical Review. *Clin. Pharmacokinet.* **2008**, *47*, 767–778. [CrossRef] [PubMed]
15. Tan, J.; Paquette, V.; Levine, M.; Ensom, M.H. Levetiracetam Clinical Pharmacokinetic Monitoring in Pediatric Patients with Epilepsy. *Clin. Pharmacokinet.* **2017**. [CrossRef] [PubMed]
16. Kuo, I.F.; Ensom, M.H. Role of Therapeutic Drug Monitoring of Voriconazole in the Treatment of Invasive Fungal Infections. *Can. J. Hosp. Pharm.* **2009**, *62*, 469–482. [CrossRef] [PubMed]
17. Ng, K.; Mabasa, V.H.; Chow, I.; Ensom, M.H. Systematic Review of Efficacy, Pharmacokinetics, and Administration of Intraventricular Vancomycin in Adults. *Neurocrit. Care* **2014**, *20*, 158–171. [CrossRef] [PubMed]
18. Stenton, S.B.; Partovi, N.; Ensom, M.H. Sirolimus: The Evidence for Clinical Pharmacokinetic Monitoring. *Clin. Pharmacokinet.* **2005**, *44*, 769–786. [CrossRef] [PubMed]

19. Ng, J.C.; Leung, M.; Wright, A.J.; Ensom, M.H. Clinical Pharmacokinetic Monitoring of Leflunomide in Renal Transplant Recipients with BK Virus Reactivation: A Review of the Literature. *Clin. Pharmacokinet.* **2017**, *56*, 1015–1031. [CrossRef] [PubMed]
20. Kendrick, J.G.; Carr, R.R.; Ensom, M.H. Pharmacokinetics and Drug Dosing in Obese Children. *J. Pediatr. Pharmacol. Ther.* **2010**, *15*, 94–109. [PubMed]
21. Strong, D.K.; Lai, A.; Primmett, D.; White, C.T.; Lirenman, D.S.; Carter, J.E.; Hurley, R.M.; Virji, M.; Ensom, M.H. Limited Sampling Strategy for Cyclosporine (Neoral) Area under the Curve Monitoring in Pediatric Kidney Transplant Recipients. *Pediatr. Transplant.* **2005**, *9*, 566–573. [CrossRef] [PubMed]
22. Teng, J.F.; Mabasa, V.H.; Ensom, M.H. The Role of Therapeutic Drug Monitoring of Imatinib in Patients with Chronic Myeloid Leukemia and Metastatic or Unresectable Gastrointestinal Stromal Tumors. *Ther. Drug Monit.* **2012**, *34*, 85–97. [CrossRef] [PubMed]
23. Schwenger, E.; Dumontet, J.; Ensom, M.H. Does Olanzapine Warrant Clinical Pharmacokinetic Monitoring in Schizophrenia? *Clin. Pharmacokinet.* **2011**, *50*, 415–428. [CrossRef] [PubMed]
24. Seto, K.; Dumontet, J.; Ensom, M.H. Risperidone in Schizophrenia: Is there a Role for Therapeutic Drug Monitoring? *Ther. Drug Monit.* **2011**, *33*, 275–283. [CrossRef] [PubMed]
25. Raju, K.S.; Taneja, I.; Singh, S.P.; Wahajuddin. Utility of Noninvasive Biomatrices in Pharmacokinetic Studies. *Biomed. Chromatogr.* **2013**, *27*, 1354–1366. [CrossRef] [PubMed]
26. Haeckel, R.; Hanecke, P. The Application of Saliva, Sweat and Tear Fluid for Diagnostic Purposes. *Ann. Biol. Clin.* **1993**, *51*, 903–910.
27. Aps, J.K.; Martens, L.C. Review: The Physiology of Saliva and Transfer of Drugs into Saliva. *Forensic Sci. Int.* **2005**, *150*, 119–131. [CrossRef] [PubMed]
28. Nunes, L.A.; Mussavira, S.; Bindhu, O.S. Clinical and Diagnostic Utility of Saliva as a Non-Invasive Diagnostic Fluid: A Systematic Review. *Biochem. Med.* **2015**, *25*, 177–192. [CrossRef] [PubMed]
29. Mullangi, R.; Agrawal, S.; Srinivas, N.R. Measurement of Xenobiotics in Saliva: Is Saliva an Attractive Alternative Matrix? Case Studies and Analytical Perspectives. *Biomed. Chromatogr.* **2009**, *23*, 3–25. [CrossRef] [PubMed]
30. Anizan, S.; Huestis, M.A. The Potential Role of Oral Fluid in Antidoping Testing. *Clin. Chem.* **2014**, *60*, 307–322. [CrossRef] [PubMed]
31. Haeckel, R. Factors Influencing the saliva/plasma Ratio of Drugs. *Ann. N. Y. Acad. Sci.* **1993**, *694*, 128–142. [CrossRef] [PubMed]
32. Levy, G.; Ellis, E.F.; Koysooko, R. Indirect Plasma-Theophylline Monitoring in Asthmatic Children by Determination of Theophylline Concentration in Saliva. *Pediatrics* **1974**, *53*, 873–876. [PubMed]
33. Jusko, W.J.; Gerbracht, L.; Golden, L.H.; Koup, J.R. Digoxin Concentrations in Serum and Saliva. *Res. Commun. Chem. Pathol. Pharmacol.* **1975**, *10*, 189–192. [PubMed]
34. Neu, C.; DiMascio, A.; Williams, D. Saliva Lithium Levels: Clinical Applications. *Am. J. Psychiatry* **1975**, *132*, 66–68. [PubMed]
35. McAuliffe, J.J.; Sherwin, A.L.; Leppik, I.E.; Fayle, S.A.; Pippenger, C.E. Salivary Levels of Anticonvulsants: A Practical Approach to Drug Monitoring. *Neurology* **1977**, *27*, 409–413. [CrossRef] [PubMed]
36. Kiang, T.K.; Ensom, M.H. A Qualitative Review on the Pharmacokinetics of Antibiotics in Saliva: Implications on Clinical Pharmacokinetic Monitoring in Humans. *Clin. Pharmacokinet.* **2016**, *55*, 313–358. [CrossRef] [PubMed]
37. Patsalos, P.N.; Berry, D.J. Therapeutic Drug Monitoring of Antiepileptic Drugs by use of Saliva. *Ther. Drug Monit.* **2013**, *35*, 4–29. [CrossRef] [PubMed]
38. Ter Heine, R.; Beijnen, J.H.; Huitema, A.D. Bioanalytical Issues in Patient-Friendly Sampling Methods for Therapeutic Drug Monitoring: Focus on Antiretroviral Drugs. *Bioanalysis* **2009**, *1*, 1329–1338. [CrossRef] [PubMed]
39. Pichini, S.; Papaseit, E.; Joya, X.; Vall, O.; Farre, M.; Garcia-Algar, O.; de laTorre, R. Pharmacokinetics and Therapeutic Drug Monitoring of Psychotropic Drugs in Pediatrics. *Ther. Drug Monit.* **2009**, *31*, 283–318. [CrossRef] [PubMed]
40. Venkatesh, B.; Morgan, T.J.; Cohen, J. Interstitium: The Next Diagnostic and Therapeutic Platform in Critical Illness. *Crit. Care Med.* **2010**, *38*, S630–S636. [CrossRef] [PubMed]
41. Wiig, H.; Swartz, M.A. Interstitial Fluid and Lymph Formation and Transport: Physiological Regulation and Roles in Inflammation and Cancer. *Physiol. Rev.* **2012**, *92*, 1005–1060. [CrossRef] [PubMed]

42. Poulin, P. Drug Distribution to Human Tissues: Prediction and Examination of the Basic Assumption in in Vivo Pharmacokinetics-Pharmacodynamics (PK/PD) Research. *J. Pharm. Sci.* **2015**, *104*, 2110–2118. [CrossRef] [PubMed]
43. Poulin, P. A Paradigm Shift in Pharmacokinetic-Pharmacodynamic (PKPD) Modeling: Rule of Thumb for Estimating Free Drug Level in Tissue Compared with Plasma to Guide Drug Design. *J. Pharm. Sci.* **2015**, *104*, 2359–2368. [CrossRef] [PubMed]
44. Poulin, P.; Haddad, S. Advancing Prediction of Tissue Distribution and Volume of Distribution of Highly Lipophilic Compounds from a Simplified Tissue-Composition-Based Model as a Mechanistic Animal Alternative Method. *J. Pharm. Sci.* **2012**, *101*, 2250–2261. [CrossRef] [PubMed]
45. Poulin, P.; Schoenlein, K.; Theil, F.P. Prediction of Adipose Tissue: Plasma Partition Coefficients for Structurally Unrelated Drugs. *J. Pharm. Sci.* **2001**, *90*, 436–447. [CrossRef]
46. Konings, I.R.; Sleijfer, S.; Mathijssen, R.H.; de Bruijn, P.; Ghobadi Moghaddam-Helmantel, I.M.; van Dam, L.M.; Wiemer, E.A.; Verweij, J.; Loos, W.J. Increasing Tumoral 5-Fluorouracil Concentrations during a 5-Day Continuous Infusion: A Microdialysis Study. *Cancer Chemother. Pharmacol.* **2011**, *67*, 1055–1062. [CrossRef] [PubMed]
47. Konings, I.R.; Engels, F.K.; Sleijfer, S.; Verweij, J.; Wiemer, E.A.; Loos, W.J. Application of Prolonged Microdialysis Sampling in Carboplatin-Treated Cancer Patients. *Cancer Chemother. Pharmacol.* **2009**, *64*, 509–516. [CrossRef] [PubMed]
48. Muller, M.; Mader, R.M.; Steiner, B.; Steger, G.G.; Jansen, B.; Gnant, M.; Helbich, T.; Jakesz, R.; Eichler, H.G.; Blochl-Daum, B. 5-Fluorouracil Kinetics in the Interstitial Tumor Space: Clinical Response in Breast Cancer Patients. *Cancer Res.* **1997**, *57*, 2598–2601. [PubMed]
49. Muller, M.; Brunner, M.; Schmid, R.; Mader, R.M.; Bockenheimer, J.; Steger, G.G.; Steiner, B.; Eichler, H.G.; Blochl-Daum, B. Interstitial Methotrexate Kinetics in Primary Breast Cancer Lesions. *Cancer Res.* **1998**, *58*, 2982–2985. [PubMed]
50. Blochl-Daum, B.; Muller, M.; Meisinger, V.; Eichler, H.G.; Fassolt, A.; Pehamberger, H. Measurement of Extracellular Fluid Carboplatin Kinetics in Melanoma Metastases with Microdialysis. *Br. J. Cancer* **1996**, *73*, 920–924. [CrossRef] [PubMed]
51. Thompson, J.F.; Siebert, G.A.; Anissimov, Y.G.; Smithers, B.M.; Doubrovsky, A.; Anderson, C.D.; Roberts, M.S. Microdialysis and Response during Regional Chemotherapy by Isolated Limb Infusion of Melphalan for Limb Malignancies. *Br. J. Cancer* **2001**, *85*, 157–165. [CrossRef] [PubMed]
52. Quist, S.R.; Quist, J.; Birkenmaier, J.; Stauch, T.; Gollnick, H.P. Pharmacokinetic Profile of Methotrexate in Psoriatic Skin Via the Oral Or Subcutaneous Route using Dermal Microdialysis Showing Higher Methotrexate Bioavailability in Psoriasis Plaques than in Non-Lesional Skin. *J. Eur. Acad. Dermatol. Venereol.* **2016**, *30*, 1537–1543. [CrossRef] [PubMed]
53. Zhou, Q.; Gallo, J.M. In Vivo Microdialysis for PK and PD Studies of Anticancer Drugs. *AAPS J.* **2005**, *7*, E659–E667. [CrossRef] [PubMed]
54. Chu, J.; Gallo, J.M. Application of Microdialysis to Characterize Drug Disposition in Tumors. *Adv. Drug Deliv. Rev.* **2000**, *45*, 243–253. [CrossRef]
55. Roberts, J.A.; Udy, A.A.; Jarrett, P.; Wallis, S.C.; Hope, W.W.; Sharma, R.; Kirkpatrick, C.M.; Kruger, P.S.; Roberts, M.S.; Lipman, J. Plasma and Target-Site Subcutaneous Tissue Population Pharmacokinetics and Dosing Simulations of Cefazolin in Post-Trauma Critically Ill Patients. *J. Antimicrob. Chemother.* **2015**, *70*, 1495–1502. [CrossRef] [PubMed]
56. Tegeder, I.; Schmidtko, A.; Brautigam, L.; Kirschbaum, A.; Geisslinger, G.; Lotsch, J. Tissue Distribution of Imipenem in Critically Ill Patients. *Clin. Pharmacol. Ther.* **2002**, *71*, 325–333. [CrossRef] [PubMed]
57. Dahyot, C.; Marchand, S.; Bodin, M.; Debeane, B.; Mimoz, O.; Couet, W. Application of Basic Pharmacokinetic Concepts to Analysis of Microdialysis Data: Illustration with Imipenem Muscle Distribution. *Clin. Pharmacokinet.* **2008**, *47*, 181–189. [CrossRef] [PubMed]
58. Varghese, J.M.; Jarrett, P.; Wallis, S.C.; Boots, R.J.; Kirkpatrick, C.M.; Lipman, J.; Roberts, J.A. Are Interstitial Fluid Concentrations of Meropenem Equivalent to Plasma Concentrations in Critically Ill Patients Receiving Continuous Renal Replacement Therapy? *J. Antimicrob. Chemother.* **2015**, *70*, 528–533. [CrossRef] [PubMed]
59. Housman, S.T.; Bhalodi, A.A.; Shepard, A.; Nugent, J.; Nicolau, D.P. Vancomycin Tissue Pharmacokinetics in Patients with Lower-Limb Infections Via in Vivo Microdialysis. *J. Am. Podiatr. Med. Assoc.* **2015**, *105*, 381–388. [CrossRef] [PubMed]

60. Hamada, Y.; Kuti, J.L.; Nicolau, D.P. Vancomycin Serum Concentrations do Not Adequately Predict Tissue Exposure in Diabetic Patients with Mild to Moderate Limb Infections. *J. Antimicrob. Chemother.* **2015**, *70*, 2064–2067. [CrossRef] [PubMed]
61. Skhirtladze, K.; Hutschala, D.; Fleck, T.; Thalhammer, F.; Ehrlich, M.; Vukovich, T.; Muller, M.; Tschernko, E.M. Impaired Target Site Penetration of Vancomycin in Diabetic Patients Following Cardiac Surgery. *Antimicrob. Agents Chemother.* **2006**, *50*, 1372–1375. [CrossRef] [PubMed]
62. Ito, Y.; Inagaki, Y.; Kobuchi, S.; Takada, K.; Sakaeda, T. Therapeutic Drug Monitoring of Vancomycin in Dermal Interstitial Fluid using Dissolving Microneedles. *Int. J. Med. Sci.* **2016**, *13*, 271–276. [CrossRef] [PubMed]
63. Linder, C.; Andersson, M.; Wide, K.; Beck, O.; Pohanka, A. A LC–MS/MS Method for Therapeutic Drug Monitoring of Carbamazepine, Lamotrigine and Valproic Acid in DBS. *Bioanalysis* **2015**, *7*, 2031–2039. [CrossRef] [PubMed]
64. Stahle, L.; Alm, C.; Ekquist, B.; Lundquist, B.; Tomson, T. Monitoring Free Extracellular Valproic Acid by Microdialysis in Epileptic Patients. *Ther. Drug Monit.* **1996**, *18*, 14–18. [CrossRef] [PubMed]
65. Lindberger, M.; Tomson, T.; Stahle, L. Validation of Microdialysis Sampling for Subcutaneous Extracellular Valproic Acid in Humans. *Ther. Drug Monit.* **1998**, *20*, 358–362. [CrossRef] [PubMed]
66. Lindberger, M.; Tomson, T.; Wallstedt, L.; Stahle, L. Distribution of Valproate to Subdural Cerebrospinal Fluid, Subcutaneous Extracellular Fluid, and Plasma in Humans: A Microdialysis Study. *Epilepsia* **2001**, *42*, 256–261. [PubMed]
67. Lindberger, M.; Tomson, T.; Stahle, L. Unbound Valproate Fraction in Plasma and Subcutaneous Microdialysate in Steady State and After a Single Dose in Humans. *Ther. Drug Monit.* **2003**, *25*, 378–383. [CrossRef] [PubMed]
68. Lindberger, M.; Tomson, T.; Lars, S. Microdialysis Sampling of Carbamazepine, Phenytoin and Phenobarbital in Subcutaneous Extracellular Fluid and Subdural Cerebrospinal Fluid in Humans: An In Vitro and In Vivo Study of Adsorption to the Sampling Device. *Pharmacol. Toxicol.* **2002**, *91*, 158–165. [CrossRef] [PubMed]
69. Lindberger, M.; Tomson, T.; Ohman, I.; Wallstedt, L.; Stahle, L. Estimation of Topiramate in Subdural Cerebrospinal Fluid, Subcutaneous Extracellular Fluid, and Plasma: A Single Case Microdialysis Study. *Epilepsia* **1999**, *40*, 800–802. [CrossRef] [PubMed]
70. Boschmann, M.; Nussberger, J.; Engeli, S.; Danser, A.H.; Yeh, C.M.; Prescott, M.F.; Dahlke, M.; Jordan, J. Aliskiren Penetrates Adipose and Skeletal Muscle Tissue and Reduces Renin-Angiotensin System Activity in Obese Hypertensive Patients. *J. Hypertens.* **2012**, *30*, 561–566. [CrossRef] [PubMed]
71. Stahle, L.; Arner, P.; Ungerstedt, U. Drug Distribution Studies with Microdialysis. III: Extracellular Concentration of Caffeine in Adipose Tissue in Man. *Life Sci.* **1991**, *49*, 1853–1858. [CrossRef]
72. Stetina, P.M.; Madai, B.; Kulemann, V.; Kirch, W.; Joukhadar, C. Pharmacokinetics of Scopolamine in Serum and Subcutaneous Adipose Tissue in Healthy Volunteers. *Int. J. Clin. Pharmacol. Ther.* **2005**, *43*, 134–139. [CrossRef] [PubMed]
73. Groenendaal, W.; von Basum, G.; Schmidt, K.A.; Hilbers, P.A.; van Riel, N.A. Quantifying the Composition of Human Skin for Glucose Sensor Development. *J. Diabetes Sci. Technol.* **2010**, *4*, 1032–1040. [CrossRef] [PubMed]
74. Ranamukhaarachchi, S. Skin Mechanics, Intradermal Delivery and Biosensing with Hollow Metallic Microneedles. Ph.D. Thesis, University of British Columbia, Vancouver, BC, Canada, December 2016.
75. Wang, P.M.; Cornwell, M.; Prausnitz, M.R. Minimally Invasive Extraction of Dermal Interstitial Fluid for Glucose Monitoring using Microneedles. *Diabetes Technol. Ther.* **2005**, *7*, 131–141. [CrossRef] [PubMed]
76. Sakaguchi, K.; Hirota, Y.; Hashimoto, N.; Ogawa, W.; Sato, T.; Okada, S.; Hagino, K.; Asakura, Y.; Kikkawa, Y.; Kojima, J.; et al. A Minimally Invasive System for Glucose Area Under the Curve Measurement using Interstitial Fluid Extraction Technology: Evaluation of the Accuracy and Usefulness with Oral Glucose Tolerance Tests in Subjects with and without Diabetes. *Diabetes Technol. Ther.* **2012**, *14*, 485–491. [CrossRef] [PubMed]
77. Donnelly, R.F.; Mooney, K.; Caffarel-Salvador, E.; Torrisi, B.M.; Eltayib, E.; McElnay, J.C. Microneedle-Mediated Minimally Invasive Patient Monitoring. *Ther. Drug Monit.* **2014**, *36*, 10–17. [CrossRef] [PubMed]

78. Caffarel-Salvador, E.; Brady, A.J.; Eltayib, E.; Meng, T.; Alonso-Vicente, A.; Gonzalez-Vazquez, P.; Torrisi, B.M.; Vicente-Perez, E.M.; Mooney, K.; Jones, D.S.; et al. Hydrogel-Forming Microneedle Arrays Allow Detection of Drugs and Glucose in Vivo: Potential for use in Diagnosis and Therapeutic Drug Monitoring. *PLoS ONE* **2015**, *10*, e0145644. [CrossRef] [PubMed]
79. Romanyuk, A.V.; Zvezdin, V.N.; Samant, P.; Grenader, M.I.; Zemlyanova, M.; Prausnitz, M.R. Collection of Analytes from Microneedle Patches. *Anal. Chem.* **2014**, *86*, 10520–10523. [CrossRef] [PubMed]
80. Mukerjee, E.V.; Collins, S.D.; Isseroff, R.R.; Smith, R.L. Microneedle Array for Transdermal Biological Fluid Extraction and in Situ Analysis. *Sens. Actuators A Phys.* **2004**, *114*, 267–275. [CrossRef]
81. Strambini, L.M.; Longo, A.; Scarano, S.; Prescimone, T.; Palchetti, I.; Minunni, M.; Giannessi, D.; Barillaro, G. Self-Powered Microneedle-Based Biosensors for Pain-Free High-Accuracy Measurement of Glycaemia in Interstitial Fluid. *Biosens. Bioelectron.* **2015**, *66*, 162–168. [CrossRef] [PubMed]
82. Jina, A.; Tierney, M.J.; Tamada, J.A.; McGill, S.; Desai, S.; Chua, B.; Chang, A.; Christiansen, M. Design, Development, and Evaluation of a Novel Microneedle Array-Based Continuous Glucose Monitor. *J. Diabetes Sci. Technol.* **2014**, *8*, 483–487. [CrossRef] [PubMed]
83. Chang, H.; Zheng, M.; Yu, X.; Than, A.; Seeni, R.Z.; Kang, R.; Tian, J.; Khanh, D.P.; Liu, L.; Chen, P.; et al. A Swellable Microneedle Patch to Rapidly Extract Skin Interstitial Fluid for Timely Metabolic Analysis. *Adv. Mater.* **2017**, *37*. [CrossRef] [PubMed]
84. Zimmermann, S.; Fienbork, D.; Flounders, A.W.; Liepmann, D. In-Device Enzyme Immobilization: Wafer-Level Fabrication of an Integrated Glucose Sensor. *Sens. Actuators B Chem.* **2004**, *99*, 163–173. [CrossRef]
85. Chua, B.; Desai, S.P.; Tierney, M.J.; Tamada, J.A.; Jina, A.N. Effect of Microneedles Shape on Skin Penetration and Minimally Invasive Continuous Glucose Monitoring In Vivo. *Sens. Actuators A Phys.* **2013**, *203*, 373–381. [CrossRef]
86. Heinemann, L.; Glucose Monitoring Study Group. Continuous Glucose Monitoring by Means of the Microdialysis Technique: Underlying Fundamental Aspects. *Diabetes Technol. Ther.* **2003**, *5*, 545–561. [CrossRef] [PubMed]
87. Tiessena, R.G.; Kapteinab, W.A.; Venemaa, K.; Korf, J. Slow Ultrafiltration for Continuous In Vivo Sampling: Application for Glucose and Lactate in Man. *Anal. Chim. Acta* **1999**, *379*, 327–335. [CrossRef]
88. Tamada, J.A.; Bohannon, N.J.; Potts, R.O. Measurement of Glucose in Diabetic Subjects using Noninvasive Transdermal Extraction. *Nat. Med.* **1995**, *1*, 1198–1201. [CrossRef] [PubMed]
89. Kost, J.; Mitragotri, S.; Gabbay, R.A.; Pishko, M.; Langer, R. Transdermal Monitoring of Glucose and Other Analytes using Ultrasound. *Nat. Med.* **2000**, *6*, 347–350. [CrossRef] [PubMed]

15

Bioavailability of Eurycomanone in its Pure Form and in a Standardised *Eurycoma longifolia* Water Extract

Norzahirah Ahmad [1,*], Dodheri Syed Samiulla [2], Bee Ping Teh [1], Murizal Zainol [1], Nor Azlina Zolkifli [1], Amirrudin Muhammad [1], Emylyn Matom [1], Azlina Zulkapli [3], Noor Rain Abdullah [1], Zakiah Ismail [1] and Ami Fazlin Syed Mohamed [1]

1 Herbal Medicine Research Centre, Institute for Medical Research, Jalan Pahang, Kuala Lumpur 50588, Malaysia; bpteh_km@yahoo.com (B.P.T.); murizal@imr.gov.my (M.Z.); norazlina@imr.gov.my (N.A.Z.); amiruddin@imr.gov.my (A.M.); emylynm@gmail.com (E.M.); noorrain@imr.gov.my (N.R.A.); drzakiah@gmail.com (Z.I.); ami@imr.gov.my (A.F.S.M.)

2 Aurigene Discovery Technologies Limited, Electronic City, Hosur Road, Bangalore 560100, Karnataka, India; samiulla_d@aurigene.com

3 Medical Resource Research Centre, Institute for Medical Research, Jalan Pahang, Kuala Lumpur 50588, Malaysia; azlina@imr.gov.my

* Correspondence: norzahirah@imr.gov.my

Abstract: *Eurycoma longifolia* is one of the commonly consumed herbal preparations and its major chemical compound, eurycomanone, has been described to have antimalarial, antipyretic, aphrodisiac, and cytotoxic activities. Today, the consumption of *E. longifolia* is popular through the incorporation of its extract in food items, most frequently in drinks such as tea and coffee. In the current study, the characterisation of the physicochemical and pharmacokinetic (PK) attributes of eurycomanone were conducted via a series of in vitro and in vivo studies in rats and mice. The solubility and chemical stability of eurycomanone under the conditions of the gastrointestinal tract environment were determined. The permeability of eurycomanone was investigated by determining its distribution coefficient in aqueous and organic environments and its permeability using the parallel artificial membrane permeability assay system and Caco-2 cultured cells. Eurycomanone's stability in plasma and its protein-binding ability were measured by using an equilibrium dialysis method. Its stability in liver microsomes across species (mice, rat, dog, monkey, and human) and rat liver hepatocytes was also investigated. Along with the PK evaluations of eurycomanone in mice and rats, the PK parameters for the Malaysian Standard (MS: 2409:201) standardised water extract of *E. longifolia* were also evaluated in rats. Both rodent models showed that eurycomanone in both the compound form and extract form had a half-life of 0.30 h. The differences in the bioavailability of eurycomanone in the compound form between the rats (11.8%) and mice (54.9%) suggests that the PK parameters cannot be directly extrapolated to humans. The results also suggest that eurycomanone is not readily absorbed across biological membranes. However, once absorbed, the compound is not easily metabolised (is stable), hence retaining its bioactive properties, which may be responsible for the various reported biological activities.

Keywords: eurycomanone; *Eurycoma longifolia*; bioavailability; pharmacokinetic

---

1. Introduction

Eurycomanone is uniquely found in *Eurycoma longifolia* Jack (family Simaroubaceae), which is a herbaceous tree found mainly in Southeast Asia. Eurycomanone is reported to be the most abundant phytochemical quassinoid in *E. longifolia* roots [1–8]. The MS: 2409:201 of producing a freeze-dried standardised water extract of *E. longifolia* uses eurycomanone as the chemical marker.

The eurycomanone level must be consistently present at 0.80–1.50% *w*/*v*, alongside other markers such as total polysaccharides, total protein, and total glycosaponin, where their levels are expected at >20%. Traditionally, *E. longifolia* was used for ailments such as fever, wounds, and ulcers, as well as an afterbirth remedy or as a general tonic [9,10]. Biological activities of *E. longifolia* previously reported, such as male fertility enhancement [4,11] and antimalarial [12–17], cytotoxic [14,15,18], antiproliferative [19,20], and antiulcer [21] effects, are largely attributed to the quassinoids group, specifically eurycomanone.

Studies identifying eurycomanone as the compound responsible for these reported activities mainly focused on in vitro systems. Previous investigation into the physicochemical properties of several quassinoids of *E. longifolia* [16] revealed that eurycomanone and 13-α-(21)-epoxyeurycomanone possessed the necessary characteristics contributing to *E. longifolia*'s effect. Favourable physicochemical properties such as solubility, lipophilicity, chemical stability, permeability, plasma stability, and plasma protein binding act as indicators of the marker's behavior in the body. The behaviour of eurycomanone in the body is of interest as the consumption of *E. longifolia* in the forms of water extracts incorporated into health supplements and beverages are the common strategies for marketed *E. longifolia*-based products. Oral consumption of *E. longifolia* in these various forms exposes its active ingredients to varying environment, which may affect their bioavailability in the body.

Bioavailability measures the delivery of an active ingredient to its site of action in order to cause the predicted effect(s). First-pass metabolism in the liver can markedly reduce the amount of eurycomanone available to the site of action, which can be predicted in vitro by assessing its metabolic stability prior to its administration orally. Previously reported eurycomanone bioavailability in rats was studied using extracts with differing amounts of eurycomanone [7,22,23].

Experimentally based data on eurycomanone's bioavailability will be highly essential if a standardised extract is to be clinically tested. Nevertheless, to date, no bioavailability study on the standardised water extract form has been previously conducted. This study investigates the bioavailability of eurycomanone in its pure form and in a standardised water extract of *E. longifolia*.

2. Materials and Methods

2.1. Chemicals and Reagents

Standardised water extract of *E. longifolia* used conformed to the MS: 2409:201 and contained eurycomanone (1.36%), total protein (30.5%), total polysaccharide (37.8%), and glycosaponin (52%). Eurycomanone (94.8% purity) was obtained from ChromaDex Inc. (Irvine, CA, USA). Propranolol, estriol, metoprolol tartrate, diethylstil bestrol, erythromycin, atenolol, carbamazepine, propantheline bromide, enalapril, dasatinib, midazolam, terfinadine, alamethicin, uridine 5′-diphospho-glucuronosyltransferase (UDPGA), nicotinamide adenine dinucleotide phosphate (NADPH), *N*-methyl-2-pyrrolidone (NMP), 2-hydroxypropyl-beta-cyclodextrin (HPCD), and chemicals used in reagents and buffer preparations were purchased from Sigma Chemical Co. (St. Louis, MO, USA). Plasma and microsomes from mice and rats were prepared in-house, whilst plasma and microsomes from dog, monkey, and human were purchased from Thermo Fisher Scientific (Waltham, MA, USA). Solvents such as methanol, formic acid, acetonitrile (ACN), and DMSO used were of LC-MS and HPLC grade and were purchased from Fisher Chemicals (Waltham, MA, USA).

2.2. Animal Experiments

2.2.1. Eurycomanone Assessment

The ethical approval for the animal experiments conducted in India was granted from the Animal Ethics Committee, Aurigene Discovery Technologies, Bangalore, India. Eight male Wistar rats (12 weeks old; weighing 250–350 g) and eight Caeserean Derived-1 (CD-1) mice (weighing 20–30 g) were obtained from the Animal House, Aurigene Discovery Technologies, Bangalore, India. They were supplied with standard rodent diets and drinking water ad libitum. Each rodent species (i.e., rats and mice) were divided into two groups. One group ($n = 3$ for each rodent species) was administered with eurycomanone via the intravenous route (IV) and another group ($n = 3$ for each rodent species) via the oral route (PO) using oral gavage intubation needle. Two animals of each of the species were used as a control and they received reverse osmosis water. All rats underwent jugular vein cannulation surgery 72 h prior to the administration of the eurycomanone.

2.2.2. Standardised Water Extract of *E. longifolia* (SWE) Assessment

The animal experiment conducted in Malaysia was approved by the Animal Care and Use Committee, Ministry of Health Malaysia (ACUC Number: ACUC/KKM/02(1/2014)). Ten male Sprague Dawley rats (12 weeks old; weighing 250–400 g) were obtained from the Laboratory Animal Resource Unit, Institute for Medical Research, Kuala Lumpur, Malaysia. They were supplied with standard rodent diets and drinking water ad libitum. One group ($n = 4$) was administered with SWE via the IV route and another group ($n = 4$) via the PO route using oral gavage intubation needle. Two rats were used as the control and they were administered reverse osmosis water. All rats underwent jugular vein cannulation surgery 72 h prior to the administration of SWE. All animals were maintained in a 12-h light and dark cycle, the temperature was maintained between 22 ± 3 °C, and the relative humidity between 50–65%.

2.3. *Sample Preparation*

Eurycomanone (rats: 1.5 mg/mL for IV route and 3.0 mg/mL for PO route; mice: 0.5 mg/mL for IV route and 1.0 mg/mL for PO route) samples were prepared fresh on the day of dosing. For the IV administration, eurycomanone was dissolved in 3% NMP and 97% of 10% HPCD in saline. For the oral administration, eurycomanone was dissolved in 3% NMP and 97% of 30% HPCD in saline. Both samples were sonicated before use. The SWE (5 mg/mL for IV route, 10 mg/mL for PO route) was prepared fresh on the day of dosing. For the IV administration, the SWE was dissolved in reverse osmosis water and filtered (0.2 μm pore size) before administration. The SWE for the PO administration was prepared using the same method, except without filtering. The animals were not fasted and doses given were based on the body weights prior to dosing.

2.4. *Specimen Collection*

Blood specimens (approximately 0.30–0.40 mL via the jugular vein cannula for rats and 0.10–0.20 mL via submanibular bleeding for mice) were collected at time points 0.083 (IV group only), 0.25, 0.5, 1, 2, 4, 6, and 8 h post-dosing with eurycomanone. At the experiment end point, the animals were euthanized by excess isoflurane inhalation followed by cervical dislocation. In the experiment using SWE, the rats were placed in metabolic cages (Techniplast, West Chester, PA, USA) and blood (approximately 0.30–0.40 mL collected via the jugular vein cannula), urine, and faeces specimens were collected at the same time points with the above plus one additional time point of 24 h. Kidney and liver specimens were collected at necropsy, where the rats were euthanized by CO_2 inhalation followed by cervical dislocation. All blood specimens were centrifuged (10,000 rpm, 10 min) to obtain plasma and were stored at −80 °C until processed. Urine and faeces specimens were collected into plastic containers on wet ice while the organ specimens were snap-frozen in liquid nitrogen and maintained at −80 °C until processed.

2.5. *Specimen Preparation for LC-MS/MS Analysis*

Plasma specimens (100 μL), collected from the eurycomanone experiment were added with the internal standard solution (10 μL). Plasma proteins were precipitated with ACN (300 μL), vortex-mixed for 5 min, and centrifuged at 4000 rpm for 7 min. The supernatant was collected and evaporated using a nitrogen evaporator for 20 min at 50 °C. Thereafter, they were reconstituted with the mobile phase (500 μL) and transferred into LC-MS vials for analysis.

Plasma specimens (200 μL) from the SWE experiment were added with the internal standard solution (50 μL). Plasma proteins were precipitated with ACN (400 μL), vortex-mixed for 5 min, and centrifuged at 4000 rpm for 7 min. The supernatant was collected and evaporated to dryness using nitrogen evaporator at 60 °C. Thereafter, they were reconstituted with 80 μL of 30% methanol: 70% (0.1% formic acid) and transferred into LC-MS vials for analysis.

Urine specimens (200 μL) were added with ACN (400 μL), vortex-mixed for 5 min, and centrifuged at 4000 rpm for 7 min. The supernatant was collected and evaporated to dryness using a nitrogen evaporator at 60 °C. Thereafter, they were reconstituted with 80 μL of 10% methanol: 90% (0.1% formic acid) and transferred into LC-MS vials for analysis.

Faeces specimens were weighed, ultrapure water (at 8 times the weighed samples) was added, and samples were homogenised. The homogenised faeces samples (200 μL) were added with ACN (400 μL), vortex-mixed for 5 min, and centrifuged at 4000 rpm for 7 min. The supernatant was collected and evaporated to dryness using a nitrogen evaporator at 60 °C. Thereafter, they were reconstituted with 80 μL of 5% methanol: 95% (0.1% formic acid) and transferred into LC-MS vials for analysis.

Tissue specimens (kidneys and livers) were blotted with filter paper, weighed, and minced. Ultrapure water (at 3 times the weighed tissue samples) were added and samples were homogenised. The homogenised tissue specimens (200 μL) were added with ACN (400 μL), vortex-mixed for 5 min, and centrifuged at 4000 rpm for 7 min. The supernatant was collected and evaporated to dryness using a nitrogen evaporator at 60 °C. Thereafter, they were reconstituted with 80 μL of 5% methanol: 95% (0.1% formic acid) and transferred into LC-MS vials for analysis.

2.6. LC-MS/MS Analysis

Eurycomanone detection in the pure eurycomanone experiments was done via the LC-MS/MS system consisting of an Agilent 1260 Infinity HPLC system and an AB SCIEX API 4000™ Triple-Quadrupole mass spectrometer equipped with TurboIonSpray® probe and atmospheric pressure chemical ionization (APCI) (AB Sciex LLC, Framingham, MA, USA). Electrospray ionization (ESI) was performed in positive ion mode. The analytical column was Agilent Zorbax Eclipse-C18 (4.6 mm I.D. × 150 mm, 3.5 μm). The mobile phase consisted of 0.1% formic acid (solvent A) and 90% ACN with 0.1% formic acid (solvent B). The flow rate was set at 1.2 mL/min and the injection volume was 50 μL with the run time of 3.5 min. The mass transitions, monitored using multiple-reaction monitoring (MRM) detections, were 409 → 221.1/143.1 for eurycomanone. Eurycomanone detection in the SWE experiments were done via an LC-MS system consisting of Agilent 1100 series HPLC and mass spectrometer detector system with APCI-ESI ionization mode (Agilent Technologies, Santa Clara, CA, USA).

For plasma specimens, the analytical column used was Agilent Zorbax Eclipse XDB-Phenyl (2.1 mm I.D. × 50 mm, 5 μm). The mobile phase consisted of 35% methanol: 65% (0.1% formic acid). The flow rate was set at 0.2 mL/min and the injection volume was 2 μL with the run time of 5 min. For urine samples, the analytical column was Agilent Zorbax Eclipse XDB-Phenyl (2.1 mm I.D. × 50 mm, 3.5 μm). The mobile phase consisted of 10% methanol: 90% (0.1% formic acid). The flow rate was set at 0.2 mL/min and the injection volume was 2 μL with the run time of 5 min.

For faeces, kidney, and liver specimens, the analytical column used was Agilent Zorbax Eclipse XDB-Phenyl (2.1 mm I.D. × 50 mm, 3.5 μm). The mobile phase consisted of 5% methanol: 95% (0.1% formic acid). The flow rate was set at 0.2 mL/min and the injection volume was 2 μL with the run time of 6 min. The identification of eurycomanone and internal standard for plasma matrix were achieved by comparing the ion sets in selected ion monitoring (SIM) for eurycomanone with sodium adduct (m/z 431.0) and metronidazole (172.0 g/mol) in samples with the standard solution, at a similar retention time using LC-MS analysis. The concentration of the specimens analysed were determined by using an inverse prediction method for the best-fit regression curve using the weighted least-square (WLS) of $\frac{1}{x^2}$, obtained from the standard concentrations.

In the analytical run, each standard in the calibration curve for each matrix was checked for the accuracy to be in the range of 80–120% for the lower limit of quantification (LLOQ) concentration and 85–115% for the remaining standards. Each quality control (QC) concentration was also checked for the accuracy to be in the range of 80–120% for the LLOQ concentration and 85–115% for the remaining QC samples. Sample matrices from the control group (blank samples) were used in the preparation of the calibration curve for determining eurycomanone concentrations. The pharmacokinetic analysis was performed using the non-compartmental analysis of Phoenix™ WinNolin®software (version 1.3, Certara, L.P., Princeton, NJ, USA).

2.7. Aqueous Solubility, Lipophilicity, and Chemical Stability of Eurycomanone

The aqueous stability was estimated by adding 10 µL of eurycomanone stock solution (10 mM) to 490 µL of aqueous buffer at pH 5.4, pH 7.4 and DMSO in triplicates in deep-well plates. Three standards (propanolol, estriol, and tamoxifen) at the same concentration were also added in the deep-well plates. The plate was kept on a shaker (300 rpm) at room temperature for 16 h. The plate was then centrifuged at 25 °C, 4000 rpm for 25 min. The supernatant was transferred and analysed using LC-MS/MS. The aqueous solubility was calculated using the following formula:

$$\text{Aqueous stability} = \frac{200\ \mu\text{M} \times \text{Peak area 1}}{\text{Peak area 2}}$$

Peak area 1 = peak area of the compound in 2% DMSO at the different pH levels.

Peak area 2 = peak area of the compound in 100% DMSO.

The lipophilicity of eurycomanone was estimated using the shake flask method with octanol and buffer (pH 7.4). Eurycomanone (5 µL) at 5 mM concentration is added to octanol (495 µL) and DMSO (495 µL) and also into the aqueous and octanol phase in a 1:1 ratio (247.4 µL of octanol phase and 247.5 µL of aqueous phase). The octanol and aqueous phases were prepared using a saturation process, where equal amounts of D-PBS (pH 7.4) and octanol were saturated (300 rpm, room temperature) for 24 h before being separated and kept at room temperature. The prepared mixtures were vortexed and kept on the shaker (300 rpm) at room temperature for 16 h. The mixtures were allowed to stand for 30 min, and 200 µL of solution was transferred and sent for HPLC analysis. The analyses were conducted along with propranolol, estriol, metoprolol tartrate, and diethylstil bestrol (5 mM) as standards and were conducted in triplicates.

The chemical stability of eurycomanone was estimated in gastric simulated fluid (GSF), pH 2; fasted simulated intestinal fluid (FASSIF), pH 6.5; fed simulated intestinal fluid (FESSIF), pH 5.0; and in 150 mM $NaHCO_3$ at pH 9.2. Eurycomanone (3 µL) at 5 mM was added to 297 µL of the respective buffers. The mixture (100 µL) was added to 100 µL of ACN at time points 1 and 3 h and sent for LC-MS/MS analysis. The test was done in triplicates with propranolol and erythromycin (5 mM) as standards.

2.8. Permeability Assay

2.8.1. Parallel Artificial Membrane Permeability Assay (PAMPA)

Eurycomanone was added to Pion buffer (Pion Inc., Billerica, MA, USA) pH 7.4 to make a 10 µM working solution. Five microlitres of the lipid mix was applied on the membrane and allowed to dry for 10 min. The working solution (200 µL) was added to the donor plate and Pion buffer (200 µL) were added to the receiver plate. The plate was kept in a moist chamber and left for 18 h at room temperature. The solution from both the donor and receiver plate and the working solution was analysed using LC-MS/MS. This test was carried out in triplicates using propranolol, atenolol, and carbamazepine as standards. The test concentration for eurycomanone is 25 µM.

2.8.2. Caco-2 Cell Permeability Assay

The Caco-2 assay was carried out after seeding the cells onto the membrane to form a confluent monolayer in 21 days. The media is removed from apical (A) and basolateral (B) chambers and the membrane is washed with HBSS buffer. Eurycomanone (10 μM, 200 μL) was added to the A compartment (which represents the intestinal lumen), and buffer (300 μL) was added to the B compartment (representing the blood), and vice versa. The plate was kept in a shaking incubator (37 °C) for 1 h. The amount of eurycomanone that had permeated across the cells was measured by LC-MS/MS, and the apparent permeability (P_{app}) values and efflux ratio were calculated. The expression of P-glycoprotein (P-gp) by differentiated Caco-2 cells was confirmed by measuring the P_{app} value and efflux ratio of vinblastine with and without the presence of a competing P-gp substrate, cyclosporine A. Eurycomanone was also measured with the presence of cyclosporine A to investigate whether eurycomanone may be transported via P-gp transporters.

2.9. *Liver Microsome Metabolic Stability Assay*

The liver microsome stability assay of eurycomanone was estimated using phase I and phase II enzymes in five types of microsomes (mice, rat, dog, monkey, and human). Eurycomanone at 1 mM (20 μL), microsomes at 0.3 mg/mL (20 μL), and 10 mg/mL of alamethicin in 1:1 DMSO and methanol (20 μL) were preincubated at 37 °C for 10 min. The cofactor, 5 mM UDPGA (20 μL), and 1 mM NADPH (20 μL) were added to make the final assay volume of 100 μL. At timepoints 0, 15, 30, 45, 60, and 90 min, 100 μL of the reaction mixture is taken out and added to the stop solution. The supernatants (10,000 rpm, 10 min, 4 °C) were collected and analysed using LC-MS/MS. The standards used for mice and rat liver microsomes were propranolol and dasatinib. The standards used with the dog and monkey liver microsomes were propranolol and midazolam, while the standards used with the human liver microsomes were propranolol and terfinadine.

2.10. *Plasma Stability*

The plasma stability was estimated by preparing 5 μM of eurycomanone in 600 μL plasma in triplicates. The plasma stability of eurycomanone was determined in five types of plasma (mice, rat, dog, monkey, and human). The reaction was kept at 37 °C and ACN (100 μL) was added at timepoints 0, 30 min, and 1, 2, and 4 h to the reaction mixture (100 μL). The supernatant (10,000 rpm, 10 min, 4 °C) was collected and analysed by LC-MS/MS. The standards (propantheline bromide and enalapril) were analysed in triplicates.

2.11. *Plasma Protein Binding Assay*

The ability of eurycomanone to bind plasma protein was analysed in five types of plasma (mice, rat, dog, monkey, and human). Each type of plasma was spiked with eurycomanone (1 mM) to make the 10 μM test concentration of eurycomanone in the plasma. Equilibrium dialysis buffer (500 μL) at pH 7.4 was added to the right chamber in rapid equilibrium dialysis (RED), while the spiked plasma (300 μL) was added to the left chamber. The Teflon base plate was covered with aluminium foil and left on the shaking incubator at 37 °C for 4 h. The matrix was balanced by mixing 100 μL of the equilibrium buffer with the spiked plasma from the left chamber in RED before adding the stop solution (350 μL) to precipitate out the protein. The supernatant (10,000 rpm, 10 min, 4 °C) was collected and analysed using LC-MS/MS. The standards (propranolol, warfarin, and acebutalol) were analysed in duplicates.

2.12. *Statistical Analysis*

The statistical analysis was performed using one-way or two-way ANOVA with either Dunnett or Tukey analysis chosen as the post-hoc analysis (GraphPad Prism, version 7.00 for Windows, GraphPad Software, La Jolla, CA, USA). Statistical significant differences were recognised at $p \leq 0.05$.

3. Results

3.1. Pharmacokinetics of Eurycomanone in Mice

A summary of the PK parameters in mice obtained following an intravenous and oral dose of eurycomanone is shown in Table 1. The plots for the mean plasma concentration of eurycomanone over time are shown in Figure 1. Following intravenous administration to mice, plasma clearance was moderate (3.85 L/h/kg) for eurycomanone. The volume of distribution was small (1.51 L/kg) for eurycomanone, with the elimination half-life of 0.30 h. Following oral administration, the absorption was moderate, where the T_{max} was observed at 2 h post-dose for the eurycomanone (C_{max} 334.7 ng/mL). The bioavailability of eurycomanone in mice was moderately high at 54.9% compared to rats. At 8 h post-dosing, the concentration of eurycomanone increased slightly in mice for both administration routes (Figure 1), which may be an indication of the enterohepatic circulation of eurycomanone in its administered form.

Table 1. Summary of pharmacokinetic parameters following an intravenous and oral dose of eurycomanone to mice.

Parameters (Mice)	Units	Eurycomanone	
		1 mg/kg	10 mg/kg
		Intravenous	Oral
AUC_{0-8}	h·ng/mL	221.0	1213
Plasma Clearance (CL)	L/h/kg	3.85	NA
Volume of Distribution at Steady State (V_{ss})	L/kg	1.51	NA
Half-life ($t_{1/2}$)	h	0.30	NA
Observed T_{max}	h	NA	2.0
Observed C_{max}	ng/mL	NA	334.7
Bioavailability (F)	%	NA	54.9

NA: Not applicable, AUC: Area under the curve, T_{max}: time taken to reach the maximum concentration, C_{max}: maximum concentration of the compound achieved in the plasma.

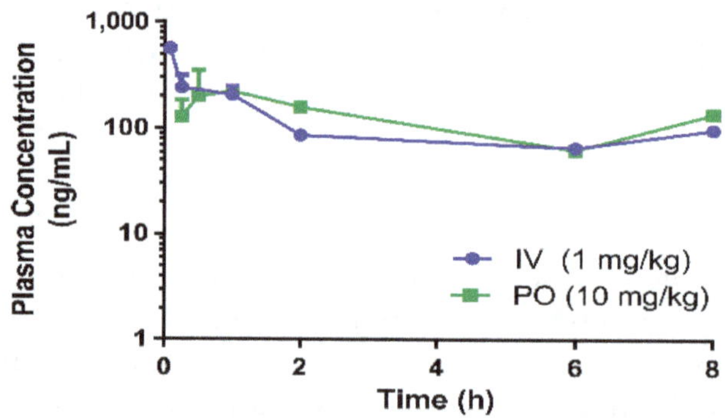

Figure 1. Pharmacokinetic profile of eurycomanone when administered as its pure compound in mice. (IV = intravenous route, PO = oral route)

3.2. Pharmacokinetics of Eurycomanone and SWE in Rats

A summary of the PK parameters in rats obtained following an intravenous and oral dose of eurycomanone and the SWE is shown in Table 2. The plots for the mean plasma concentration of eurycomanone over time are shown in Figure 2a,b. Following intravenous administration to rats, the plasma clearance was moderate (2.74 L/h/kg) for eurycomanone in the compound form and low (0.76 L/h/kg) for eurycomanone in the SWE. The volume of distribution was low (0.95 L/kg) for eurycomanone and lower (0.12 L/kg) for the SWE, while their elimination half-lives were 0.30 and 0.12 h, respectively. Following oral administration, the absorption was moderate, where the

T_{max} was observed at 2 h post-dose for the eurycomanone (C_{max} 238.3 ng/mL). The bioavailability of eurycomanone in rats was calculated to be low at 11.8%. At 6 and 8 h post-dosing of eurycomanone in the compound form, the concentration of eurycomanone increased slightly for the oral and intravenous routes, respectively (Figure 2). This may indicate that eurycomanone is recirculated via enterohepatic circulation in its unchanged administered form.

Table 2. Summary of pharmacokinetic parameters following an intravenous and oral dose of eurycomanone and SWE to rats.

Parameters (Rats)	Units	Eurycomanone		SWE	
		3 mg/kg	30 mg/kg	10 mg/kg	100 mg/kg
		Intravenous	Oral	Intravenous	Oral
AUC_{0-8}	h·ng/mL	970.0	1149.0	100.8	ND
Plasma Clearance (CL)	L/h/kg	2.74	NA	0.76	NA
Volume of Distribution at Steady State (V_{ss})	L/kg	0.95	NA	0.12	NA
Half-life ($t_{1/2}$)	h	0.30	NA	0.11	NA
Observed T_{max}	h	NA	2.0	NA	ND
Observed C_{max}	ng/mL	NA	238.3	NA	ND
Bioavailability (F)	%	NA	11.8	NA	NC
Urinary excretion 24 h post-dose	%	NA	NA	22.52	5.02
Fecal excretion 24 h post-dose	%	NA	NA	0.56	33.02
Liver accumulation	ng/mL	NA	NA	47.6	104.7
Kidney accumulation	ng/mL	NA	NA	NA	NA

NA: Not applicable, ND: Not detected, NC: Not calculated, AUC: Area under the curve, T_{max}: time taken to reach the maximum concentration, C_{max}: maximum concentration of the compound achieved in the plasma.

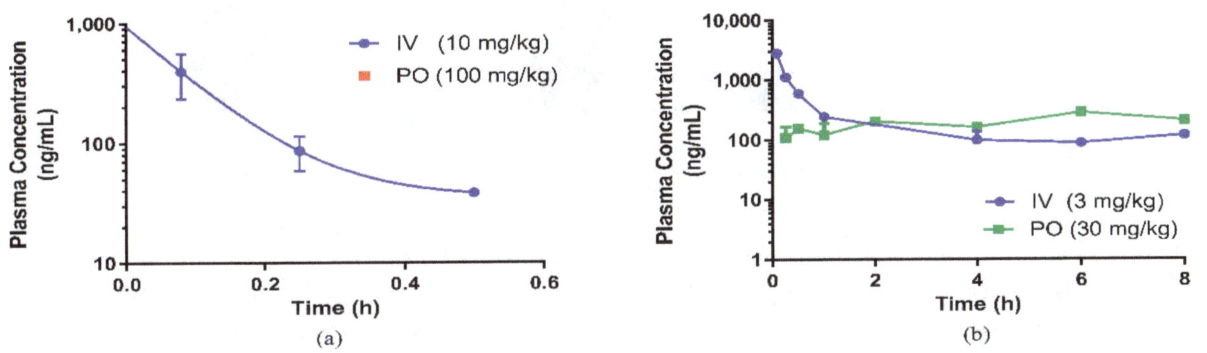

Figure 2. Pharmacokinetic profile of (**a**) standardized water extract (SWE) of *E. longifolia* and (**b**) eurycomanone compound, respectively, in rats. (IV = intravenous route, PO = oral route).

When SWE was orally administered, the plasma concentration of eurycomanone was undetectable in the plasma and it was mainly eliminated via faecal excretion. However, eurycomanone was detected in the liver samples at 47.6 ng/mL (intravenous) and 104.7 ng/mL (oral) at 24 h post-administration of SWE, indicating that a minimal amount of eurycomanone may have been absorbed, though not detectable. Intravenous administration of SWE showed that eurycomanone remains in the plasma up until 30 min and is mainly eliminated via urinary excretion.

3.3. Eurycomanone Aqueous Solubility, Lipophilicity, and Chemical Stability

Eurycomanone was highly soluble at pH 5.4 (205.5 μM) and 7.4 (205.4 μM) and was comparable to propranolol (Figure 3). Estriol, which has moderate solubility at both pHs, and tamoxifen, which was insoluble at pH 7.4 and highly soluble in pH 5.4, were used as internal controls. Due to this highly aqueous nature of eurycomanone, it is expected that its distribution coefficient log D at pH 7.4 is low (−0.35). Propranolol (0.82), estriol (2.82), metoprolol (−0.29), and diethylstilbestrol (3.18) were assayed together as internal controls as they have a wide range of log D values (Figure 4). The chemical stability of eurycomanone at the varying pH levels, mimicking changing pH environments in physiological conditions, i.e., using GSF (pH 2), FESIIF (pH 5.0), and FASSIF (pH 6.5), were also carried out. The percentage of eurycomanone remaining after 3 h of incubation showed that eurycomanone is chemically stable across all pH values tested (Figure 5).

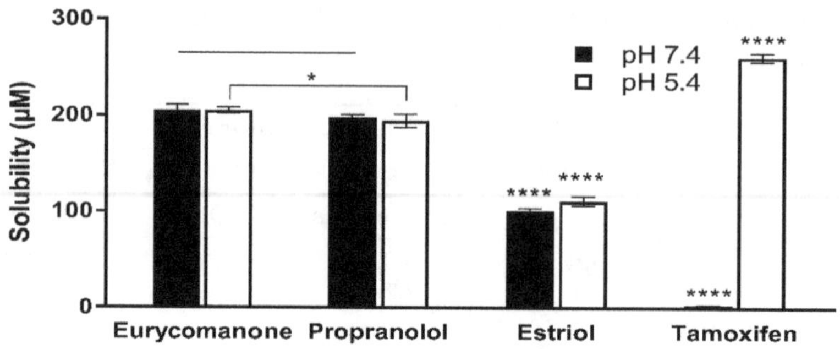

Figure 3. Aqueous solubility of eurycomanone, propranolol, estriol, and tamoxifen at pH 7.4 and pH 5.4. The values were plotted based on the mean ± standard deviation. **** denotes significant difference when compared to eurycomanone ($p \leq 0.0001$) at the two pH values. * denotes significance difference between propranolol and eurycomanone at pH 5.4 ($p \leq 0.05$). Line over bars indicates no significant difference when compared to eurycomanone ($p \geq 0.05$).

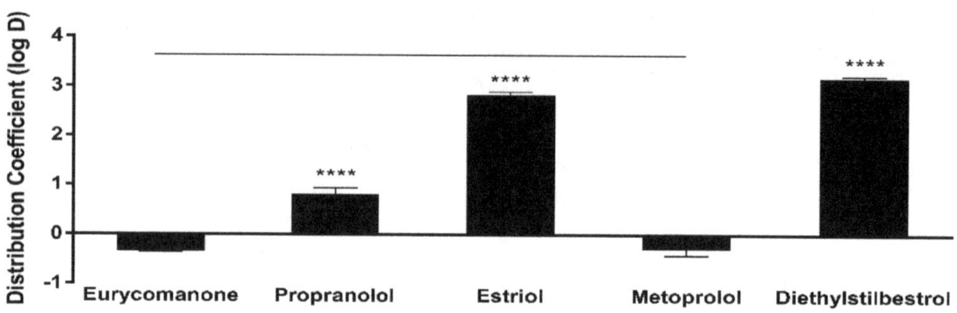

Figure 4. Lipophilicity properties of eurycomanone, propranolol, estriol, metoprolol, and diesthylstilbestrol. The distribution coefficient (log D) value for eurycomanone was −0.35. All standards showed acceptable log D values, respectively. The values were plotted based on the mean ± standard deviation. **** denotes significant difference when compared to eurycomanone ($p \leq 0.0001$). The log D value of eurycomanone is comparable to that of metoprolol. Line over bars indicates no significant difference between metoprolol and eurycomanone ($p \geq 0.05$).

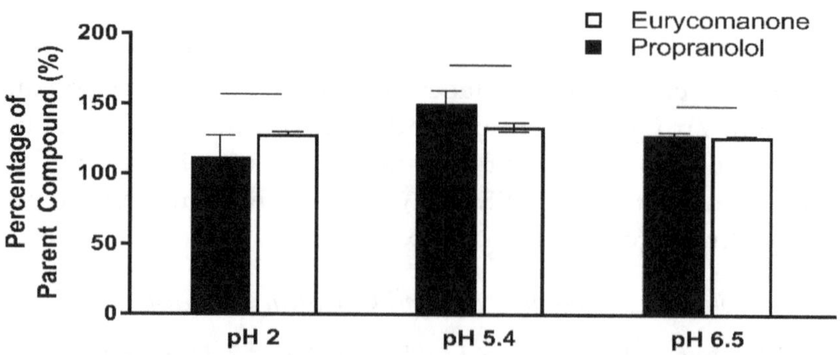

Figure 5. Eurycomanone showed high stability at pH 2, pH 5, and pH 6.5 and is comparable to the stability of propranolol. The values were plotted based on the mean ± standard deviation. There were no significant differences between propranolol and eurycomanone at all the pH levels tested. Line over bars indicates no significant difference when compared to eurycomanone ($p \geq 0.05$).

3.4. Eurycomanone Permeability

The rapid assessment of the absorption ability of eurycomanone was conducted via the PAMPA. Eurycomanone's permeation through this artificial membrane is low at 0.78×10^{-6} cm/s (Figure 6). As the PAMPA system lacks some similarity to natural membranes, i.e., lack of pores and proteins responsible for active transport such as P-gp protein, eurycomanone was also evaluated in a Caco-2 cell monolayer (Table 3). However, eurycomanone showed low permeability in Caco-2 cells at 0.45×10^{-6} cm/s (A to B direction) and 0.73×10^{-6} cm/s (B to A direction), similar to its permeation in the artificial membrane. Eurycomanone was not a substrate for efflux transporter as the efflux ratio is less than 2. Incubation of eurycomanone with cyclosporine A (a P-gp substrate) showed no changes and no competition with eurycomanone. Alongside eurycomanone, vinblastine, which is also a P-gp substrate, was also tested to ensure the Caco-2 cells were expressing P-gp transporters.

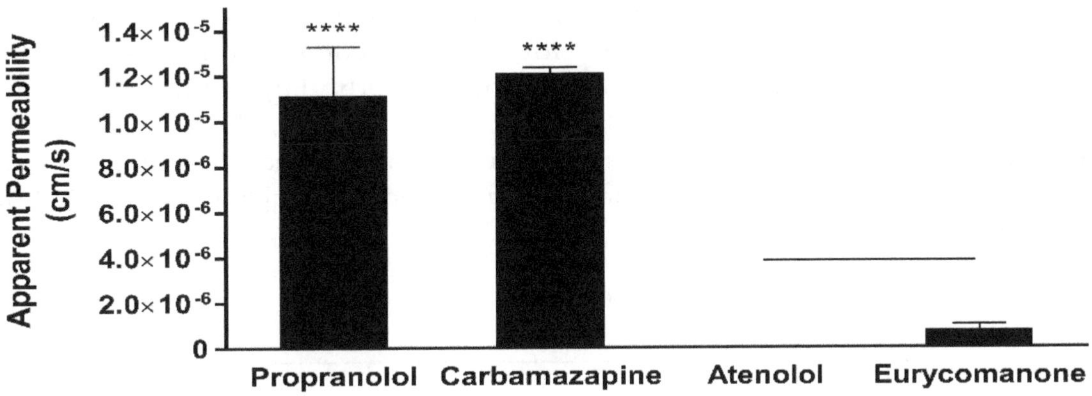

Figure 6. Eurycomanone showed low permeability as compared to propranolol and carbamazepine when assayed using the parallel artificial membrane permeability assay (PAMPA). The values were plotted based on the mean ± standard deviation. **** denotes significant difference when compared to eurycomanone ($p \leq 0.0001$). Line over bars indicates no significant difference between atenolol and eurycomanone ($p \geq 0.05$).

Table 3. Apparent permeability of eurycomanone assayed via the Caco-2 permeability assay.

Tested Compounds	Direction	P_{app} ($\times 10^{-6}$ cm/s)	Efflux Ratio
Eurycomanone	A to B B to A	0.45 0.73	1.62
Eurycomanone + Cyclosporine A	A to B B to A	1.20 1.35	1.13
Vinblastine	A to B B to A	3.76 55.34	14.72
Vinblastine + Cyclosporine A	A to B B to A	16.71 40.00	2.39

P_{app}: Apparent permeability.

3.5. Liver Microsome Metabolic Stability

Eurycomanone was relatively stable in rat liver microsomes and hepatocytes and in human liver microsomes, with the half-life of more than 90 min (Table 4). The intrinsic clearances (Cl_{int}) calculated from the rate of metabolism of eurycomanone in the liver microsomal incubations were high for rat (83.16 mL/min/kg) and slightly lower in human microsomes (52.39 mL/min/kg). Intrinsic clearance in the rat liver hepatocytes was also slow at 0.67 µL/min/million cells. These results suggest that eurycomanone is not a species-specific substrate and that is may be highly metabolised in the liver.

Table 4. Rat liver microsomes and hepatocytes and human liver microsome stability of eurycomanone.

Parameters	Units	Rat Liver Microsomes	Rat Liver Hepatocytes	Human Liver Microsomes
Half-life ($t_{1/2}$)	h	>1.5	>1.5	>1.5
Intrinsic clearance (Cl_{int})	mL/min/kg	83.16	NA	52.39
Intrinsic clearance (Cl_{int})	μL/min/million cells	NA	0.67	NA

NA: Not applicable.

3.6. Plasma Stability and Plasma Protein Binding

Eurycomanone was highly stable in the human, rat, and dog plasma, while stability was slightly lower in the monkey and mice plasma (Figure 7). The varied species used in the plasma profiling were used to assess possible differences in eurycomanone's stability as exhibited by other compounds such as propantheline bromide and enalapril. However, eurycomanone were shown to be stable in all the species tested. From the plasma protein binding study (Figure 8), it was found that the percentages of bound eurycomanone were 30.1% (rat), 35.4% (monkey), 21.6% (mice), 38.9% (human), and 67.8% (dog). Apart from in the dog plasma, eurycomanone exhibited a low plasma binding ability in all the other species' plasma, with a high fraction of unbound eurycomanone (61.1–78.4%) with free access to its target sites.

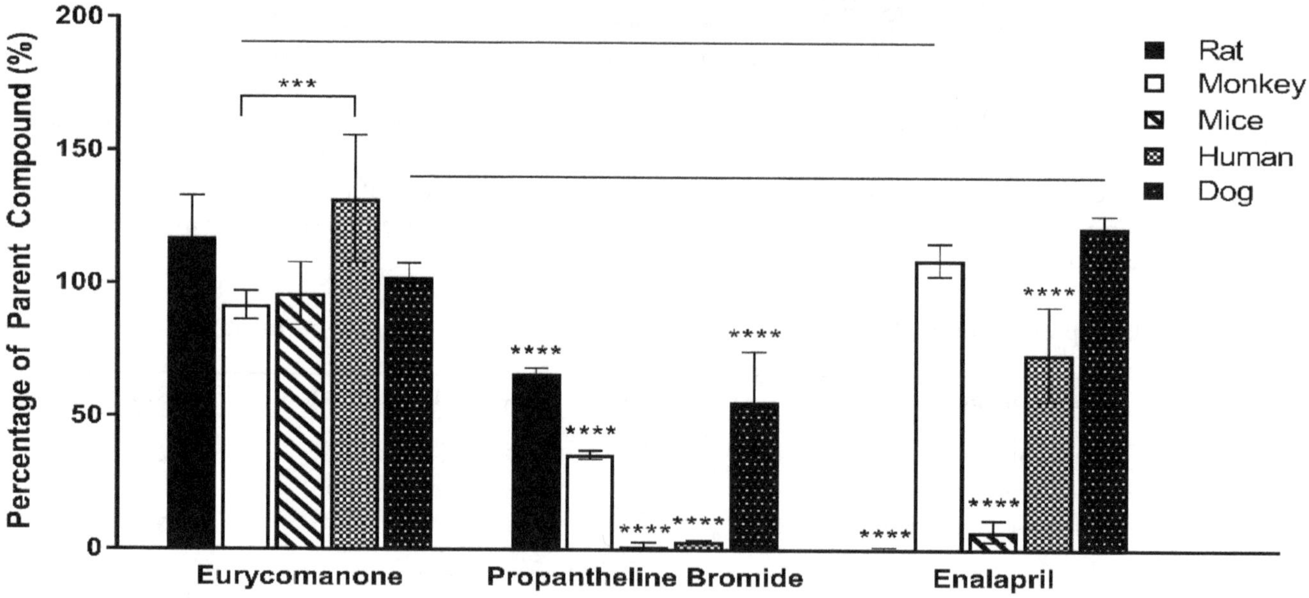

Figure 7. Eurycomanone's stability in rat, monkey, mice, human, and dog plasma as compared to propantheline bromide and enalapril. The values were plotted based on the mean ± standard deviation. **** denotes significant difference when compared to eurycomanone ($p \leq 0.0001$) in the five species tested. *** denotes significance difference ($p \leq 0.001$) in eurycomanone's stability between species monkey and human. Line over bars indicates no significant difference when compared to eurycomanone in species monkey and dog for enalapril ($p \geq 0.05$).

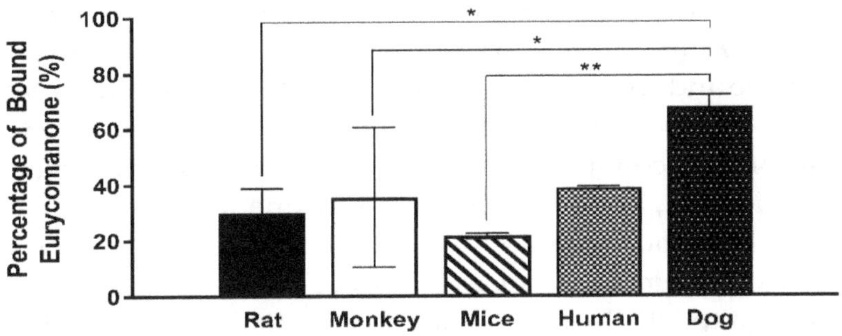

Figure 8. Eurycomanone plasma protein binding in rat, monkey, mice, human, and dog plasma. The values were plotted based on the mean ± standard deviation. ** and * denote significant difference when compared to across species ($p \leq 0.01$) and ($p \leq 0.05$) respectively. No significant difference was found between the rest of the species tested ($p \geq 0.05$) (not indicated on graph).

4. Discussion

Eurycomanone has been evaluated for its biological activities via various in vitro methods [17,20,24–27], while the extract form was mainly used in various in vivo tests [28–32]. From this study, the concentration of the pure eurycomanone in rat plasma was at its maximum (C_{max} 238.3 ng/mL) at 2 h post oral administration, and the bioavailability for the eurycomanone compound was low (11.8%). The findings in this study with regard to eurycomanone's bioavailability was similar to findings by Low et al. [22], where it was reported that the bioavailability of the orally administered fortified eurycomanone in *E. longifolia* extract was 10.5% and the C_{max} was found to be 330 ng/mL. There was no notable difference in terms of eurycomanone's bioavailability and maximum concentration when using a pure compound as in the current study and when compared to using a fortified extract as used by Low et al. [22]. Rehman and his coworkers, in their investigation, found the C_{max} to be lower at 40.43 ng/mL for the pure eurycomanone and 9.90 ng/mL for eurycomanone in *E. longifolia* extract [7]. In this study, interspecies variation in the bioavailability of eurycomanone was noted. The pure compound was found to be more bioavailable (higher absorption) in mice (54.9%) than in rats, and the C_{max} (335 ng/mL) in mice was slightly higher than the levels found in rats. This also indicates that eurycomanone may behave differently in different species and the PK values may not be able to be directly extrapolated from rodents to humans. This species-dependent characteristic of eurycomanone behaviour in rodents may be due to species differences in the metabolism and disposition of eurycomanone, as there was a variation in the absorption, distribution, and metabolism of eurycomanone, in which they were faster in mice than in rats. Two peaks were observed in the PK profiles in both the oral and intravenous profiles. The presence of these secondary peaks may indicate the occurrence of enterohepatic circulation of eurycomanone [33]; however, this must be further investigated in a separate study. Ma et al. suggest that the secondary peak of eurycomanone may be caused by eurycomanone's activity as a muscle relaxant, which caused delayed gastric emptying and hence delayed intestinal absorption, resulting in the secondary peak in the profile [23]. In the present study, the plasma concentration–time profile was only conducted for 8 h, which limits the window of analysis to confirm the second peak.

Previously, Zakaria et al. reported eurycomanone activity in vivo, where eurycomanone was orally administered at 6 mg/kg and 17 mg/kg to mice. At the dose of 17 mg/kg, tumour suppression ability was demonstrated in nude mice with HepG2 cell-induced tumours, which showed that there was sufficient or better bioavailability to exert the reported efficacy [32]. However, in relation to previous in vitro studies, the C_{max} value obtained in the current study was much lower than those shown in previous studies of eurycomanone and *E. longifolia* extracts (in the range of micrograms to miligrams) [17,20,24–27]. The reported efficacy via in vitro models may not accurately represent eurycomanone's level in vivo. Stability in plasma was measured via predetermined time incubation (0 and 30 min and 1, 2, 4 h) of eurycomanone and it was found to be highly stable; nevertheless, eurycomanone's ability to bind to proteins present in the plasma may affect its availability to its target site of action. However, the plasma protein binding in rats indicates that a low percentage of eurycomanone (30%) is bound to plasma proteins. In other words, the remaining 70% unbound fraction of eurycomanone is freely available and can possibly access the target sites [34].

The low absorption of eurycomanone in vivo correlates with findings from in vitro studies, namely the lipophilicity, solubility, and permeability assessment of eurycomanone. The lipophilicity of eurycomanone was very low and its solubility was high, which influences its permeation rate via lipid membranes as well as cell membranes such as of Caco-2 cells. The low log D value determined in this study indicates the extent to which eurycomanone was likely to stay in the aqueous environment instead of dissociating into the hydrophobic octanol. This relates to eurycomanone being highly soluble and its low permeation when assayed using the PAMPA method. When eurycomanone's permeability was assessed using the Caco-2 cells, the results also indicated that a low amount of eurycomanone permeated the cell monolayer. However, this may be due to the condition where eurycomanone, which was not lipophilic enough to be absorbed, accumulates on the cell monolayer, introducing a sink condition [35]. This accumulation then draws the compound to cross the membrane, which may not be due to the compound's innate ability to cross the membrane freely.

The ability of the compound to cross the biological membrane without the use of transporters is possible when the compound of interest is in its uncharged state. Eurycomanone is predicted to have an acid dissociation constant (pK_a) value of 11 [36]. The pH values of the environments in the stomach and small intestine vary in the different sections and depending on the fasted or fed state. The pH range in the stomach in its fasted state is between 1.4 and 2.1; while in its fed state, it is in between 4.3 and 5.4. In the small intestine, the pH values of the different segments in their fasted state are 4.9–6.4 (duodenum); 4.4–6.6 (jejunum), and 6.5–7.4 (ileum); while in their fed state, the pH values are 4.2–6.1 (duodenum); 5.2–6.2 (jejunum), and 6.8–7.5 (ileum) [37]. The changing pH values then affect the ionic state of eurycomanone. The predicted pK_a for eurycomanone was high, which means that in a lower pH environment, eurycomanone exists in its ionised form. This then prevents eurycomanone from crossing the membrane barriers passively.

As determined in the Caco-2 permeability assessment, eurycomanone was not an active transporter P-gp substrate. The chemical stability assay conducted using the fasted and fed state simulative buffer system indicates that eurycomanone was stable; however, its ionic state could not be confirmed. The plasma stability and liver metabolic stability study also showed eurycomanone to be stable in the different matrices, indicating that eurycomanone may stay intact and survive first-pass metabolism in vivo. This study hypothesised that when eurycomanone was administered orally, only a small amount crosses the membrane to enter the blood stream, while when it was administered intravenously, only a small amount of eurycomanone permeates into tissues, while most remained in the blood in its ionised form. The small amount of eurycomanone which may have been absorbed (as a low amount was detected in liver tissues) could still potentially exert the desired effects of eurycomanone or *E. longifolia* extract in general.

5. Conclusions

In conclusion, the results indicate that eurycomanone was a very polar compound with high stability at different pHs, in the plasma and in liver microsome. No major degradation of the compound in the gastrointestinal tract and blood plasma was noted and eurycomanone also exhibited low plasma protein binding ability. Despite the favourable properties of eurycomanone, its low permeability hinders its absorption, hence its bioavailability in in vivo models. The low absorptive value of eurycomanone may indicate the need to use eurycomanone at lower concentrations in assays aimed at finding its efficacy. The adoption of eurycomanone as the bioactive marker for *E. longifolia* may be considered with further evaluations of eurycomanone in in vivo models.

Author Contributions: Conceptualization, N.A. and D.S.S.; Methodology, N.A. and D.S.S.; Software, N.A. and D.S.S.; Validation, N.A. and D.S.S.; Formal Analysis, N.A. and D.S.S.; Investigation, N.A., D.S.S., B.P.T., N.A.Z., A.M., E.M. and A.Z.; Resources, N.A., D.S.S., B.P.T. and A.Z.; Data Curation, N.A. and D.S.S.; Writing–Original Draft Preparation, N.A.; Writing–Review & Editing, N.A., T.B.P., M.Z. and A.F.S.M.; Visualization, N.A. and D.S.S.; Supervision, N.R.A., Z.I. and A.F.S.M.; Project Administration, N.A. and D.S.S.; Funding Acquisition, N.A., M.Z., N.R.A, Z.I. and A.F.S.M.

Acknowledgments: This study was funded by the Ministry of Agriculture, Malaysia, under project number NH0712PC001 and the Ministry of Health, Malaysia, under project number NMRR-12-1033-13911 (JPP-IMR 12-032). We would like to thank the Director General of Health Malaysia for his permission to publish this article. The authors also would like to acknowledge those who contributed directly or indirectly to this study's accomplishment. There are no competing financial interests in this study.

References

1. Chan, K.L.; Choo, C.Y.; Morita, H.; Itokawa, H. High performance liquid chromatography in phytochemical analysis of *Eurycoma longifolia*. *Planta Med.* **1998**, *64*, 741–745. [CrossRef] [PubMed]
2. Chua, L.S.; Amin, N.A.M.; Neo, J.C.H.; Lee, T.H.; Lee, C.T.; Sarmidi, M.R.; Aziz, R.A. LC-MS/MS-based metabolites of *Eurycoma longifolia* (Tongkat Ali) in malaysia (perak and pahang). *J. Chromatogr. B* **2011**, *879*, 3909–3919. [CrossRef] [PubMed]
3. Han, Y.M.; Jang, M.; Kim, I.S.; Kim, S.H.; Yoo, H.H. Simultaneous quantitation of six major quassinoids in Tongkat Ali dietary supplements by liquid chromatography with tandem mass spectrometry. *J. Sep. Sci.* **2015**, *38*, 2260–2266. [CrossRef] [PubMed]
4. Low, B.S.; Choi, S.B.; Wahab, H.A.; Das, P.K.; Chan, K.L. Eurycomanone, the major quassinoid in *Eurycoma longifolia* root extract increases spermatogenesis by inhibiting the activity of phosphodiesterase and aromatase in steroidogenesis. *J. Ethnopharmacol.* **2013**, *149*, 201–207. [CrossRef] [PubMed]
5. Miyake, K.; Tezuka, Y.; Awale, S.; Li, F.; Kadota, S. Quassinoids from *Eurycoma longifolia*. *J. Nat. Prod.* **2009**, *72*, 2135–2140. [CrossRef] [PubMed]
6. Morita, H.; Kishi, E.; Takeya, K.; Itokawa, H.; Tanaka, O. New quassinoids from the roots of *Eurycoma longifolia*. *Chem. Lett.* **1990**, *44*, 749–752. [CrossRef]
7. Rehman, S.U.; Choi, M.S.; Han, Y.M.; Kim, I.S.; Kim, S.H.; Piao, X.L.; Yoo, H.H. Determination of eurycomanone in rat plasma using hydrophilic interaction liquid chromatography-tandem mass spectrometry for pharmacokinetic study. *Biomed. Chromatogr.* **2017**, *31*. [CrossRef] [PubMed]
8. Teh, C.H.; Murugaiyah, V.; Chan, K.L. Developing a validated liquid chromatography-mass spectrometric method for the simultaneous analysis of five bioactive quassinoid markers for the standardization of manufactures batches of *Eurycoma longifolia* Jack extract as antimalarial medicaments. *J. Chromatogr. A* **2011**, *1218*, 1861–1877. [CrossRef] [PubMed]
9. Gimlette, J.D.; Burkhill, I.H. *The Medical Book of Malayan Medicine*; The Gardens Buletin Straits Settlements: Singapore, Singapore, 1930; Volume 6, p. 329.
10. Burkill, I.H.; Haniff, M. *Malay Village Medicine*; The Gardens Bulletin Straits Settlements: Singapore, Singapore, 1930; Volume 2, p. 182.
11. Low, B.S.; Das, P.K.; Chan, K.L. Standardized quassinoid-rich *Eurycoma longifolia* extract improved spermatogenesis and fertility in male rats via the hypothalamic-pituitary-gonadal axis. *J. Ethnopharmacol.* **2013**, *145*, 706–714. [CrossRef] [PubMed]
12. Ang, H.H.; Chan, K.L.; Mak, J.W. In vitro antimalarial activity of quassinoids from *Eurycoma longifolia* against malaysian chloroquine-resistant plasmodium falcifarum isolates. *Planta Med.* **1995**, *61*, 177–178. [CrossRef] [PubMed]
13. Chan, K.L.; O'Neill, M.J.; Phillipson, J.D.; Warhurst, D.C. Plants as sources of antimalarial drugs. Part 31 *Eurycoma longifolia*. *Planta Med.* **1986**, *52*, 105–107. [CrossRef]
14. Kardono, L.B.; Angerhofer, C.K.; Tsauri, S.; Padmawinata, K.; Pezzuto, J.M.; Kinghorn, A.D. Cytotoxic and antimalarial constituents of the roots of *Eurycoma longifolia*. *J. Nat. Prod.* **1991**, *54*, 1360–1367. [CrossRef] [PubMed]

15. Kuo, P.C.; Damu, A.G.; Lee, K.H.; Wu, T.S. Cytotoxic and antimalarial constituents from the roots of *Eurycoma longifolia*. *Bioorg. Med. Chem.* **2004**, *12*, 537–544. [CrossRef] [PubMed]
16. Low, B.S.; Teh, C.H.; Yuen, K.H.; Chan, K.L. Physico-chemical effects of the major quassinoids in a standardized *Eurycoma longifolia* extract (Fr 2) on the bioavailability and pharmacokinetic properties, and their implications for oral antimalarial activity. *Nat. Prod. Commun.* **2011**, *6*, 337–341. [PubMed]
17. Wernsdorfer, W.H.; Ismail, S.; Chan, K.L.; Congpuong, K.; Wernsdorfer, G. Activity of *Eurycoma longifolia* root extract against plasmodium falciparum in vitro. *Wien. Klinische Wochenschr.* **2009**, *121*, 23–26. [CrossRef] [PubMed]
18. Rehman, S.U.; Choe, K.; Yoo, H.H. Review on a traditional herbal medicine, *Eurycoma longifolia* Jack (Tongkat Ali). Its traditional uses, chemistry, evidence-based pharmacology and toxicology. *Molecules* **2016**, *21*, 331. [CrossRef] [PubMed]
19. Hajjouli, S.; Chateauvieux, S.; Teiten, M.H.; Orlikova, B.; Schumacher, M.; Dicato, M.; Choo, C.Y.; Diederich, M. Eurycomanone and eurycomanol from *Eurycoma longifolia* Jack as regulators of signalling pathways involved in proliferation, cell death and inflammation. *Molecules* **2014**, *19*, 14649–14666. [CrossRef] [PubMed]
20. Wong, P.F.; Cheong, W.F.; Shu, M.H.; Teh, C.H.; Chan, K.L.; AbuBakar, S. Eurycomanone suppress expression of lung cancer cell tumor markers, prohibitin, annexin 1 and endoplasmic reticulum protein 28. *Phytomedicine* **2012**, *19*, 138–144. [CrossRef] [PubMed]
21. Tada, H.; Yasuda, F.; Otani, K.; Doteuchi, M.; Ishihara, Y.; Shiro, M. New antiulcer quassinoids from *Eurycoma longifolia*. *Eur. J. Med. Chem.* **1991**, *26*, 345–349. [CrossRef]
22. Low, B.S.; Ng, B.H.; Choy, W.P.; Yuen, K.H.; Chan, K.L. Bioavailability and pharmacokinetic studies of eurycomanone from *Eurycoma longifolia*. *Planta Med.* **2005**, *71*, 803–807. [CrossRef] [PubMed]
23. Ma, H.Q.; Ebrahimi, F.; Khan, N.A.K.; Chan, K.L. Investigating the double-peak phenomenon in oral pharmacokinetics of *Eurycoma longifolia* quassinoids in lipid-based solid dispersion. *J. Bioequivalence Stud.* **2015**, *1*, 1–10.
24. Pan, Y.; Tiong, K.H.; Abd-Rashid, B.A.; Ismail, Z.; Ismail, R.; Mak, J.W. Effect of eurycomanone on cytochrome P450 isoforms CYP1A2, CYP2A6, CYP2C8, CYP2C9, CYP2C19, CYP2E1 and CYP3A4 in vitro. *J. Nat. Med.* **2014**, *68*, 402–406. [CrossRef] [PubMed]
25. Purwantiningsih; Hussin, A.H.; Chan, K.L. Phase 1 drug metabolism study of the standardised extract of *Eurycoma longifolia* (TAF-273) in rat hepatocytes. *Int. J. Pharm. Pharm. Sci.* **2010**, *2*, 147–152.
26. Purwantiningsih; Hussin, A.H.; Chan, K.L. Free radical scavenging activity of the standardized ethanolic extract of *Eurycoma longifolia* (TAF-273). *Int. J. Pharm. Pharm. Sci.* **2011**, *3*, 343–347.
27. Zakaria, Y.; Rahmat, A.; Pihie, A.H.L.; Abdullah, N.R.; Houghton, P.J. Eurycomanone induce apoptosis in HepG2 cells via up-regulation of p53. *Cancel Cell Int.* **2009**, *9*, 16. [CrossRef] [PubMed]
28. Ang, H.H.; Ikeda, S.; Gan, E.K. Evaluation of the potency activity of aphrodisiac in *Eurycoma longifolia* Jack. *Phytother. Res.* **2001**, *15*, 435–436. [CrossRef] [PubMed]
29. Ang, H.H.; Ngai, T.H. Aphrodisiac evaluation in non-copulator male rats after chronic administration of *Eurycoma longifolia* Jack. *Fundam. Clin. Pharmacol.* **2001**, *15*, 265–268. [CrossRef] [PubMed]
30. Solomon, M.C.; Erasmus, N.; Henkel, R.R. In vivo effects of *Eurycoma longifolia* Jack (Tongkat Ali) extract on reproductive functions in the rat. *Andrologia* **2014**, *46*, 339–348. [CrossRef] [PubMed]
31. Teh, C.H.; Abdulghani, M.; Morita, H.; Shiro, M.; Hussin, A.H.; Chan, K.L. Comparative X-ray and conformational analysis of a new crystal of 13-alpha, 21-dihydroeurycomanone with eurycomanone from *Eurycoma longifolia* and their anti-estrogenic activity using the uterotrophic assay. *Planta Med.* **2011**, *77*, 128–132. [CrossRef] [PubMed]
32. Zakaria, Y.; Rain, A.N.; Hawariah, L.P.A. Suppression effect of eurycomanone on the growth of HepG2 tumor transplanted in mice. In Proceedings of the 1st International Congress on Natural Products, Putrajaya, Malaysia, 14–16 November 2011; pp. 51–57.
33. Roberts, M.S.; Magnusson, B.M.; Burczynski, F.J.; Weiss, M. Enterohepatic circulation: Physiological, pharmacokinetic and clinical implications. *Clin. Pharm.* **2002**, *41*, 751–790. [CrossRef] [PubMed]
34. Stern, S.T.; Martinez, M.N.; Stevens, D.M. When is it important to measure unbound drug in evaluating nanomedicine pharmacokinetics? *Drug Metab. Dispos.* **2016**, *44*, 1934–1939. [CrossRef] [PubMed]
35. Valko, K. *Physicochemical and Biomimetic Properties in Drug Discovery. Chromatographic Techniques for Lead Optimization*; John Wiley & Sons, Inc.: Hoboken, NJ, USA, 2014; pp. 150–181.

36. JChem. Chemaxon Version 17.29.0. Available online: https://chemaxon.com/ (accessed on 1 March 2018).
37. Mudie, D.M.; Amidon, G.L.; Amidon, G.E. Physiological parameters for oral delivery and in vitro testing. *Mol. Pharm.* **2010**, *7*, 1388–1405. [CrossRef] [PubMed]

Permissions

All chapters in this book were first published by MDPI; hereby published with permission under the Creative Commons Attribution License or equivalent. Every chapter published in this book has been scrutinized by our experts. Their significance has been extensively debated. The topics covered herein carry significant findings which will fuel the growth of the discipline. They may even be implemented as practical applications or may be referred to as a beginning point for another development.

The contributors of this book come from diverse backgrounds, making this book a truly international effort. This book will bring forth new frontiers with its revolutionizing research information and detailed analysis of the nascent developments around the world.

We would like to thank all the contributing authors for lending their expertise to make the book truly unique. They have played a crucial role in the development of this book. Without their invaluable contributions this book wouldn't have been possible. They have made vital efforts to compile up to date information on the varied aspects of this subject to make this book a valuable addition to the collection of many professionals and students.

This book was conceptualized with the vision of imparting up-to-date information and advanced data in this field. To ensure the same, a matchless editorial board was set up. Every individual on the board went through rigorous rounds of assessment to prove their worth. After which they invested a large part of their time researching and compiling the most relevant data for our readers.

The editorial board has been involved in producing this book since its inception. They have spent rigorous hours researching and exploring the diverse topics which have resulted in the successful publishing of this book. They have passed on their knowledge of decades through this book. To expedite this challenging task, the publisher supported the team at every step. A small team of assistant editors was also appointed to further simplify the editing procedure and attain best results for the readers.

Apart from the editorial board, the designing team has also invested a significant amount of their time in understanding the subject and creating the most relevant covers. They scrutinized every image to scout for the most suitable representation of the subject and create an appropriate cover for the book.

The publishing team has been an ardent support to the editorial, designing and production team. Their endless efforts to recruit the best for this project, has resulted in the accomplishment of this book. They are a veteran in the field of academics and their pool of knowledge is as vast as their experience in printing. Their expertise and guidance has proved useful at every step. Their uncompromising quality standards have made this book an exceptional effort. Their encouragement from time to time has been an inspiration for everyone.

The publisher and the editorial board hope that this book will prove to be a valuable piece of knowledge for researchers, students, practitioners and scholars across the globe.

List of Contributors

Mi Hye Kwon and Hee Eun Kang
College of Pharmacy and Integrated Research Institute of Pharmaceutical Sciences, The Catholic University of Korea, 43 Jibong-ro, Wonmi-gu, Bucheon 14662, Korea

Jin Seok Jeong, Jayoung Ryu and Young Woong Cho
Research Center, Dong-A ST Co., Ltd., 21 Geumhwa-ro, 105beon-gil, Giheung-gu, Yongin 17073, Korea

Jan F. Joseph
Core Facility BioSupraMol, Freie Universität Berlin, 14195 Berlin, Germany

Leonie Gronbach, Jill García-Miller, Leticia M. Cruz and Christian Zoschke
Institute of Pharmacy (Pharmacology & Toxicology), Freie Universität Berlin, 14195 Berlin, Germany

Bernhard Wuest
Agilent Technologies GmbH, 76337 Waldbronn, Germany

Ulrich Keilholz
Charité–Universitätsmedizin Berlin, corporate member of Freie Universität Berlin, Humboldt-Universität zu Berlin and Berlin Institute of Health, Comprehensive Cancer Center, 10117 Berlin, Germany

Maria K. Parr
Institute of Pharmacy (Pharmaceutical and Medicinal Chemistry), Freie Universität Berlin, 14195 Berlin, Germany

Suk-Jae Chung
College of Pharmacy, Seoul National University, Seoul 08826, Korea

Yoo-Kyung Song
College of Pharmacy, Seoul National University, Seoul 08826, Korea
Laboratory Animal Resource Center, Korea Research Institute of Bioscience and Biotechnology, Ochang 28116, Korea

Kyeong-Ryoon Lee
Laboratory Animal Resource Center, Korea Research Institute of Bioscience and Biotechnology, Ochang 28116, Korea

Jin-Ha Yoon, Jong Kyu Woo, Ju-Hee Kang, Han-Joo Maeng and Seung Hyun Oh
College of Pharmacy, Gachon University, Incheon 21936, Korea

Alanna McEneny-King, Pierre Chelle and Andrea N. Edginton
School of Pharmacy, University of Waterloo, Waterloo, ON N2L 3G1, Canada

Severine Henrard
Louvain Drug Research Institute, Clinical Pharmacy Research Group and Institute of Health and Society (IRSS), Université catholique de Louvain, 1348 Brussels, Belgium

Cedric Hermans
Haemostasis and Thrombosis Unit, Division of Haematology, Cliniques universitaires Saint-Luc, Université catholique de Louvain, 1348 Brussels, Belgium

Alfonso Iorio
Department of Health Evidence, Research Methods and Impact, McMaster University, Hamilton, ON L8S 4L8, Canada
Department of Medicine, McMaster University, Hamilton, ON L8S 4L8, Canada

Sarah Maximos
Centre de recherche du Centre hospitalier de l'Université de Montréal (CRCHUM), Montreal, QC H2X 0A9, Canada
Faculty of Medicine, Université de Montréal, Montreal, QC H3T 1J4, Canada

Sophie Gravel
Centre de recherche du Centre hospitalier de l'Université de Montréal (CRCHUM), Montreal, QC H2X 0A9, Canada
Faculty of Pharmacy, Université de Montréal, Montreal, QC H3T 1J4, Canada

Michel Chamoun
Faculty of Pharmacy, Université de Montréal, Montreal, QC H3T 1J4, Canada

Tae Hwan Kim
College of Pharmacy, Catholic University of Daegu, Gyeongsan, Gyeongbuk 38430, Korea

Subindra Kazi Thapa and Soyoung Shin
College of Pharmacy, Wonkwang University, Iksan, Jeonbuk 54538, Korea

Ju-Hyun Kim
College of Pharmacy, Yeungnam University, Gyeongsan 38541, Korea

Jacques Turgeon and Veronique Michaud
Centre de recherche du Centre hospitalier de l'Université de Montréal (CRCHUM), Montreal, QC H2X 0A9, Canada
Faculty of Medicine, Université de Montréal, Montreal, QC H3T 1J4, Canada
Faculty of Pharmacy, Université de Montréal, Montreal, QC H3T 1J4, Canada

Da Young Lee, Seung Eun Chung, Jun Young Lim, Hyeon Myeong Jeong, Chang Ho Song and Beom Soo Shin
School of Pharmacy, Sungkyunkwan University, Suwon, Gyeonggi 16419, Korea

Youn-Woong Choi, Sang-Min Cho, Kyu-Yeol Nam and Won-Ho Kang
Korea United Pharm. Inc., Seoul 06116, Korea

Deok-Kyu Hwang, Yongho Shin, Won-Gu Choi, Sunjoo Kim, Yong-Yeon Cho, Joo Young Lee, Han Chang Kang and Hye Suk Lee
BK21 PLUS Team for Creative Leader Program for Pharmacomics-based Future Pharmacy, College of Pharmacy, The Catholic University of Korea, Bucheon 14662, Korea

Samaa Alrushaid and Frank J. Burczynski
College of Pharmacy, Rady Faculty of Health Sciences, University of Manitoba, Winnipeg, MB R3E 0T5, Canada

Casey L. Sayre
College of Pharmacy, Rady Faculty of Health Sciences, University of Manitoba, Winnipeg, MB R3E 0T5, Canada
College of Pharmacy, Roseman University of Health Sciences, South Jordan, UT 84096, USA

Jaime A. Yáñez
YARI International Group, New Brunswick, NJ 08901 and INDETEC Corp., Lima, Peru

M. Laird Forrest and Sanjeewa N. Senadheera
Department of Pharmaceutical Chemistry, School of Pharmacy, University of Kansas, Lawrence, KS 66047, USA

Raimar Löbenberg and Neal M. Davies
Faculty of Pharmacy and Pharmaceutical Sciences, University of Alberta, Edmonton, AB T6G 2R3, Canada

Munawar A. Mohammed, Jaweria T. M. Syeda, Kishor M. Wasan and Ellen K. Wasan
College of Pharmacy and Nutrition, University of Saskatchewan, Saskatoon, SK S7N 2Z4, Canada

Yuri Park, Nahye Kim, Jangmi Choi, Min-Ho Park, Byeong ill Lee, Seok-Ho Shin, Jin-Ju Byeon and Young G. Shin
College of Pharmacy and Institute of Drug Research and Development, Chungnam National University, Daejeon 34134, Korea

Min-Koo Choi
College of Pharmacy, Dankook University, Cheon-an 31116, Korea

So Jeong Nam and Im-Sook Song
College of Pharmacy and Research Institute of Pharmaceutical Sciences, Kyungpook National University, Daegu 41566, Korea

Hye-Young Ji, Mi Jie Park and Ji-Soo Choi
Life Science Institute, Daewoong Pharmaceutical, Yongin, Gyeonggido 17028, Korea

Young A. Choi and Min-Koo Choi
College of Pharmacy, Dankook University, Cheon-an 31116, Korea

Yuejian Liu and Michael W. H. Coughtrie
Faculty of Pharmaceutical Sciences, The University of British Columbia, Vancouver, BC V6T 1Z3, Canada

Tony K.L. Kiang
Faculty of Pharmacy and Pharmaceutical Sciences, University of Alberta, Edmonton, AB T6G 2E1, Canada

Sahan A. Ranamukhaarachchi
Department of Electrical and Computer Engineering, University of British Columbia, Vancouver, BC V6T 1Z4, Canada

Mary H.H. Ensom
Faculty of Pharmaceutical Sciences, University of British Columbia, Vancouver, BC V6T 1Z3, Canada

Norzahirah Ahmad, Bee Ping Teh, Murizal Zainol, Nor Azlina Zolkifli, Amirrudin Muhammad, Emylyn Matom, Noor Rain Abdullah, Zakiah Ismail and Ami Fazlin Syed Mohamed
Herbal Medicine Research Centre, Institute for Medical Research, Jalan Pahang, Kuala Lumpur 50588, Malaysia

Dodheri Syed Samiulla
Aurigene Discovery Technologies Limited, Electronic City, Hosur Road, Bangalore 560100, Karnataka, India

Azlina Zulkapli
Medical Resource Research Centre, Institute for Medical Research, Jalan Pahang, Kuala Lumpur 50588, Malaysia

Index

www.ingramcontent.com/pod-product-compliance
Lightning Source LLC
LaVergne TN
LVHW082146200926
848484LV00008B/2115
* 9 7 9 8 8 8 7 4 0 0 7 8 5 *